Seminars in Old

College Seminars Series

Series Editors

Professor Hugh Freeman, Honorary Professor, University of Salford, and Honorary Consultant Psychiatrist, Salford Health Authority

Dr Ian Pullen, Consultant Psychiatrist, Dingleton Hospital, Melrose, Roxburghshire

Dr George Stein, Consultant Psychiatrist, Farnborough Hospital, and King's College Hospital

Professor Greg Wilkinson, Editor, *British Journal of Psychiatry*, and Professor of Liaison Psychiatry, University of Liverpool

Other books in the series

Seminars in Alcohol and Drug Misuse. Edited by Jonathan Chick & Roch Cantwell

Seminars in Basic Neurosciences. Edited by Gethin Morgan & Stuart Butler

Seminars in Child and Adolescent Psychiatry. Edited by Dora Black & David Cottrell

Seminars in Clinical Psychopharmacology. Edited by David King

Seminars in General Adult Psychiatry. Edited by George Stein & Greg Wilkinson

Seminars in Liaison Psychiatry. Edited by Elspeth Guthrie & Francis Creed

Seminars in Practical Forensic Psychiatry. Edited by Derek Chiswick & Rosemarie Cope

Seminars in Psychiatric Genetics. By Peter McGuffin, Michael J. Owen, Michael C. O'Donovan, Anita Thapar & Irving Gottesman

Seminars in the Psychiatry of Learning Disabilities. Edited by Oliver Russell

Seminars in Psychology and the Social Sciences. Edited by Digby Tantam & Max Birchwood

Seminars in Psychosexual Disorders. Series editors: Hugh Freeman, Ian Pullen, George Stein & Greg Wilkinson

Forthcoming titles

Seminars in Psychotherapy. Edited by Sandra Grant & Jane Naismith

Seminars in Old Age Psychiatry

Edited by
Rob Butler & Brice Pitt

GASKELL

British Library Cataloguing-in-Publication Data
A catalogue record for this book is available from the British Library.

ISBN 1 901242 21 8

Distributed in North America
by American Psychiatric Press, Inc.
ISBN 0 88048 591 4

Gaskell is an imprint of the Royal College of Psychiatrists,
17 Belgrave Square, London SW1X 8PG
The Royal College of Psychiatrists is a registered charity, number 228636

The views presented in this book do not necessarily reflect those of
the Royal College of Psychiatrists, and the publishers are not
responsible for any error of omission or fact. College Seminars are
produced by the Publications Department of the College; they should
in no way be construed as providing a syllabus or other material for
any College examination.

Printed by Bell & Bain Ltd, Thornliebank, Glasgow

Contents

Contributors

Osvaldo P. Almeida, Queen Elizabeth II Medical Centre, Perth, Australia.

Robert Baldwin, Consultant Old Age Psychiatrist and Honorary Senior Lecturer, Manchester Royal Infirmary, Manchester.

John Besson, Consultant Psychiatrist, St Thomas' Hospital, London.

Carol Brayne, Lecturer in Epidemiology, Addenbrooke's Hospital, Cambridge.

Jerry Brown, Consultant Neurologist, Addenbrooke's Hospital, Cambridge.

Alistair Burns, Professor of Old Age Psychiatry, University of Manchester, Manchester.

Rob Butler, Lecturer in Old Age Psychiatry, Imperial College, London.

Simon Dixey, Consultant Old Age Psychiatrist, Penn Hospital, Wolverhampton.

Hans Forstl, Professor of Psychiatry, University of Western Australia.

Chris Gilleard, Senior Lecturer in the Psychology of Old Age, St George's Hospital Medical School, London.

Colin Godber, Thornhill Unit, Moorgreen Hospital, Southampton

Tony Hope, Honorary Consultant Psychiatrist and Reader in Medicine, University of Oxford.

Peter Jeffreys, Consultant Psychiatrist, Northwick Park and St Mark's Hospital, London.

David Jolley, Professor of Old Age Psychiatry, Penn Hospital, Wolverhampton.

Dee Jones, Director, Research Team for Care of Elderly People, University of Wales College of Medicine, Cardiff.

James Lindesay, Professor of Psychiatry for the Elderly, Leicester General Hospital, Leicester.

Brice Pitt, Emeritus Professor of Old Age Psychiatry, Imperial College, London.

Kate Read, Planning and Development Officer, Social Services, Wolverhampton.

Henry Rosenvinge, Thornhill Unit, Moorgreen Hospital, Southampton.

Martin Rossor, Consultant Neurologist, National Hospital for Neurology and Neurosurgery, London.

Ken Shulman, Professor of Psychiatry, Sunnybrook Health Science Centre, University of Toronto, Ontario.

Charles Twining, Consultant Clinical Psychologist, Whitchurch Hospital, Cardiff.

John Wattis, Senior Lecturer, Psychiatry for Older Adults, University of Leeds School of Clinical Medicine.

Foreword

Series Editors

The publication of *College Seminars*, a series of textbooks covering the breadth of psychiatry, is very much in line with the Royal College of Psychiatrists' established role in education and in setting professional standards.

College Seminars are intended to help junior doctors during their training years. We hope that trainees will find these books useful, on the ward as well as in preparation for the MRCPsych examination. Separate volumes will cover clinical psychiatry, each of its sub-specialities, and also the relevant non-clinical academic disciplines of psychology and sociology.

College Seminars will make a contribution to the continuing professional development of established clinicians.

Psychiatry is concerned primarily with people, and to a lesser extent with disease processes and pathology. The core of the subject is rich in ideas and schools of thought, and no single approach or solution can embrace the variety of problems a psychiatrist meets. For this reason, we have endeavoured to adopt an eclectic approach to practical management throughout the series.

The College can draw on the collective wisdom of many individuals in clinical and academic psychiatry. More than a hundred people have contributed to this series; this reflects how diverse and complex psychiatry has become.

Frequent new editions of books appearing in the series are envisaged, which should allow *College Seminars* to be responsive to readers' suggestions and needs.

Hugh Freeman
Ian Pullen
George Stein
Greg Wilkinson

Preface

When this book was first commissioned, the editors were Mohsen Naguib and Brice Pitt, who welcomed the opportunity to write a succinct, up to the minute text, which would appeal to all professionals working in the mental health of older age.

The contributors had been identified, and most had sent in their chapters, when Mohsen died suddenly and unexpectedly of a heart attack, at the age of forty-four. This devastating loss set the book back by three years. Much of it was in Mohsen's filing cabinets, or on computer, and all the contributors (and a few new ones) were asked to update their manuscripts. We are most grateful for their forbearance, goodwill and hard work in producing finished texts. We also appreciate the faith of Professor Greg Wilkinson and Dave Jago that the book would come to fruition.

Rob Butler
Brice Pitt

Dedication

Mohsen Naguib, MD PhD MRCPsych, 1949–1993

1 Assessment

Rob Butler & Brice Pitt

Location of assessment ● *History* ● *Mental state* ● *Physical examination*
● *Investigations* ● *Formulation* ● *Rating instruments* ● *Conclusion*

Old age psychiatry is general adult psychiatry adapted to later life, and has come into being chiefly because of the spectacular increase in the proportion of the population surviving into the senium (over the age of 65 and beyond)(Box 1.1). Many people become mentally ill for the first time in late life, partly because of vicissitudes such as bereavement and infirmity, and partly because of pathological changes in the brain reflected in delirium and the dementias.

In old age, psychiatry is modified by the frequency of physical illness (including sensory deficits) and organic mental changes. Organic and functional illness often coexist. Older people present their troubled feelings as physical symptoms more often than younger patients. Some others are complained of, rather than as presenting complaints in their own right. So, it is necessary to evaluate the history given by relatives and carers as well as the patients themselves. Because of the growth of dependency with advancing years, the complex situations arising from the needs of patients and their carers (not necessarily identical) need appraisal. In practical terms this means that cognitive assessment and physical examination are essential. Since many patients are unable, or unwilling, to come to a surgery or an out-patient department, there is an important place for domiciliary assessment. Finally, as with general medicine, unusual presentations of disorders encountered in younger people, such as pseudo-dementia and somatisation, are more common.

Box 1.1 Features of old age psychiatry

The older population is growing
Older people may have more losses and be more isolated
Physical illness is more common
Carers often play key roles
Cognitive testing and physical examination are very important
Assessments are usually carried out at home

Location of assessment

Old age psychiatrists, at least in the UK, often see the patient in the first instance at home. This saves the patient from having to come to the hospital and enables the problem to be assessed where it presents. Assets and liabilities, such as a lunch club two doors away, a loose stair rod or a hole in the carpet, are readily identified. Evidence of dysfunction such as squalor, rotting food, an empty larder and the taps left on, can all be noted. It is particularly useful to look at the medications that the patient is currently taking, or has taken, or which belong to other members of the household (Box 1.2). Evidence of help provided by the family, or home helps, with the management of correspondence or accounts, evidence of enjoyment of TV or recorded music and availability of a telephone or alarm system, all help to indicate the quality of life and amenities. If neighbours or family are in attendance, their attitudes, feelings and readiness to cope can be ascertained. Although domiciliary visits are sometimes seen as time-consuming and costly, it may be possible to reach a decision at the time of the best action (which of course includes inaction). It is, as a rule, inappropriate to have more than two people visit a patient at home. Brice Pitt recalls an occasion when he visited a patient, accompanied by several medical students, and a neighbour called the police believing she was being invaded by a gang!

By contrast, out-patient departments suffer from the vagaries of ambulance transport, the unwillingness of many patients to attend, and their being unsettled by the journey and a strange clinical environment if they do so. Physical examination and blood taking are a little easier than at home, but less information may be forthcoming. A good compromise is attendance at a day hospital for assessment, which allows activities of daily living and social behaviour to be observed and a medical assessment to be conducted under less pressure of time. The day hospital is a good setting for multi-disciplinary assessment. Of course, it is sometimes necessary to admit a patient to hospital. This offers the advantages of a safe environment, day and night nursing observations and a complete

---

Box 1.2 Advantages of home assessments

More convenient (usually) for the patient
More relaxing for the patient
Living conditions can be seen
Activities and social activities can be assessed
Medications can be examined

break for the patient and their carer. Liaison assessments are an important part of old age psychiatry, and are covered in Chapter 14.

Interviewing relatives and carers

In old age psychiatry, it is often particularly helpful to interview a carer, or another involved individual. This initial meeting can establish a rapport which will prove important for future help and support. The carer needs to be asked questions about the patient and themselves, and their relationship with the patient (Box 1.3). This will help to establish how much the information may be influenced by the relationship or situation. Useful addresses are listed in the Appendix (see also Chapter 18).

History

Setting

Usually, it is best to see patients on their own first. It is important to recognise and respect the patient's right to tell their own story. Indeed, unless severely cognitively impaired and unwilling to cooperate, patients must be asked for their permission for information to be given by others. Older people may be deaf or dysarthric and these deficits need to be recognised and allowed for if they cannot be remedied, e.g. by finding a hearing aid (even an ear trumpet) or retrieving false teeth. Very old people may be somewhat over-awed by respect for doctors and will be helped to be at their ease if the doctor does not take up too commanding a position (e.g. sitting by the patient rather than behind a desk) and is friendly and informal. Sitting slightly below the patient (rather than looming intimidatingly), with the light on one's

---

Box 1.3 Questions for carers

Relationship to the patient
Amount of care provided
Degree of stress they are under
What help they can be offered
Understanding of the patient's illness
What expectations they have from services
Their awareness of support or voluntary organisations
Their knowledge of the illness

Box 1.4 Key features of the history

The patient must be at ease, seeing and hearing the doctor
Why is the individual presenting now?
Activities of daily living
Is there a carer? What is their situation?
What was the patient's highest level of functioning?
What is the housing and income position?

---

face, enables the patient to feel less threatened and helps the hard of hearing to read lips (Box 1.4).

History of presenting complaint

As always in medicine, we want to know not only the nature of the presenting complaint, but why it is presenting now. Is this a new problem, or have circumstances altered so that an old problem has come to the fore (e.g. a wife with dementia whose husband has recently died)? The history is likely to include disturbance of feelings, cognition (especially memory) and activities of daily living. It is important to establish how patients usually cope with the latter, and to what extent they rely on others. For those who rely heavily on others, there may have been a change in the pattern of care, such as a new home help or the suspension of a day service.

Family history

There may be a relevant history of psychiatric illness, e.g. dementia (having to go into a home in late life) or depression (taking a long time to recover from childbirth, unexplained time off work, electroconvulsive therapy, suicide). A history of early deprivation, such as the death of the patient's mother, may be relevant to subsequent coping. Siblings may still be alive and in contact with the patient.

Personal history

A personal history puts the patient and their problems in context. Events which happened many years ago may have important implications for the present. The patient's level of education and occupational history are useful indications of what might be expected by way of recreational interest (e.g. reading, playing bridge or doing crossword puzzles). It is recognised that the less well educated, and ostensibly less intelligent, perform less well on cognitive tests such as the Abbreviated Mental Test

Score (AMTS; Hodkinson, 1973) or the Mini-Mental State Examination (MMSE; Folstein *et al*, 1975). It is worth asking how the patient spent the Second World War years (e.g. evacuation, refugee or national service). The ability to cope with five years active service in the army without incident is one indication of stability and resilience. Few older people are still at work, so work difficulties are rare, although forced retirement may have been distressing and couples may have problems in adjusting to seeing more of each other when neither is at work.

Past psychiatric history

A previous history of psychiatric illness may be informative, though this is frequently not volunteered, or the details are highly obscure, either because the patient or the family are not very keen on disclosing them or because it was all a long time ago and much has been forgotten.

Medical history

Old people have, of course, lived a long time and their present general practitioner may have little or no awareness of past disorders, though some information may be buried in bulky packages of notes. Where the previous record is exceedingly slender, the fact that a patient is presenting at all is likely to be highly significant.

Medications

With a multiplicity of disorders, or symptoms, may come polypharmacy. Patients are often perplexed about what the different drugs they take are for, and when they should be taking them. It may be evident that they comply well with some medications and not others. On the whole, for example, analgesics are more readily taken than antipsychotics. Despite the general aversion to benzodiazepine tranquillisers, there is still a great willingness to take and prescribe benzodiazepine hypnotics, which may either have side-effects or withdrawal effects if suddenly discontinued (e.g. on admission to hospital). Iatrogenic falling, drowsiness and confusion are all common in old age. A wide range of over-the-counter medications are ever more available and there is the possibility of ill effects from interactions.

Alcohol history

Admission to hospital for alcohol-related disorder declines with ageing, but alcohol misuse is not unknown in older people (see Chapter 11). A long habit may continue and become difficult when medications are added, or some lonely, depressed older people may start drinking for the first time. Since this information is rarely volunteered it must be asked for (e.g. the four CAGE screening questions; Ewing, 1984).

Activities of daily living

Is the patient independent or in sheltered housing? Is their environment clean and are they well nourished? How often, if at all, does a carer (family, friend or home help) need to shop, draw a pension, pay the rent, cook meals, do laundry or escort the patient?

Social history

Though poverty is rarer in old age than it used to be, many older people need to live frugally to eke out their retirement or occupational pension, and such savings as they may have. They are more likely to have lived in their own homes a long time, and to own them. Any threat to this security by pressure to move because of infirmity, or a landlord's desire to increase the rent, may be extremely stressful, as may income tax and local tax demands. Sometimes there are relatives in financial need with expectations of their aged parents which may colour their attitudes to nursing home care. Some of the oldest people have bad memories from before the Second World War of means testing, or 'the workhouses', which may make them very reluctant to consider going into a home, even when the need is great. For all these reasons, judicious inquiry about income, assets, obligations and expenditures is useful. In the morbidly depressed, fears of privation and ruin may be unjustified. A very important question is who owns the property or who holds the tenancy. Is the old lady living with her daughter, or her daughter with her? Even now, the oldest people are likely to be living in the least suitable accommodation, with ancient and unsafe wiring, poor lighting and heating, insufficient hot water, outdoor lavatories, many levels and steep steps. Yet, understandably, there is a considerable attachment to the home they are familiar with.

What does the patient do for leisure and pleasure? Have they any hobbies, do they socialise? Are there any particularly close friends or confidants? Very isolated old people are at considerable risk if they become infirm.

Premorbid personality

It is difficult to establish the premorbid personality reliably, but the effort to do so by recourse to the opinions of others may be useful. For example, learning that chronically miserable and hypochondriacal Mrs Jones was by no means always like this, but on the contrary was, until three years ago, lively, sociable and neighbourly, may sharpen therapeutic endeavours. It is probably easier to get accurate information about how outgoing or otherwise the patient was than other aspects of personality.

Mental state

Appearance and behaviour

The mental state examination will first take account of the patient's appearance (Box 1.5). Are there obvious signs of neglect such as dirty clothes, features and fingers, matted hair, or is the patient clean and well groomed? Is the manner confident, sociable, exuding bonhomie and well-being, or the opposite, with extravagant 'illness behaviour' – stumbling, shaking, subsiding helplessly? Is the patient fully alert, animated and articulate, or clouded, placid and lacking in spontaneity? Are there any impairments of vision, hearing or mobility?

Speech

Is the history spontaneous, pertinent, consistent and insightful, or hesitant, circumstantial, unfocused? Are questions understood and answers adequate, relevant and informative? If not, is the patient deaf, dysphasic, demented, delirious or disaffected?

Mood

Depressed older people may well not say they are miserable, but worry about physical disorders, poverty, mugging, loneliness or, if specifically asked, admit that they are unable to enjoy themselves. Suicide is relatively common in later life and the inquiry is incomplete without questions about whether life seems worth living and whether there is, or has been, suicidal intent. Anxiety in older people is often regarded as natural or appropriate and is underestimated. It is particularly likely to cause the sufferer to become house bound, so an inquiry about whether the subject goes out and if not, why not, is important.

Box 1.5 Key features of the mental state examination

Establish sight or hearing difficulties
Anxiety symptoms are common
Be aware of masked depression
Ask about suicidal ideation
A full cognitive examination is essential

Abnormal beliefs

Paranoia may compound deafness, be a phase of dementia, colour severe depression or be a prime symptom of schizophrenia. In dementia or delirium, strangers may be recognised warmly as friends or family, and those nearest and dearest may be perceived as alien.

Abnormal perceptions

Auditory hallucinations are common in paraphrenia, but less so in dementia. Visual hallucinations, however, especially towards evening, are not uncommon in dementia and may be taken so seriously that patients believe they have to make provision for the intruder (e.g. providing meals!).

Cognition

Cognitive assessment should include orientation in time, place and person; recent and long-term memory; concentration; language; praxis and simple calculation. These are incorporated in a brief form in the MMSE (Folstein *et al*, 1975). An estimation should also be made of intelligence and judgement. Even in those who appear cognitively intact it is important to test cognition, but try not to alienate or alarm the patient by direct or challenging questions. It can be helpful to warn patients not to be insulted by some of the questions, and not to worry about the ones they can not answer. Deaf, drugged and disaffected older people tend to perform less well than they should.

Insight

People with early dementia may admit that their memory is faulty but later revert to defensive denial. Depressed older people tend to emphasise their infirmity and incompetence. Anxiety may be attributed to physical illness or environmental hazards (stairs, mugging). Insight is rare in mania and paraphrenia.

Physical examination

The assessment is incomplete without a physical examination. This may not be appropriate in the patient's home, although at the very least vision, hearing, speech and mobility should be noted. At out-patients, day hospital or on admission, a full physical examination should be undertaken. Pay particular attention to the patient's general state of nutrition, health, signs of injury or self-neglect, and disability limiting function or causing distress and affecting mood or cognition.

Investigations

In a clinical setting, investigations include weight, TPR (temperature, pulse and respiration rate), urine testing, blood tests for haematology, B12, folate, syphilis serology and chemical profile (urea and electrolytes, liver function tests and thyroid function tests) and a chest X-ray. Brain imaging is required where there is cognitive impairment, especially when it takes a rapid or unusual form, and to exclude space occupying lesions, including haematoma, hydrocephalus and cerebral infarction (see Chapter 12).

Formulation

The history, mental state, physical examination and investigations conclude with a formulation. This includes: a brief resume of the above; differential diagnosis; aetiology; management plans; and prognosis.

Diagnosis

The current diagnostic systems are the *International Classification of Diseases and Related Health Problems* (ICD–10; World Health Organization, 1993) and the *Diagnostic and Statistical Manual of Mental Disorders* (DSM–IV; American Psychiatric Association, 1994). The ICD–10 criteria for mental disorders are covered in the relevant chapters of the book. Neither classification includes a separate section for mental disorders of older age nor a diagnosis of paraphrenia (see Chapter 10). ICD–10 has one axis (for mental disorders) while DSM–IV has five axes: I, clinical syndromes; II, personality disorders and mental retardation; III, physical disorders or conditions; IV, psychosocial and environmental problems; V, global assessment of functioning.

Rating instruments

Rating instruments are often used in old age psychiatry. They should be used in addition to, rather than instead of, a history, mental state and physical examination. They offer the advantages of being comprehensive (they do not forget to ask things) and repeatable (particularly useful to look back at). For example, it is important to remember that a diagnosis of dementia is not made just on a score of less than 24 on the MMSE (Folstein *et al*, 1975), but is arrived at after taking the full range of clinical information into account. That being said, a score of less than 24 on the MMSE is a useful measure. It is a good idea to complete a cognitive scale, and a depression scale where appropriate, as part of every assessment.

Cognitive scales

Cognitive rating instruments are a means of organising the assessment of cognition, and giving a numerical value to overall function (Box 1.6). Scores are affected by previous levels of education and intelligence, as well as familiarity with the culture and language in which they are given. Ceiling and floor effects mean that patients with severe cognitive impairment (floor) or mild (ceiling), lose discrimination. In clinical practice, it is probably best to use one instrument routinely and become familiar with it, since they all have strengths and weaknesses. In research, shorter cognitive instruments are often used for screening, so that subjects with less than a cut-off score can be identified for further assessment.

Abbreviated Mental Test Score

One of the simplest and longest established cognitive tests is the Abbreviated Mental Test Score (AMTS; Hodkinson, 1973). This is widely used in geriatric departments in the UK and, being short, is quite popular in general practice. It is designed for use in hospital and needs some adaptation for subjects at home (e.g. identification of a doctor and a nurse and the name of the hospital are inappropriate questions). It is almost entirely an orientation and memory test, although counting backwards from 20 may be regarded as a test of concentration. For all its limitations it is of some value, particularly

---

Box 1.6 Summary of cognitive tests

AMTS – cut-off 7 or 8/10, a few minutes to use but only covers memory and orientation

MMSE – cut-off 24/30, takes 5–10 minutes to complete, a standard baseline test

CAPE – information/orientation sub-scale has 12 questions

CAMCOG – wide ranging test of cognition takes approximately 40 minutes to complete

Clock drawing test – a revealing test of praxis, offers qualitative as well as quantitative information

when repeated. Scores of seven or less in a cooperative patient suggest cognitive impairment.

Mini-Mental State Examination

Probably the most widely used cognitive test in old age psychiatry is the MMSE (Folstein *et al*, 1975). Its main strengths are that it covers the basic cognitive functions reasonably comprehensively in 10 minutes or so, and is well established internationally. It covers the following areas of cognition.

Orientation – the MMSE begins with five items of orientation in time and five in place, but does not test orientation in person. How much credit to give to approximately correct answers is a matter of common sense, for example to be one day out on the date is normal, and should not be marked incorrect unless it is a notable date such as Christmas or the patient's birthday. It is not generally known that the seasons change on 21 March, June, September and December. Ignorance of the month is more allowable if it has only just changed. Ignorance of location may be more significant when patients do not know they are at home, than in an accident and emergency department after a road traffic accident.

Memory – apple, book and coat are easier to register and therefore preferable to an address. Their initial letters provide a mnemonic for the more observant. If alternative words are then used the loss of the mnemonic aid may affect performance. The MMSE measures registration and recall, but not long-term memory.

Concentration – the MMSE gives the same mark of five points if the patient can do five successive serial seven subtractions or spell 'world' backwards, even though these tasks are complicated and the skills rather different. Simple calculation can be tested using an easier sum (e.g. 15 – 8), while concentration can be tested by reciting the months of the year backwards. The Cambridge Examination for Mental Disorders of the Elderly (CAMCOG) (see below) only uses the numerical test.

Language – naming a pencil and watch may be too easy to detect nominal aphasia and should be followed by questions about less common names (e.g. a watch face or hands). Repetition of the sentence 'no ifs, ands or buts' is more appropriate for someone familiar with this warning from childhood than someone who has never heard it before. The paper folding task should not be prompted after the initial instructions. It tests understanding of language as well as praxis and memory.

Praxis – copying the intersecting pentagons tests constructional apraxia. It is quite a difficult test and can be followed by an easier test or the clock drawing test

Gnosis – recognition is tested in the more extensive CAMCOG by using pictures, small objects and commands.

Other cognitive scales

The comprehensive Clifton Assessment Procedures for the Elderly (CAPE; Pattie & Gilleard, 1979) and Cambridge Examination for Mental Disorders of the Elderly (CAMDEX; Roth *et al*, 1988) each include a cognitive sub-scale: the information/orientation sub-scale and CAMCOG, respectively. The information/orientation sub-scale has 12 questions, is easy to administer and widely used. CAMCOG is a more comprehensive cognitive test which covers a wide range of ability. It gives a score out of 104. With all these tests, qualitative information is often as important as scores. This is certainly the case with the clock drawing test (Ainslie *et al*, 1993). The subject is asked to draw a circle, put in the numbers and set the hands at ten minutes past eleven. It is interesting to note whether the patient starts by establishing the four poles of 12, 3, 6 and 9 and then fills in the numbers, or starts with 12 and then laboriously goes round to 11. It is surprising how often those who can tell the time will turn out to have a lot of difficulty in deciding which of the clock hands should be the longer or shorter.

Depression scales

Depression questionnaires and scales help to collate symptoms and signs for screening and can be used as an aid to diagnosis. Scales are particularly useful for monitoring the course of depressive symptoms, and for research (Box 1.7).

Geriatric Depression Scale

The Geriatric Depression Scale (GDS; Yesavage *et al*, 1983) is designed to avoid questions concerning somatic symptoms and functions which in older patients might be accounted for by physical disorders (e.g.

Box 1.7 Summary of depression scales

GDS: brief, 15 items, avoids somatic questions so good for older patients

BASDEC: for liaison, a series of questions on cards, particularly useful with deaf subjects

Hamilton Rating Scale: general adult scale, quantifies depression but is not a diagnostic tool

MADRS: sensitive to change in depressive illness

Depressive Sign Scale: nine items to help detect depression in people with dementia

sleep disturbance or weight loss). Originally a 30-item test, it now has 15 items, which enables most subjects to be scored for depression in four to five minutes. An overall score of five or more suggests the possibility of a depressive illness, though further inquiry is needed to establish a diagnosis.

Brief Assessment Schedule Depression Cards

The BASDEC (Adshead *et al*, 1992) consist of a series of statements in large print on cards which are shown to the patient, one at a time, and answered 'true' or 'false'. Each true answer scores one point except 'I've given up hope' and 'I've seriously considered suicide' which score two. A score of seven or more raises the likelihood of a depressive disorder. The BASDEC was initially designed for use in liaison psychiatry where a visual aid to verbal enquiry is often helpful.

Other depression scales

The Hamilton Rating Scale for depression (Hamilton, 1960), although widely used, has a number of somatic items which render it less appropriate for older subjects than the Montgomery–Åsberg Depression Rating Scale (MADRS; Montgomery & Åsberg, 1979). The MADRS, however, may not be reliably answered by patients with dementia. In this case depression may be better recognised through observing behaviours such as going off food, becoming withdrawn or poorer sleep. The Depressive Signs Scale (Katona & Aldridge, 1985) is a useful means of quantifying such phenomena.

Comprehensive assessments

Clifton Assessment Procedures for the Elderly

CAPE (Pattie & Gilleard, 1979) is intended to assess level of disability and estimate need for care. It consists of a short cognitive scale and a behavioural rating scale. The latter has four sub-scales: physical disability, apathy, communication difficulties and social disturbance. It is quick and easy to administer, and is widely used by professional staff and care workers (Box 1.8).

Geriatric Mental State

The Geriatric Mental State (GMS), based on a semi-structured interview, and computerised as AGECAT (Copeland *et al*, 1986), is a useful epidemiological tool which can also be used to find levels of caseness for all psychiatric disorders in old age, ranging from zero to five. Levels one and two are sub-clinical while five is the

---

Box 1.8 Comprehensive assessments

CAPE: has a 12 question information/orientation sub-scale
GMS: for psychiatric diagnoses, computerised as AGECAT
CAMDEX: includes CAMCOG for cognitive testing
CARE: shortened version has 143 items and takes about 30
    minutes to administer

---

most severe. It has an optional informant section: the History and Aetiology Schedule (HAS).

Cambridge Examination for Mental Disorders of the Elderly

The CAMDEX (Roth *et al*, 1988) incorporates the MMSE, the Blessed Dementia Rating Scale (BDRS; Blessed *et al*, 1968) and the Hachinski Ischaemia Score (Hachinski *et al*, 1975), in a comprehensive inquiry from the subject and informant. BDRS is a measure of activities of daily living. The Hachinski Ischaemia Score helps differentiate between vascular and Alzheimer's dementia (see Chapter 5). A notable feature of CAMDEX is CAMCOG, which is the cognitive sub-scale. CAMDEX is mainly used in research by trained non-doctors.

Comprehensive Assessment and Referral Evaluation

The Comprehensive Assessment and Referral Evaluation (CARE; Gurland *et al*, 1984) has a shortened version, the Short-CARE, which is a semi-structured interview designed to identify and assess depression and dementia for research purposes.

Conclusion

The thorough assessment of an older person is an essential first step in offering the best management for their mental illness. Experience helps a professional know which parts of an assessment are particularly useful for the individual patient. However, a multi-disciplinary assessment will almost invariably offer more information. Not only does it help to view complex problems from many angles, but it also involves those offering support in management decisions. This allows a team of professionals to offer consistent and effective care.

References

Adshead, F., Day Code, D. & Pitt, B. (1992) BASDEC: a novel screening instrument for depression in elderly medical inpatients. *British Medical Journal*, 305, 397.

Ainslie, N. & Murden, R. (1993) Effect of education on the clock-drawing dementia screen in non-demented elderly persons. *Journal of the American Geriatrics Society*, 41, 429–452.

American Psychiatric Association (1994) *Diagnostic and Statistical Manual of Mental Disorders* (4th edn) (DSM–IV). Washington, DC: APA.

Blessed, G., Tomlinson, B. & Roth, M. (1968) Association between quantitative measures of dementing and senile change in cerebral grey matter of elderly subjects. *British Journal of Psychiatry*, 114, 797–811.

Copeland, J., Dewey, M. & Griffiths-Jones, H. (1986) Psychiatric case nomenclature and a computerised diagnostic system for elderly subjects: GMS and AGECAT. *Psychological Medicine*, 16, 89–99.

Ewing, J. (1984) Detesting alcoholism: The CAGE questionnaire. *Journal of the American Medical Association*, 252, 1905–1907.

Folstein, M., Folstein, S. & McHugh, P. (1975) Mini-Mental State. A practical method for grading the cognitive state of patients for the clinician. *Journal of Psychiatric Research*, 12, 189–198.

Gurland, B., Golden, R., Teresi, J., *et al* (1984) The Short-CARE: an efficient instrument for the assessment of depression, dementia and disability. *Journal of Gerontology*, 39, 166–169.

Hachinski, V., Iliff, L., Zilkha, E., *et al* (1975) Cerebral blood flow in dementia. *Archives of Neurology*, 32, 632–637.

Hamilton, M. (1960) A rating scale for depression. *Journal of Neurology, Neurosurgery and Psychiatry*, 23, 56–62.

Hodkinson, M. (1973) Mental impairment in the elderly. *Journal of the Royal College of Physicians of London*, 7, 305–317.

Katona, C. & Aldridge, D. (1985) The DST and depression signs in dementia. *Journal of Affective Disorders*, 8, 83–89.

Montgomery, S. & Åsberg, M. (1979) A new depression scale designed to be sensitive to change. *British Journal of Psychiatry*, 134, 382–389.

Pattie, A. & Gilleard, C. (1979) *Manual of the Clifton Assessment Procedures for the Elderly* (CAPE). Sevenoaks: Hodder and Stoughton.

Roth, M., Huppert, F., Tym, E., *et al* (1988) *CAMDEX: The Cambridge Examination for Mental Disorders of the Elderly*. Cambridge: Cambridge University Press.

World Health Organization (1993) *The ICD–10 Classification of Mental and Behavioural Disorders. Diagnostic Criteria for Research*. Geneva: WHO.

Yesavage, J., Brink, T., Rose, T., *et al* (1983) Development and evaluation of a geriatric depression screening scale: a preliminary report. *Journal of Psychiatric Research*, 17, 37–49.

2 Epidemiology

Rob Butler & Carol Brayne

Demographic trends ● *Epidemiological terms* ● *Sources of information*
● *Types of study* ● *Stages in epidemiological studies* ● *Quality control*
● *Conclusion*

The increase in the proportion of old people in the population has given prominence to mental illness in old age. Society is forced to make decisions about how many and which services to provide to the older community. Mental illness is one of the largest areas of activity in the health service, with mental disorders of the elderly an important part of it.

Demographic trends

The population of the UK is roughly 58 million, 16% of whom are over the age of 65. By the year 2034, the total population is projected to be around 60 million and 24% will be aged 65 or over (Government Actuary's Department, 1996). The number of people aged over 85 will have risen from one to two million. At the beginning of this century the population was much smaller (33 million) and the proportion of older people much less (5% aged over 65) (Central Statistical Office, 1979).

This substantial ageing of the population is a new phenomenon, occurring over the last century following reduction in infant mortality, control of infectious diseases and improvement in sanitation, living standards and nutrition. These changes, along with declining birth rates in developed countries, have resulted in the sharp increase in the proportion of elderly in the population. This increase is projected to continue for the UK (Table 2.1), which has among the highest proportion of elderly in Europe. Although the overall increase has slowed down, this conceals the continuing increase in the very oldest age groups. This is of major importance to health and social services because of the concomitant increase in chronic disease and disability and their cost.

The fourth age

The change in demographic pattern in developed countries has led to the concept of the third age, a time of fulfilment of potential after

16

Table 2.1 Projected population in hundred thousands (adapted from Government Actuary's Department, 1996)

	1994	2004	2014	2024	2034
65–74	52	49	60	65	79
75–84	30	33	33	43	47
85+	10	11	13	15	20
Total > 65	92	93	107	123	147
Total population	583	598	608	612	603
% > 65	15.7	15.6	17.6	20.2	24.3

retirement, followed by the fourth age, a period of dependence and pre-terminal illness (Laslett, 1990). This view remains controversial but is consistent with the suggestion that the elderly might suffer less morbidity as mortality is reduced (Fries, 1989). This means that a large proportion of the population would survive to a given point and then suffer a short period of illness followed by death; prolonging the third age and shortening the fourth. In fact, while life expectancy has increased slightly over the past 20 years, it is not yet clear whether disability-free life expectancy is correspondingly longer.

Implications of the demographic trends

Financial

As the proportion of pensioners increases and the proportion of the working population decreases, it follows that each member of the workforce will have to find more money to contribute to those on state support. This may occur without great strain to the economy (as occurred during the earlier part of this century) by adjustments to present working conditions. These could include raising the retirement age, or encouraging more people to take out private pensions. Alternatively, a drop in living standards may be acceptable for society to care for its older members, or a growing standard of living may be shared across all groups of society.

Health

There is little doubt that the changes in demography will have major implications for health services. The very old have more disability (Office of Population Censuses and Surveys, 1988) and more psychiatric illness than the old. A meta-analysis by Jorm *et al* (1987) found that the prevalence of dementia doubles for every 5.1 years above the age of 65. It is likely that there will be a need for more services for the elderly mentally ill.

Social services

Recent years have seen an increase in the number of elderly cared for in residential and nursing homes (see Chapter 15). Presently, the vast majority of older people live independently, or are looked after by informal carers such as wives or daughters. However, the very old, those living alone and those limited in activity are the most likely to require help from statutory services (Livingston *et al*, 1990*b*). It is therefore likely that the number of people requiring support from the social services will continue to increase.

Epidemiological terms

Epidemiology

Epidemiology is the study of the distribution of illness in populations and its application to the control of health problems (Last, 1988). This information can be used by clinicians, managers and politicians in planning and running effective health care services. Epidemiological studies can be used to:

(a) identify the causes and contributory factors of disorders (including genetic and environmental risk);
(b) provide data on morbidity and mortality;
(c) assess the effectiveness of interventions in defined populations.

Prevalence

This is the number of cases of a disorder in a population. It is a proportion, expressed as cases per unit population. It is dependent on incidence, recovery and survival, as well as other factors relating to population movement such as migration.

Incidence

This is the number of new cases of a disorder in a population, developing over time. It is expressed as cases per unit population per unit time.

Standardised rates

When populations have different age and gender distributions, it is important to deal with standardised rates. These are rates adjusted to take account of these differences. If rates are standardised, it reduces the chance of interpreting differences between groups, when only the age or gender structure differ.

Sources of information

Routine sources

(a) Census information from the 10 yearly censuses carried out by the Office of Population Censuses and Surveys (OPCS). This includes socio-demographic details but little information directly relevant to mental health.
(b) Mortality statistics, which includes data about suicides.
(c) Local morbidity data from hospitals or districts. The quality of data has been poor but is improving.
(d) General practice data. This is also of variable quality.

Recently, there has been an increasing availability of morbidity data in the UK as a result of the changes in the National Health Service. These data are mainly of use in examining the process, rather than the outcome of health service activity, and are not easily broken down into accurate diagnostic groups.

Non-routine sources

Research

Most of the information on mental illness in the elderly has been collected in research carried out by academic or service researchers. The methods used in these studies are described below.

Surveys

Sources such as the General Household Survey, or ad hoc surveys set up by the OPCS (e.g. the Disability Survey) can provide useful data, but none are capable of including detailed enough information to answer questions about mental disorder. National surveys have included components on mental health and provide important information on samples chosen to be representative of the population of the country, but they have been somewhat limited by brevity and lack of follow-up and have not provided information on older populations. There are data emerging from large scale population studies of the older population which will be of value (Anonymous, 1997).

Case registers

In some areas case registers for specific conditions in defined populations have been set up (e.g. in Camberwell for Alzheimer's disease and schizophrenia). These are usually limited to those cases known to services. Criteria for the disorder covered by the register

---

Box 2.1 Sources of epidemiological information

Censuses
Mortality statistics and coroners courts
Hospital or trust figures
General practitioner data
Case registers
Surveys

---

may change over time, as may fashions in referral and treatment, which hampers time comparisons.

Types of study

Descriptive studies

Cross-sectional studies

Cross-sectional studies provide estimates of the magnitude of a disorder in the population. They are particularly appropriate for more common disorders such as dementia. For rarer disorders such as schizophrenia, alternative strategies including admissions, prescribing patterns or community service contact may be more appropriate. Conditions which relapse and remit, such as depression, are best examined by current mental state and mental state over a specified period before the interview. These studies are particularly useful for service planning.

Longitudinal studies

A limitation of cross-sectional studies is that prevalence is affected by survival and recovery, which may differ from population to population. Longitudinal studies follow cohorts of individuals who are initially disease free, to measure how many develop the disorder. If accurate records are available on a known cohort, retrospective studies can be carried out, for example, birth cohort studies. However, longitudinal studies present the difficulties of establishing and keeping track of a cohort and are often not helpful in the elderly, or in conditions that remit and relapse. More recent longitudinal studies, such as the Caerphilly Study (Chadwick, 1992), have multiple measurements at baseline and multiple end-points, including cardiovascular outcomes and cognitive and service measures.

Case-control studies

Case-control studies compare groups with and without disease for exposures or risk factors.

Ecological studies

Comparisons of populations can provide important insights into aetiology. This can be achieved by looking across regions within countries, across countries, across ethnic groups and geographical setting, by looking at migrants and comparing them with those who do not migrate, and by comparing those born between certain years (cohorts) or across time (periods). This can be done retrospectively or prospectively.

Expression of risk

(a) Relative risk: odds ratios (estimates of relative risk) calculate how much more likely a case is to have a given risk factor than a control. Relative risk is calculated as the incidence in the exposed population, divided by the incidence in the non-exposed population. It provides evidence of temporal association, but not causation.

(b) Absolute risk: this measures the absolute increase in risk of developing a disorder given a particular exposure or risk factor.

(c) Attributable risk: this is a measure of the risk of disease for an individual who has been exposed, or who has a risk factor. It is the difference in incidence rates for those exposed and those not exposed.

There are three major sources of error:

(a) Confounding variables: these variables have their own relationship to the risk factors and can therefore cause a spurious result or hide a positive association.

(b) Selection bias: the control group should reflect the study group, except for the risk factor studied.

(c) Information bias: it is often easier to obtain risk factor information from cases than controls.

Stages in epidemiological studies

The question

Studies are carried out to answer different questions and the results must be interpreted accordingly. An illustration of this is a survey to assess the requirement for long-stay geriatric beds. Such a survey only needs to examine a given population, in a fashion which identifies people with severe dependency or with behavioural difficulties. This does not provide, for example, an estimate of the prevalence of dementia.

Case definition

Having identified the question, the next step is clarifying the definition of caseness. There is a tendency for the literature to dichotomise normality and illness, whereas most disorders lie on a continuum of severity (Barker & Rose, 1990). Therefore, not only can the detailed criteria of case definition be different between studies, but also the severity defined as case level. A particular difficulty is the definition of suicide and attempted suicide. Criteria become increasingly elaborate in order to formalise arbitrary decisions about whether an individual is a case. The blurring of normality and caseness is particularly apparent in mental illness and in the elderly, where many factors interact such as physical illness, psychological illness and social well-being.

Increasingly, standardised criteria are being used. ICD–10 (World Health Organization, 1993) and DSM–IV (American Psychiatric Association, 1994) are used widely in epidemiological studies. The Diagnostic Interview Schedule (Robins *et al*, 1981) and the Canberra Interview contain information specifically to fulfil current diagnostic criteria (Social Psychiatry Research Unit, 1992). DSM–IV grappled with cross-cultural issues, which are a considerably source of difficulty with current criteria (Fabrega, 1992).

Sampling

Studies are only interpretable if it is clear who has been studied. There are a variety of possible sampling frames which have been used to estimate the importance of a disorder to the community. These include hospitals (Adelstein *et al*, 1968); nursing homes (Ames *et al*, 1988); total populations using the electoral register (Lindesay *et al*, 1989); age-selected populations from family health service authority lists (Chadwick 1992); or the door-to-door census approach (Livingston *et al*, 1990*a*). The sample can be complete, randomly selected or systematic (e.g. every third person on a list). If not complete, the sample may be stratified by age or gender, or other selected characteristics such as occupation or socio-economic group, so that some groups are not relatively over-represented.

Screening versus diagnosis

For some studies it is sufficient to collect a limited amount of information such as a cognitive scale, but for others a full diagnostic work-up is required. Because this is time-consuming and expensive, this type of interview is rarely applied to whole populations. A sampling procedure, on the basis of answers to a screening interview, allows the selection of individuals with a high probability of diagnosis (e.g. O'Connor *et al,* 1989). Occasionally diagnostic interviews are applied by clinicians to whole populations but this is unusual (e.g. Brayne & Calloway, 1989). An alternative method is for trained non-medical interviewers to apply an interview, which can be run through a computerised algorithm to provide a standardised 'diagnosis'. This approach is used in the Canberra Interview and the Geriatric Mental State Examination (AGECAT; Copeland *et al,* 1986).

Interviews

The information necessary to make a diagnosis can be collected from an individual in a face-to-face or telephone interview, collected by written questionnaire or extracted from case records. The data collection can be highly structured, which limits the qualitative nature of the data but eases standardisation, or it can be semi-structured which can increase qualitative data but cause problems with standardisation. The Cambridge Examination for Mental Disorders of the Elderly (Roth *et al,* 1988) and the Geriatric Mental State Examination (Copeland *et al,* 1986) are examples of highly structured questionnaires which contain most elements of a full psychiatric interview.

Interviewers

Data collection can be carried out by a variety of interviewers. These can be trained lay interviewers or qualified professionals. The choice of interviewer depends on the requirements of the interview, for example a physical examination will usually require a doctor. High

---

Box 2.2 Stages in epidemiological studies

Establishing the question(s)
Defining caseness
Sampling
Interviewing
Analysis and presentation of data

interrater reliability is achieved by the use of highly structured data collection and training and continuous monitoring of data collectors.

Quality control

Repeatability

There is a variation in the way that raters apply the same set of diagnostic criteria or interview schedule. This can be reduced by training, but not eliminated. Interrater reliability is more likely to be systematic than intra-interviewer variability, which is more likely to be random. There is, of course, variability in the respondent also. All these issues are well recognised in psychiatry, but make difficulties for comparative and aetiological studies since the error caused by such variation can obscure any real effects (Eaton *et al*, 1989).

Validity

The gold standard against which most instruments are compared is the clinical diagnosis. In the US this is often a consensus diagnosis, which is more reliable than individual diagnosis. If alternatives are available, such as neuropathological measures or progression of a disorder to a level where the diagnosis is not in doubt, they are preferred but have seldom been used to date. For example, in Alzheimer's disease where a pathological measure of disease is available, it is often difficult to obtain brain specimens.

Response rates

Response rates are important in understanding whether results truly represent the basic population, or whether they may be biased. Some studies report on the demographic characteristics of non-responders, but it is rarely possible to infer accurately what bias may have been introduced, unless further information is collected such as recorded admissions or general practitioners' notes. In practice this is often not possible and results are taken at face value.

Conclusion

Epidemiology involves the systematic study of disease in the population. The difficulties in old age psychiatry of defining disorders and populations have meant that studies have often had apparently conflicting results. More recently, bigger, systematic studies have helped to reach a consensus on the prevalence of depression and dementia. Larger cohort and case-control studies should help clarify aetiological and service issues.

References

Adelstein, A. M., Downham, D. Y., Stein, Z., *et al* (1968) The epidemiology of mental illness in an English city. *Social Psychiatry*, 3, 47–59.

American Psychiatric Association (1994) *Diagnostic and Statistical Manual of Mental Disorders* (4th edn) (DSM–IV). Washington, DC: APA.

Ames, D., Ashby, D., Mann, A. H., *et al* (1988) Psychiatric illness in elderly residents of Part III homes in one London Borough. *Age and Ageing*, 17, 249–256.

Anonymous (1997) *Cognitive Functioning and Ageing Study (CSAS), MRC Update no 2*, Spring. London: Medical Research Council.

Barker, D. J. P & Rose, G. (1990) *Epidemiology in Medical Practice*. London: Churchill Livingstone.

Brayne, C. & Calloway, P. (1989) An epidemiological study of dementia in a rural population of elderly women. *British Journal of Psychiatry*, 155, 214–219.

Central Statistical Office (1979) *Social Trends*, Vol. 9. London: Central Statistical Office.

Chadwick, C. (1992) The MRC multicentre study of cognitive function and ageing: a EURODEM incidence study in progress. *Neuroepidemiology*, 11 (suppl. 1), 37–43.

Copeland, J. R. M., Dewey, M. E. & Griffiths-Jones, H. M. (1986) A comprehensive diagnostic system and case nomenclature for elderly subjects: GMS and AGECAT. *Psychological Medicine*, 16, 89–99.

Eaton, W. W., Kramer, M., Anthony, J. C., *et al* (1989) Conceptual and methodological problems in estimation of the incidence of mental disorders from field survey data. In *Epidemiology and the Prevention of Mental Disorders* (eds B. Cooper & R. Helgason). London and New York: Routledge.

Fabrega, H. (1992) Diagnosis interminable: towards a culturally sensitive DSM–IV. *Journal of Nervous and Mental Disorder*, 180, 5–7.

Government Actuary's Department (1996) *1994-Based National Population Projections*. Series PP2, no. 20. London: HMSO.

Fries, J. F. (1989) Compression of morbidity: near or far? *Millbank Quarterly*, 208–232.

Jorm, A. F., Korten, A. E. & Henderson, A. S. (1987) The prevalence of dementia: a quantitative integration of the literature. *Acta Psychiatrica Scandinavica*, 76, 469–479.

Laslett, P. (1990) *A Fresh Map of Life*. Cambridge: Cambridge University Press.

Last, J. M. (1988) *A Dictionary of Epidemiology IEA*. Oxford: Oxford University Press.

Lindesay, J., Briggs, K. & Murphy, E. (1989) The Guys/Age Concern Survey. Prevalence rates of cognitive impairment, depression and anxiety in an urban elderly community. *British Journal of Psychiatry*, 155, 317–329.

Livingston, G., Hawkins, A., Graham, N., *et al* (1990*a*) The Gospel Oak study. Prevalence rates of dementia and depression and activity limitation among elderly residents in inner London. *Psychological Medicine*, 20, 137–146.

——, ——, ——, *et al* (1990*b*) The Gospel Oak Study. Use of health and social services by the dependent elderly in the community. *Health Trends*, 22, 70–73.

O'Connor, D. W., Pollitt, P. A., Hyde, J. B., *et al* (1989) The prevalence of dementia as measured by the Cambridge Examination for Mental Disorders of the Elderly. *Acta Psychiatrica Scandinavica*, 79, 190–198.

Office of Population Censuses and Surveys (1988) *The Prevalence of Disability Among Adults*. London: HMSO.

Robins, L. N., Helzer, J. E. Croughan, J., *et al* (1981) National Institute of Mental Health Diagnostic Interview Schedule. *Archives of General Psychiatry*, 38, 381–389.

Roth, M., Huppert, F. A., Tym, E., *et al* (1988) *CAMDEX. The Cambridge Examination for Mental Disorders of the Elderly*. Cambridge: Cambridge University Press.

Social Psychiatry Research Unit (1992) The Canberra Interview for the Elderly: a new field instrument for the diagnosis of dementia and depression by ICD–10 and DSM–III–R. *Acta Psychiatrica Scandinavica*, 85, 105–113.

World Health Organization (1993) *The ICD–10 Classification of Mental and Behavioural Disorders. Diagnostic Criteria for Research*. Geneva: World Health Organization.

3 Delirium

Brice Pitt

---

*Historical context ● Classification ● Epidemiology ● Clinical features
● Natural history ● Aetiology ● Mechanisms of delirium ● Differential
diagnosis ● Diagnosis ● Management ● Prognosis ● Conclusions*

Delirium is a common accompaniment of physical illness in old age, affecting about one in five of those admitted to medical wards and a higher number of those with fractured femurs. Its existence has long been recognised and recorded in general literature. It is a 'final common pathway disorder', the prime feature of which is altered arousal.

Historical context

Before the public health measures and the advent of antibiotics, infectious diseases were rife. Consequently delirium was a common experience in survivors, as was frequently reflected in the literature of the day. The Latin verb 'delire' (to be deranged, crazy, out of one's wits) appears in the Coventry mystery plays in 1400: "God wyl be vengyd on man.... That wyl nevyr be schrevyn, but evermore doth delyre". Other accounts from literature include:

(a) Shakespeare's death of Falstaff ("a babbled of green fields").
(b) Lady Macbeth sleepwalking (compounded by guilt and insomnia).
(c) Tolstoy's depiction of Anna Karenina's post-partum delirium.
(d) Dickens' account of Fagin's, presumably psychogenic, pre-execution fantasising.

One of the best known literary deliria is that from which King Lear emerges to recognise his discarded daughter Cordelia; this is not only the most moving moment in the least sparing of Shakespeare's tragedies, but the culmination of an extraordinarily astute and perceptive series of clinical observations of madness in old age. Lear begins the play with his judgement deranged, perhaps by cerebral vascular disease. After being rejected by his daughters and exposed to the storm, he becomes delirious as a result of hypothermia, pneumonia, or both? Then (as is the best outcome of delirium) he

27

recovers and is reconciled with his youngest daughter. The tragedy becomes even more bitter and she is killed, Lear only briefly outliving her. The play indicates some important features of delirium:

(a) Older patients are especially liable to delirium.
(b) Exposure and infection are common causes, so is severe emotional disturbance.
(c) The premorbid personality contributes to its content.
(d) It is reversible.
(e) There is a high mortality.

Classification

Definitions

The *Oxford English Dictionary* (1971) defines delirium as: "a disordered state of the mental faculties resulting from disturbance of the functions of the brain, and characterised by incoherent speech, hallucinations, restlessness and frenzied or manic excitement".

Etymologically, the word is a metaphor, derived from the Latin 'lira', a ridge or furrow in ploughing, meaning 'to go out of one's furrow'. 'Delirium' is a long-established term, expressing in a single word a concept, which is preferable to alternatives, such as 'acute confusional state', 'acute brain syndrome', 'acute brain failure', 'acute encephalopathy' and even 'intensive care unit psychosis' (Roca, 1988).

Lishman (1978) defines delirium as "a syndrome of impaired consciousness along with intrusive abnormalities derived from the fields of perception and affect". Mesulam's (1985) definition is: "a change of mental state in which the most salient features occur in overall attentional tone", while Lipowski (1987) describes: "acute onset of a fluctuating state of awareness, accompanied by sleep–wake disruption, lethargy or agitation and nocturnal worsening of symptoms are diagnostic".

ICD–10

The Tenth Revision of the International Classification of Diseases and Related Health Problems (ICD–10; World Health Organization, 1992) describes delirium (not induced by alcohol and other psychoactive substances) as: "an aetiologically non-specific syndrome characterised by concurrent disturbances of consciousness and attention, perception, thinking, memory, psychomotor behaviour and the sleep–wake cycle" (Box 3.1). It may occur at any age but is most common after the age of 60. The delirious state is transient and of fluctuating intensity; most cases recover within four weeks or less.

**Box 3.1 The ICD–10 criteria features of delirium
(World Health Organization, 1992)**

Impairment of consciousness and attention (on a continuum
from clouding to coma; reduced ability to direct, focus,
sustain and shift attention)

Global disturbance of cognition (perceptual distortions, illusions
and hallucinations most often visual; impairment of abstract
thinking and comprehension with or without transient
delusions, but typically with some degree of incoherence;
impairment of immediate recall and of recent memory but
with relatively intact remote memory; distortion of time as
well as, in more severe cases, of place and person)

Psychomotor disturbances (hypo- or hyperactivity and
unpredictable shifts from one to the other; increased reaction
time; increased or decreased flow of speech; enhanced startle
reaction)

Disturbance of the sleep-wake cycle (insomnia or, in severe
cases, total sleep loss or reversal of the sleep–wake cycle;
daytime drowsiness; nocturnal worsening of symptoms;
disturbing dreams or nightmares which may continue as
hallucinations after awakening)

Emotional disturbances, (e.g. depression, anxiety or fear,
irritability, euphoria, apathy or wondering perplexity)

Epidemiology

Being a transient disorder, usually associated with physical illness
affecting brain function, delirium has a low prevalence in the
community and does not appear in epidemiological studies. Even in
general hospitals its prevalence is lower than that of dementia, which
increases the risk of admission by dependency and self-neglect and
is then associated with delayed discharge. Complementary incidence
studies are therefore appropriate and informative for delirium.

A number of studies have looked at the incidence and prevalence
of delirium in older patients on medical wards (Pitt, 1995). These have
found a prevalence of between 10 and 20%, and new cases in 4–10%
of medical admissions. O'Keefe & Lavan (1997) found delirium in 18%
of patients admitted to an acute geriatric unit, and it arose in a further
24% in the course of their stay.

The nature of the ward, acute or less so, and the procedures
undertaken there (e.g. medical or surgical), may well relate to the
frequency of delirium. Gustafson *et al* (1988) found an incidence of
delirium in over 60% of consecutive patients undergoing surgery for
fractured neck of femur.

Clinical features

Impaired consciousness

'Clouding' of consciousness is a classic sign of delirium, but is not of great diagnostic value because it is only intermittently present. Although Rabins & Folstein (1982) claimed to use clouding alone to distinguish patients with dementia from those with delirium, rating them on a continuum from 'accessible' to 'inaccessible' and validating the distinction by the outcome, in clinical practice it is of far less importance in establishing the diagnosis than the length of the history of confusion. Old people with dementia may be drowsy because they are bored, replete, have been awake all night or are sedated. Where cognition is grossly impaired it is not always easy to determine whether there is also any diminution of consciousness.

Impaired consciousness ranges from failure to maintain attention and distractibility, through drowsiness to unconsciousness, all of which fluctuate. The milder degrees of impairment are the most common, and are very easily missed. Rockwood *et al* (1994) found that before training in the recognition of delirium, house staff diagnosed delirium in 3% of patients over 65 admitted to general medical wards, though after training it was recognised in three times as many. However, Harwood *et al* (1997) found that physicians in Oxford recorded the diagnosis in 14 out of 15 patients in whom psychiatrists had diagnosed delirium by DSM–III–R (American Psychiatric Association, 1987) criteria.

Fairweather (1991) points out that there is a paradoxical contrast between a reduced level of consciousness and increased arousal; a sleepy old person may be startled into sudden apprehensive or aggressive vigilance.

Perceptual disturbances

There is a difficulty overall in making sense of what is perceived (Lipowski, 1994). Dreams and reality are muddled, and patients may take personally what is unrelated to them (ideas of reference) or feel distanced and detached from what concerns them closely.

Visual hallucinations (for example, of insects, strange people, shadowy presences, fronds that cannot be brushed away) or illusions (the flecks on the wall or the pattern on the counterpane perceived as mites, ants or beetles on the move) typically predominate. Distortions include increased, diminished or distanced sights and sounds. According to Fairweather (1991), disturbances of body image are not uncommon: some parts feel shrunk, others enlarged or there may be a sensation of floating. Time, too, may be distorted; a day may seem like a week, a week like a few hours.

These phenomena are neither invariably present nor diagnostic. They are sometimes present in dementia, even when uncomplicated by delirium. Even when they are present in delirium they may not be reported by patients who have enough insight to fear that they may be regarded as evidence of madness!

Impairment of abstract thinking and comprehension

Logic, reason and judgement are all jeopardised by delirium, and 'getting hold of the wrong end of the stick' is a basis of the, not infrequent, paranoid delusions. Sometimes talk that almost makes sense is nevertheless unrelated to the present situation and it is hard to 'get on the patient's wavelength'. A son visiting his sick mother in a nursing home found her talking with animation to an empty room; both before, and after, she caught sight of him. She was discussing domestic arrangements and appointments for her late husband's patients, and the son could not get her to address current issues at all, such as her health and his news. Instead, everything he said was grist to the mill of her preoccupation.

Talk may be rapid and hard to follow, or hesitant, repetitive, stammering, laboured and dysarthric – not unlike that of someone who is drunk. Disconnected, muttered, dysphasic ramblings characterise the patient who is seriously ill with delirium. Incoherence (a late, and then fixed, feature of dementia) is a common but fluctuating accompaniment of delirium.

Memory impairment

The impairment of memory in delirium is the most constant sign and is fairly readily elicited by the judicious use of such cognitive tests as the Abbreviated Mental Test Score (AMTS; Hodkinson, 1973) and the Mini-Mental State Examination (MMSE; Folstein *et al*, 1975) (see Chapter 1). Ni-Chonchubhair *et al* (1995) found a drop of two points on the AMTS, from the pre-operative to the third post-operative day, to diagnose delirium with a specificity of 84% and a sensitivity of 93%. Registration is especially affected by inattention, distractibility and clouding of consciousness, so that many patients, after recovery from delirium, recall very little of the experience – except, perhaps, the more horrific or bizarre hallucinations. Recent memory suffers more than remote and contributes to the disorientation, which, at some time or other, is always found in delirium (of time and place most commonly, but also of person).

Psychomotor disturbances

Excited or agitated over-activity is less common in delirium in old age than apathetic inactivity, although one may suddenly give way to the other. Tremor is apparent, especially when the patient tries to hold a cup or glass, and the sickest patients pluck at the bedclothes (the 'typhoid state' of the past century). Lipowski (1990) distinguishes three types of delirium according to the state of alertness and psychomotor behaviour:

(a) Hyperalert–hyperactive: the patient is agitated, distractible, emotional, more likely to hallucinate and show such autonomic features as tremor, sweating, a rapid pulse and breathing, dry mouth, raised blood pressure and dilated pupils.
(b) Hypoalert–hypoactive: lethargic, withdrawn, slow to respond and frequently incontinent.
(c) Mixed, with unpredictable rapid shifts from vigilant restlessness to inactivity.

Disorder of the sleep–wake cycle

Lipowski (1980) describes "disorder of wakefulness" as the second core feature of delirium (the first being cognitive impairment). He points out the similarity of the sense of unreality, illusions and hallucinations in the delirious patient to a 'waking dreamer'. Likewise, the reversal of the sleep–wake cycle is similar to the sleepiness by day and restless insomnia at night. The 'waking dream' state has been related to stage one rapid eye movement sleep, from malfunction of serotoninergic neurones in the raphe nuclei and/or noradrenergic neurones in the locus caeruleus (Hishikawa, 1981).

Emotional disturbance

While apathy is the most common emotional accompaniment of delirium in old age, anger, irritation, terror, apprehension, bewilderment, depression and even euphoria are also seen, although not usually for long. Lability is characteristic of emotional states other than apathy, laughter giving way to tears, tears to rage, rage to fear, and fear again to laughter, or any of these ending in sudden sleep. Anger may be associated with aggression or paranoia, fear with attempts to escape, euphoria to sexual disinhibition, all of which may cause problems in management. It is worth bearing in mind that however troubled or troublesome the patient is, the state may well not last long.

Natural history

Typically the onset of delirium is acute; one day it is not present, the next it is (or it even develops in the evening, not having been there

---

Box 3.2 Physical: mnemonic for the clinical features of delirium

Perplexity: because the onset of delirium is so acute the patient is often bemused and bewildered, which may better distinguish it from dementia than, say, clouding of consciousness
Hallucinations: mainly visual
Yawning: by day, because of lack of sleep at night
Suspicion: misapprehensions and frank delusions, secondary to cognitive disorder
Illusions: distorted perceptions
Cognitive impairment: memory, communication, comprehension, judgement
Apathy or agitation: psychomotor disturbances
Lability of mood: laughter, tears, anger, terror

---

during the day). The prodromal symptoms described by Roca (1988), restlessness, nocturnal agitation, daytime drowsiness, irritability, hypersensitivity to noise and light for a few days before the frank disorder, are probably delirium itself writ somewhat small.

Delirium usually lasts up to a week or two, subsiding as the underlying disorder abates, although cognitive recovery often lags behind physical recovery. Rockwood (1989) found that 18 out of 24 delirious states lasted less than a day (and could, therefore, very easily have been overlooked), while of the rest, the longest was for a week. Koponen *et al* (1989), on the other hand, found that the average duration in 70 elderly subjects in a psychiatric setting was 20 days, with a range of three to 81 days.

ICD–10 states:

> "However, delirium lasting, with fluctuations, for up to six months is not uncommon, especially when arising in the course of chronic liver disease, carcinoma or subacute bacterial endocarditis. The distinction that is sometimes made between acute and subacute delirium is of little clinical relevance; the condition should be seen as a unitary syndrome of variable duration and severity ranging from mild to very severe."

Aetiology

Why does one old person with pneumonia become delirious while another does not? The severity of the infection may differ, but so may susceptibility to delirium. Box 3.3 lists factors which increase the liability of elderly people to delirium (Lipowski, 1987).

Predisposing factors

Age

Seymour and colleagues (Seymour & Pringle, 1983; Seymour & Vaz, 1987) found higher rates of post-operative delirium in patients over 75 years than in those aged 65–74. Burrows *et al* (1985) gave a battery of psychological tests (sorting shapes, recall of an address after 10 minutes, digit span, random reaction time included) to patients before and after cataract extraction, comparing a younger group of subjects (mean age 50) with an older group (mean age 74). Transient cognitive impairment was significantly greater in the older group, who were significantly worse at performing the tests mentioned during the first three days after surgery.

Brain damage

Dementia is a major risk factor for delirium, which sets the clinician the taxing task of distinguishing one cause of confusion from another. Koponen *et al* (1989) found predisposing brain disease in 81% of delirious elderly patients admitted to a psychiatric hospital, and 30% of Rockwood's (1989) delirious old people admitted to medical wards had had dementia previously. Dementia was identified as one of three major risk factors for delirium by O'Keefe & Lavan (1996). Other forms of brain damage than dementia (stroke, Parkinson's disease, head injury, learning difficulties) may also lower the threshold for delirium.

Sensory deprivation

Blindness and deafness limit sensory information and may predispose to the perceptual disturbances of delirium.

Environment

Sudden inadequately explained removal of an old person from one place to another (usually within an institutional setting) might facilitate delirium, especially when cognition is already somewhat impaired. Stories of mentally frail old people who become acutely confused on holiday or when moved from one ward to another are all too common. Inouye & Charpentier (1996) identified the use of physical restraints as a risk factor.

Sleep disturbance

This may contribute to and warn of imminent delirium. Sleep may be disturbed by worry, depression, noisiness, excessive heat or cold, discomfort, pain, itching, shortness of breath and a full bladder or bowel, among other causes, some of which are easily preventable.

Drugs and alcohol

Foy *et al* (1986) studied patients, aged over 65, admitted to the department of medicine at the Royal Newcastle Hospital. They found that the half who were using benzodiazepine hypnotics had a greater risk of developing a confusional state during the admission, especially if the drugs were stopped abruptly. Habituation to hypnotics may be a more frequent risk factor for delirium in old people than alcohol misuse, which is of great importance in younger adults. Any 'iatrogenic event', notably the prescription of three or more drugs, is implicated as putting the patient at risk of delirium according to Inouye & Charpentier (1996).

Personal characteristics

While it is unlikely that there is any personality susceptibility to delirium, the classic paper by Wolff & Curran (1935) showed that people having a subsequent episode of delirium, even for a different cause, repeated the clinical pattern and content of the first, suggesting a 'host' component.

Precipitating factors

Any physical illness has the potential to cause delirium in a susceptible old person but some seem especially liable to do so. O'Keefe & Lavan (1996) found a raised serum urea and severe illness to be important risk factors. Inouye & Charpentier (1996) identified the use of a bladder catheter. Rockwood (1989) listed the most common causes of delirium, in older patients on admission, as: congestive cardiac failure, gram-negative sepsis (mainly associated with pyelonephritis) and pneumonia.

Box 3.3 Predisposing factors

Ageing or disease of the brain
Impairment of vision and hearing
Reduced synthesis of neurotransmitters (especially acetylcholine)
Changes in pharmacokinetics and dynamics of drugs
High prevalence of chronic diseases
High susceptibility to acute diseases
Reduced capacity for homeostatic regulation

Heart disease

Cardiac causes other than congestive cardiac failure include myocardial infarction (often painless) and transient arrhythmias (notably paroxysmal supraventricular tachycardia) which can cause recurrent delirium and may be revealed by an ambulatory electrocardiograph (ECG). Another cause of recurrent delirium is cerebral emboli from a fibrillating left atrium or carotid atheromatous plaque. Sudden bleeding (e.g. from esophageal varices or a peptic ulcer) may present with delirium, as may other states of acute hypotension, perhaps induced by drugs. Temporal arteritis should not be overlooked (Pascuzzi *et al*, 1989).

Infection

Levkoff *et al* (1988) found a urinary tract infection to be the major risk factor in delirium, while I have found cellulitis (not always apparent until the patient is properly undressed) to be another infection often associated with the syndrome.

Respiratory failure

Respiratory failure, perhaps precipitated by further infection in a patient already crippled by chronic obstructive airways disease, must be mentioned: the patient's wretched plight is compounded by fluctuating confusion from hypoxia and respiratory acidosis or alkalosis. Whitney & Gannon (1966) described obstructive sleep apnoea presenting as acute delirium.

Falls

Many old people fall over and do not remember having done so, so the possibility of concussion, a subdural hematoma or even a fractured femur (in a patient who is anyway not very ambulant) should be considered even if there is no history of a fall. Neglected, impoverished, infirm, depressed, eccentric or miserly old people are at risk of malnutrition and hypothermia, both of which may present with delirium (Inouye & Charpentier, 1996).

Endocrine disorders

Diabetes may be associated with delirium (ketosis, vascular and renal complications, hypoglycaemia from insulin treatment). Hyper-parathyroidism (Peterson, 1968), hyperthyroidism and hypothyroidism ('myxoedematous madness'; Asher, 1949) are other endocrine disorders that occasionally present with delirium.

Drug reactions

Delirium may present as a serious adverse drug reaction. Grimley Evans (1982) points out that illness may result from an adverse reaction to a drug previously well tolerated (e.g. digitalis toxicity following a decline in renal function). Anticholinergic drugs, present in eye drops and anaesthesia and used in the treatment of Parkinson's disease and depression, are especially 'deliriogenic' (Tune *et al*, 1981; Blazer *et al*, 1983). Potential precipitants of delirium are listed in Box 3.4.

Mechanisms of delirium

The blood–brain barrier to corporeal toxins may be impaired by ageing (Fairweather, 1991) and dementias are associated with increased vascular permeability (Alafuzoff *et al*, 1983; Elovara *et al*, 1985), which may help to explain the susceptibility of the demented brain to delirium.

Engel & Romano (1959) postulated that there is a widespread reduction of cerebral metabolism, reflected in slowing of background activity on the electroencephalogram (EEG). Blass & Plum (1983) suggested that the synthesis of acetylcholine is especially affected. Delirium has been induced clinically by anticholinergic drugs, and reversed by the anticholinesterase physostigmine (Greene, 1971; Summers & Reich, 1979). Itil & Fink (1966) proposed an imbalance between central cholinergic and noradrenergic activity. Banki & Vojnik (1978) have also implicated serotonin, and Hebenstreit *et al* (1989) claim to have mitigated delirium both prospectively and currently by L-tryptophan transfusions.

Grimley Evans (1982) saw delirium as the consequence of an exacerbation of 'neural noise' distorting attention, memory and perception. Noise, already somewhat increased by age, is increased further by disordered neurotransmitter activity, from anoxic or toxic effects on neurones, while perception is impaired by sensory deprivation (Slade, 1984).

Diffferential diagnosis

Dementia

I have pointed out elsewhere (Pitt, 1987) the many similarities between delirium and dementia (thereby agreeing with Isaacs (1992) and others, who talk of brain failure, acute or chronic). Macdonald & Treloar (1996), in an elegant essay about validating concepts of dementia, suggest that the only definite difference between dementias

Box 3.4 Precipitating factors (adapted from Davison, 1989; Fairweather, 1991)

Intracerebral
Vascular: transient ischaemic attack, stroke (infarction or haemorrhage), subarachnoid haemorrhage
Head injury: concussion, subdural haematoma
Infection: meningitis, encephalitis, cerebral abscess
Epileptic: ictal or post-ictal
Neoplasm: primary (glioma), secondary (carcinoma of breast, bronchus)

Extra-cerebral
Vascular: myocardial infection, heart failure, arrhythmia, aortic stenosis, temporal arteritis, haemorrhage, severe anaemia, hypotension
Trauma: surgery, fractures, burns
Infection: respiratory, urinary tact, cellulitis, subacute bacterial endocarditis, herpes zoster, AIDS
Neoplastic: carcinomatosis
Metabolic: hypoxia (heart or lung disease), hepatic failure, renal failure
Endocrine: hyperthyroidism, hypothyroidism, hyperparathyroidism, hypoparathyoidism, hypoglycaemia, diabetic precoma
Electrolyte imbalance: diarrhoea, vomiting, dehydration
Body temperature: Pyrex, hypothermia
Starvation: hypoglycaemia, vitamin deficiency

Drugs
Alcohol use, misuse and withdrawal of alcohol
Benzodiazepines and their withdrawal
Anticholinergics: tricyclic antidepressants, some antipsychotics, old anti-Parkinsonian drugs
Dopamine agonists: levodopa, bromocriptine, amantidine, selegiline
Anticonvulsants: phenytoin, barbiturates,
Cardiovascular: digoxin, diuretics, beta-blockers
Miscellaneous: lithium carbonate, cimetidine, non-steroidal, anti-inflammatory drugs

and deliria is that the latter recover – or do they? (see below). However, the traditional distinctions between the syndromes are of prime importance to the clinician (Table 3.1).

Without a history, the distinction is not always easy. Impairment of cognition, affective reactions (Farrell & Gauzini, 1995) and perceptual disturbances are common to both, and clouding of consciousness is neither always present in the delirious nor always absent in those who have dementia. People with dementia hallucinate sometimes and when they do they see rather than hear things. They may also develop (mainly paranoid) delusions, although these tend to be much more sustained than those of delirium. Delirium is not associated with a manifest physical cause in a quarter of sufferers, who, on other grounds, seem likely to be delirious (Lipowski, 1980), while people with dementia are not infrequently physically ill. Even the duration of the delirium, as long as six months (World Health Organization, 1992), overlaps with that of dementia (three months according to Marsden, 1978). The distinction of prolonged delirium from Lewy body dementia (McKeith, 1995) may present problems, though complete lucidity during the fluctuating course of the latter is unusual.

However, the onset of delirium is acute, within a day or two, and even in those who already have dementia an acute change in the level of cognition and functioning is usually reported. Clouding of consciousness is nearly always evident at some time during any 24-hour period, and most of the time there is an obvious physical illness (or prescription) to account for the delirium. Hallucinations and illusions dominate the scene more than is usual in dementia. And (although this is a bit late in the day for a diagnosis) the outcome is

Table 3.1 Features of delirium and dementia (adapted from Lipowski, 1987)

Feature	Delirium	Dementia
Onset	Acute	Insidious
Course	Fluctuating	Consistent
Duration	Hours to weeks	Months to years
Lucid spells	Common	Early – occasional
Sundowning	Always	Often
Awareness	Reduced	Clear
Alertness	Heightened or reduced	Usually normal
Attention	Fitful, distractible	More sustained
Sleep–wake cycle	Always disrupted	Occasionally disrupted
Orientation	Variably impaired	More consistently impaired
Memory	Immediate and recent impairment	Recent and remote impairment
Speech	Variably rambling and incoherent	Early – losing words Late – incoherent
Hallucinations	Common, visual	Occasional
Delusions	Fleeting	Early – more sustained Late – absent
Affect	Labile, intense	Often normal or apathetic
Physical illness	Usual	Occasional
Recovery	Common	Very rare

likely to be death or recovery: only the former is usually available to people with dementia.

Mania

Acute mania may take the form of pseudodelirium (Lipowski, 1980). Flights of ideas, especially where the associations are loose, are not unlike delirious ramblings, and manic patients are both inattentive and distractible. Cognition is not easily tested in mania, although the occasional remark may reveal that the patient is quite 'au fait' with matters personal and general. Euphoria is not always part of mania in old age (Pitt, 1982) and there may not always be a past history of affective disorder. However, the absence of an underlying physical disorder and the patient's continuing volubility, over-activity and disinhibition will generally make the diagnosis clear in a week or two. There is, of course, no reliable biochemical test for mania.

Depression

Agitated or retarded depression superficially resembles Lipowski's (1990) hyperalert–hyperactive and hypoactive forms of delirium. Farrell & Gauzini (1995) found that 42% of 'delirious' medically ill old people referred to a consultation–liaison service, were in fact depressed. There is some cognitive impairment in severe depression, but the onset is more gradual than is usual in delirium (except in the recurrent bipolar form of the illness, when the history should be known), and the depth and persistence of the depression, with ideas of profound despair, guilt, poverty or nihilistic delusions, far exceed what is occasionally experienced in delirium. Any refusal of food or fluids is far more resolute, and could actually cause delirium, complicating the depression, through dehydration.

Schizophrenia

Now that so many 'graduate' people with schizophrenia, who are not always able to take proper care of themselves, are back in the community; sick, thought-disordered elderly people appearing in acute medical and geriatric wards could be thought to be delirious by those unfamiliar with schizophrenia. Acute schizophrenia (apart from paraphrenia, in which cognition and personality are well preserved) is rare in later life, but may at first resemble delirium: organic incoherence and schizophrenic thought-disorder are not so easily distinguished. However, lucid spells are lacking in schizophrenia; hallucinations are mainly auditory; the affect may be flat or incongruous rather than labile; rapport may be elusive; and, unless there is a superimposed delirium, the psychosis will persist without psychopharmacological treatment.

Diagnosis

History

As in every medical diagnosis, the history and examination are paramount. Cognitively impaired patients cannot give a reliable history, so information from others must be sought at the earliest opportunity. This will include when and how the condition developed; what seemed to precipitate it (especially any recent medication); its subsequent course; and any risk factors, especially dementia.

Mental state examination

Mental state examination includes a cognitive test such as the AMTS (Hodkinson, 1973) or the MMSE (Folstein *et al*, 1975) (see Chapter 1).

Specific scales

A number of specific scales have been introduced, mainly for the purpose of research:

(a) The Delirium Rating Scale (DRS; Trzepacz *et al*, 1988), developed as a complement to DSM criteria to indicate the severity of delirium, has items which refer to aetiology and course. Rockwood *et al* (1996) found that a cut off point of 10 on the DRS diagnosed delirium with a sensitivity of 82% and a specificity of 94%.

(b) The Delirium Symptom Interview (Albert *et al*, 1992), based on DSM–III, assesses three 'critical' symptoms (disorientation, disturbance of consciousness, perceptual disturbance), as well as disruption of the sleep–wake cycle, incoherence, altered psychomotor behaviour and fluctuations. There is a behavioural sub-scale for patients who do not communicate. The instrument is designed to be usable by other than doctors.

(c) The Confusion Assessment Method Questionnaire (Inouye *et al*, 1990) requires the following features for the diagnosis of delirium (based upon DSM–III): acute change in mental state, fluctuating course, inattention and either disorganised thinking or altered level of consciousness.

(d) The Confusional State Evaluation (CSE) has been introduced by Robertson *et al* (1997) in the hope that it will supersede its predecessors. There are 12 core items: disorientation in four modes, thought, memory and concentration disturbance, distractibility, perseveration, impaired contact, paranoid ideation and hallucinations. There are seven associated symptoms: irritability, lability, wakeful disturbance, increased/reduced psychomotor activity, unease and disturbance of the sleep–wake pattern. Three items relate to the duration and intensity of the delirium.

(e) The Informant Questionnaire on Cognitive Decline in the Elderly (IQCDE; Jorm, 1994) is a useful means of recording information from informants.

Physical examination

A thorough physical examination will usually indicate the most likely cause of the problems suggested by the history. Such an examination may not be all that easy in an uncooperative or resistant patient, and tact, persuasiveness and opportunism may be demanded to bring it to a conclusion. It is tempting, but not good practice, to wait until the patient is more compliant, because the sooner the diagnosis is made and appropriate treatment started the better. Physical signs suggestive of delirium, fever, tachycardia (Rabins & Folstein, 1982), dysarthria, tremor, asterixis and myoclonus (Fairweather, 1991), may be detected at this time.

Investigations

Body temperature, urine analysis, full blood count and erythrocyte sedimentation rate, biochemical profile including plasma glucose, liver function tests, thyroid function tests, ECG and chest X-ray are always indicated, and serum B12, serology, blood culture, blood gases and ambulatory ECG are often also required. More invasive investigations, such as lumbar puncture and cerebral imaging, are sometimes necessary.

EEG typically shows slowing of alpha rhythms, the emergence of theta waves, and eventually bilaterally symmetrical predominantly frontal delta waves (Davison, 1989). Rabins & Folstein (1982) found diffusely slow EEGs in 81% of their delirious subjects but in only 33% of their patients with dementia. While it is rarely appropriate to use EEG in the diagnosis of delirium per se, it can help to identify focal lesions: infarcts, tumours and epilepsy.

Management

Delirium is an ominous syndrome with a high mortality, so unless it is a terminal event in a patient with a long illness in continuing care it demands active treatment, which usually means in a well-equipped general hospital. Apart from specific treatment for the underlying disorder, the patient needs:

Fluids

A fluid balance chart; subcutaneous or intravenous fluids if oral intake is inadequate.

Nourishment

Nutritious and high calorie drinks are needed until an appetising balanced diet is accepted; weighing is a useful check. Routine administration of vitamin supplements is not necessary.

Excretion

Urinary output of less than 1 litre a day suggests possible dehydration or retention (needing catheterisation), while constipation may warrant laxatives or a gentle enema.

Information

This, par excellence, is a situation for reality orientation (Holden & Woods, 1988); a large clock and calendar and a familiar photograph may help (Macdonald *et al*, 1989).

Reassurance

Reassurance should be combined with reorientation. "Mr Jones, you're here in St Saviour's Hospital on Ward Nine and I'm nurse Brown; you've got a nasty chest infection and it's made you a bit confused. You came in the day before yesterday, and it's 10 o'clock in the morning of Thursday the 14th of April; your wife was here last evening and she'll be here this afternoon. I'm just going to ask you to take these antibiotic capsules which will soon put you right; here are some 'Get well' cards, for you to look at when you're ready. Ring that bell if you need me for anything – nurse Brown: all right?" (Pitt, 1995). Such an approach requires well-trained, well-supported, patient, empathic and accepting staff. They are still to be found, but not always and not everywhere. Anxious, rejecting staff, more concerned about potentially disruptive behaviour than what underlies it, are quick to shunt the patient into a side-room, use cot-sides and call for sedation or transfer, which may be to the patient's detriment.

Rest

Bright, plain, well-lit surroundings, ready access to the nursing team, quiet, physical comfort and a regular routine all tend to lessen anxiety and promote rest without recourse to sedation.

Sedation

Sedation is sometimes needed, especially when agitation and restlessness are causing exhaustion. Major tranquillisers are useful (see chapter 16). Phenothiazines, like chlorpromazine and thioridazine are anticholinergic, and chlorpromazine is hypotensive too. Drugs with a high affinity for dopamine receptors are preferable. One is haloperidol, 0.5–3 mg orally (tablets or liquid) up to four times a day (or by intramuscular injection). Extrapyramidal side-effects (stiffness, tremor, akathisia, drooling) may rarely require an anti-Parkinsonian (and anticholinergic) drug such as orphenadrine, 100 mg thrice a day by mouth or procyclidine two or three times a day by injection. However, reducing the dose or stopping the neuroleptic is to be preferred. Newer antipsychotics such as risperidone or olanzapine may prove useful.

Minor tranquillisers (benzodiazepines) also have a place in withdrawal syndromes, partly because they are anticonvulsant, although they themselves can cause delirium when withdrawn from those who are habituated to them. The longer-acting are the most suitable (Davison, 1989), e.g. diazepam up to 20 mg a day in divided doses by mouth or intravenous injection. Temazepam (10–20 mg at night) or zopiclone are useful hypnotics.

Meagher *et al* (1996) found that only four of eight potential environmental modifications were used in over 50% of delirious patients referred for consultation–liaison, and these were for the more severely delirious, agitated and emotionally labile patients with sleep–wake disturbance rather than (as might have been more appropriate) those who were disorientated or suffered altered perceptions and disturbed thinking.

Prognosis

There is good evidence that the presence of delirium worsens the chances of surviving the underlying illness (Pitt, 1985). A third of Bedford's (1959) huge series of 4000 patients, delirious on admission to hospital, died within a month. Of the survivors, 80% made a full mental recovery but after six months 5% were still confused. Rockwood (1993) found that after a year, recovery from delirium was complete in only 59% of their sample; prolonged memory impairment was common. While it is most clinicians' experience that delirious patients who survive, recover, there is a dearth of good studies to demonstrate that this is so, or that if there is continuing cognitive impairment it is part of previous dementia and not the consequence of the delirium.

Saravay & Lavin (1994), reviewing 11 outcome studies, concluded that impaired cognition associated with delirium was a major factor leading to longer stay in hospital and increased use of medical resources. O'Keefe & Lavan (1997) found delirium in patients admitted to an acute geriatric unit to be independently associated with longer stay, functional decline, increased risk of hospital-acquired complications and long-term care

Conclusions

Age and dementia are major predisposing factors of delirium. Infections, anoxic, vascular, metabolic and drug-induced disorders the most common precipitants. Mechanisms include impairment of the blood–brain barrier, neurotransmitter derangement (especially acetylcholine) and increased 'neural noise'. Delirium carries a serious risk of mortality – much greater than dementia, and up to 20 times greater than that of like illness without delirium. It is mainly differentiated from dementia by its abrupt onset and brief duration; otherwise the disorders are strikingly similar. Fluids, nourishment, excretion, information, reassurance, rest and judicious sedation are part of the general management, best undertaken in a general hospital. Mental recovery in survivors is thought to be the rule.

Acknowledgement

This chapter is revised and brought up-to-date from 'Delirium in old age: causes diagnosis and treatment' (1995), in *Acute Medical Illness in Old Age* (eds A. J. Sinclair & K. W. Woodhouse), pp. 259–274. London: Chapman and Hall Medical.

References

Alafuzoff, L., Adolfsson, R., Bucht, G., *et al* (1983) Albumin and immunoglobulin in plasma and cerebrospinal fluid and blood–cerebrospinal fluid barrier function in patients with dementia of Alzheimer type and multi-infarct dementia. *Journal of Neurological Science*, 60, 465–472.

Albert, M. S., Levkoff, M. E., Reilly, C., *et al* (1992) The delirium symptom interview: an interview for the detection of delirium symptoms in hospitalised patients. *Journal of Geriatric Psychiatry and Neurology*, 5, 14–21.

46   *Pitt*

American Psychiatric Association (1987) *Diagnostic and Statistical Manual of Mental Disorders* (3rd edn, revised) (DSM–III–R). Washington, DC: APA.

Asher, R. (1949) Myxoedematous madness. *British Medical Journal*, 2, 555–562.

Banki, C. M. & Vojnik, M. (1978) Comparative simultaneous measurement of cerebrospinal fluid 5-hydroxyindoleacetic acid and blood serotonin levels in delirium tremens and clozapine-induced delirious reaction. *Journal of Neurology, Neurosurgery and Psychiatry*, 41, 420–424.

Bedford, P. D. (1959) General medical aspects of confusional states in elderly people. *British Medical Journal*, 2, 185–188.

Blass, J. P. & Plum, F. (1983) Metabolic encephalopathies. In *The Neurology of Aging* (eds I. Z. Katzman & R. D. Terry). Philadelphia, PA: Davis.

Blazer, D., Federspiel, C. F. & Ray, W. A. (1983) The risk of anticholinergic toxicity in the elderly: a study of prescribing practices in two populations. *Journal of Gerontology*, 38, 31–35.

Burrows, J., Briggs, R. S. & Ewington, A. R. (1985) Cataract extraction and confusion in elderly patients. *Journal of Clinical and Experimental Gerontology*, 7, 51–70.

Davison, K. (1989) Acute organic brain-syndromes. *British Journal of Hospital Medicine*, 41, 89–92.

Elovara, I., Icen, A., Paolo, J., *et al* (1985) CSF in Alzheimer's disease – studies on blood–brain barrier function and intrathecal protein synthesis. *Journal of Neurological Science*, 70, 73–80.

Engel, G. L. & Romano, J. (1959) A syndrome of cerebral insufficiency. *Journal of Chronic Diseases*, 9, 260–270.

Fairweather, J. S. (1991) Delirium. In *Psychiatry in the Elderly* (eds R. Jacoby & C. Oppenheimer), pp. 647–675. Oxford: Oxford University Press.

Farrell, K. R. & Gauzini, L. (1995) Misdiagnosing delirium as depression in medically ill elderly patients. *Archives of Internal Medicine*, 155, 2459–2464.

Folstein, M. F., Folstein, S. E. & McHugh, P. R. (1975) Mini-mental state: a practical method for grading the cognitive state of patients for clinicians. *Journal of Psychiatric Research*, 12, 189–198.

Foy, A., Drinkwater, V., March, S., *et al* (1986) Confusion after admission to hospital in elderly patients using benzodiazepines. *British Medical Journal*, 293, 1072.

Greene, L. T. (1971) Physostigmine treatment of anticholinergic drug delirium in post-operative patients. *Anaesthesia and Analgesia*, 50, 222–226.

Grimley Evans, J. (1982) The psychiatric aspects of physical disease. In *The Psychiatry of Late Life* (eds R. Levy & F. Post), pp. 114–142. Oxford: Blackwell.

Gustafson, Y., Berggren, D., Brinnstrbm, B., *et al* (1988) Acute confusional states in elderly patients treated for femoral neck fracture. *Journal of the American Geriatrics Society*, 36, 525–530.

Harwood, D. M. Y., Hope, T. & Jacoby, R. (1997) Do physicians miss cognitive impairment? *Age and Ageing*, 26, 37–39.

Hebenstreit, G. F., Fellerer, K., Twerdy, B., *et al* (1989) L-tryptophan in pre-delirium and delirium conditions. *Infusionstherapie*, 16, 92–96.

Hishikawa, Y. (1981) A dissociated sleep-state 'stage 1-REM' and its relation to delirium. In *Actualites en medicine experimentale* (ed. M. Baldy-Moulnier). Montpellier: Euromed.

Hodkinson, M. (1973) Mental impairment in the elderly. *Journal of the Royal College of Physicians*, 7, 305–317.

Holden, U. P. & Woods, R. T. (1988) *Reality-Orientation: Psychological Approaches to the 'Confused' Elderly* (2nd edn). Edinburgh: Churchill Livingstone.

Inouye, S. K. & Charpentier, P. A (1996) Precipitating factors for delirium in hospitalized elderly patients. Predictive model and interrelationship with baseline vulnerability. *Journal of the American Medical Society,* 275, 852–857.

—, van Dyck, C. H., Alessi, C. A., *et al* (1990) Clarifying confusion: the confusion assessment method. *Annals of Internal Medicine,* 113, 941–948.

Isaacs, B. (1992) *The Challenge of Geriatric Medicine.* Oxford: Oxford University Press.

Itil, T. & Fink, M. (1966) Anticholinergic drug induced delirium: experimental modification, quantitive EEG and behavioural correlations. *Journal of Nervous and Mental Diseases,* 143, 492–507.

Jorm, A. F. (1994) A short form of the Informant Questionnaire on Cognitive Decline in the Elderly (IQCODE): development and validation. *Psychological Medicine,* 24, 145–153.

Koponen, H., Stenback, U., Mattila, E., *et al* (1989) Delirium among elderly persons admitted to a psychiatric hospital: clinical course during the acute stage and a one-year follow-up. *Acta Psychiatrica Scandinavica,* 79, 579–585.

Levkoff, S. E., Safrajn, C., Cleary, P. D., *et al* (1988) Identification of factors associated with diagnosis of delirium in elderly hospitalized patients. *Journal of the American Geriatrics Society,* 36, 1099–1104.

Lipowski, Z. J. (1980) Delirium updated. *Comprehensive Psychiatry,* 21, 190–196.

— (1987) Delirium (acute confusional states). *Journal of the American Geriatrics Society,* 258, 1789–1792.

— (1990) *Delirium: Acute Confusional States.* New York: Oxford University Press.

— (1994) Delirium (acute confusional states). In *Principles and Practice of Geriatric Psychiatry* (eds J. M. Copeland, M. T. Abou-Saleh & D. Blazer). Chichester: Wiley.

Lishman, W. A. (1978) *Organic Psychiatry.* Oxford: Blackwell.

Macdonald, A. J. D., Simpson, A. & Jenkins, D. (1989) Delirium in the elderly: a review and a suggestion for a research programme. *International Journal of Geriatric Psychiatry,* 4, 311–319.

— & Treloar, A. (1996) Delirium and dementia – are they distinct? *Journal of the American Geriatrics Society,* 44, 1001–1002.

Marsden, C. (1978) The diagnosis of dementia. In *Studies in Geriatric Psychiatry* (eds B. Isaacs & F. Post), pp. 99–118. New York: Wiley.

McKeith, I. (1995) Lewy body disease. *Current Opinion in Psychiatry,* 8, 252–257.

Meagher, D. J., O'Hanlon, D., O'Mahony, E., *et al* (1996) The use of environmental strategies and psychotropics in the management of delirium. *British Journal of Psychiatry,* 168, 512–515.

Mesulam, M. M. (ed.) (1985) Attention, confusional states and neglect. In *Principles of Behavioural Neurology.* Philadelphia, PA: Davis.

Ni-Chonchubhair, A., Valacio, R., Kelly, J., *et al* (1995) Use of the abbreviated mental test score to detect post-operative delirium in elderly people. *British Journal of Anaesthsia,* 75, 481–482.

O'Keefe, S. & Lavan, J. (1996) Predicting delirium in elderly patients: development and validation of a risk-stratification model. *Age and Ageing,* 25, 317–321.

— & — (1997) Prognostic significance of delirium in older patients. *Journal of the American Geriatrics Society,* 45, 174–178.

Oxford English Dictionary (1971) *Oxford English Dictionary*. Oxford: Oxford University Press.

Pascuzzi, R. M., Roos, K. L. & Davis Jr, T. E. (1989) Mental state abnormalities in temporal arteritis: a treatable cause of dementia in the elderly. *Arthritis and Neurology*, 32, 1308–1311.

Peterson, P. (1968) Psychiatric disorders in primary hyperparathyroidism. *Journal of Clinical Endocrinological Metabolism*, 28, 1491–1495.

Pitt, B. (1982) *Psychogeriatrics: An Introduction to the Psychiatry of Old Age* (2nd edn), pp. 5–38. Edinburgh: Churchill Livingstone.

— (ed.) (1987) *Delirium and Dementia, Dementia in Old Age*. Edinburgh: Churchill Livingstone.

— (1995) Delirium in old age: causes, diagnosis and treatment. In *Acute Medical Illness in Old Age* (eds A. J. Sinclair & K. W. Woodhouse). London: Chapman and Hall Medical.

Rabins, P. & Folstein, M. F. (1982) Delirium and dementia: diagnostic criteria and fatality rates. *British Journal of Psychiatry*, 140, 149–153.

Robertsson, B., Karlsson, E., Styrud, E., *et al* (1997) Confusional State Evaluation (CSE): an instrument for measuring severity of delirium in the elderly. *British Journal of Psychiatry*, 170, 565–570.

Roca, R. P. (1988) Delirium: a diagnostic dilemma. *Clinical Reports on Ageing (American Geriatrics Society)*, 2(4), 3–5.

Rockwood, K. (1989) Acute confusion in elderly medical patients. *Journal of the American Geriatrics Society*, 37, 150–154.

— (1993) The occurrence and duration of symptoms in elderly patients with delirium. *Journal of Gerontology*, 48, 162–166.

—, Cosway, S., Stolee, P., *et al* (1994) Increasing the recognition of delirium in elderly patients. *Journal of the American Geriatrics Society*, 42, 252–256.

—, Goodman, J., Flynn, M., *et al* (1996) Cross-validation of the Delirium Rating Scale (DRS). *Journal of the American Geriatrics Society*, 44, 839–842.

Saravay, S. M. & Lavin, M. (1994) Psychiatric morbidity and length of stay in the general hospital: a critical review of outcome studies. *Psychosomatics*, 35, 233–252.

Seymour, D. G. & Pringle, R. (1983) Post-operative complications in the elderly surgical patient. *Gerontology*, 29, 262–270.

Seymour, D. G. & Vaz, F. G. (1987) Aspects of surgery in the elderly: pre-operative medical management. *British Journal of Hospital Medicine*, 37, 102–104, 106–108.

Slade, P. D. (1984) Sensory deprivation and clinical psychiatry. *British Journal of Hospital Medicine*, 32, 256–260.

Summers, W. K. & Reich, T. C. (1979) Delirium after cataract surgery: review of two cases. *American Journal of Psychiatry*, 136, 386–391.

Trzepacz, P. T., Baker, R. W. & Greenhouse, J. (1988) A symptom rating scale for delirium. *Psychiatric Research*, 23, 89–97.

Tune, L. E., Holland, A., Folstein, M., *et al* (1981) Association of post-operative delirium with raised levels of anticholinergic drugs. *Lancet*, *ii*, 651–653.

Whitney, J.F. & Gannon, D. E. (1996) Obstructive sleep apnea presenting as acute delirium. *American Journal of Emergency Medicine*, 14, 270–271.

Wolff, H. G. & Curran, D. (1935) Nature of delirium and allied states: the dysergastic reaction. *Archives of Neurology and Psychiatry*, 33, 1175–1193.

World Health Organization (1992) *The Tenth Revision of the International Classification of Diseases and Related Health Problems* (ICD–10). Geneva: WHO.

4 Alzheimer's disease

Alistair Burns & Hans Forstl

Epidemiology ● *Clinical features* ● *Differential diagnosis* ● *Diagnostic criteria* ● *Assessment* ● *Prognosis* ● *Aetiology* ● *Neuropathology* ● *Neurochemistry* ● *Conclusion*

Alzheimer's disease is a common condition in the elderly. In the past 20 years knowledge about the dementias in general, and Alzheimer's disease in particular, has increased rapidly.

Epidemiology

Dementia

There is no shortage of information on the epidemiology of dementia. Many studies and several reviews have been published. The difficulty is integrating the results because:

(a) The types of population vary enormously in parameters such as place of residence (e.g. community versus hospital-based samples) and age range (as dementia is much more common in the very elderly, a sample stratified towards the upper age ranges will contain numerically more cases).

(b) The diagnostic procedures vary, some involve personal examination by trained staff, others rely on second-hand information.

(c) The use of ancillary investigations and diagnostic categories vary.

(d) Many reports simply talk of cognitive impairment, some diagnose dementia, but relatively few attempt accurate subtyping of cases into Alzheimer's disease or vascular dementia.

In view of these problems, it has been claimed that the simple question "what is the prevalence of dementia?" is not answerable (Jorm, 1990). However, it is important to know the available evidence, as well as the methodological problems.

Prevalence

Ineichen (1987) uses the rule of thumb, dementia affects 1% of those aged 65 to 74, and 10% of those 75 and above. While the actual number of affected cases varies from study to study, Jorm (1990) has shown that the prevalence rate increases with age with remarkable uniformity across studies – prevalence doubles every 5.1 years. The EURODEM project (Hofman *et al*, 1991; Rocca *et al*, 1991) pooled data from a number of studies around Europe which employed standardised diagnostic criteria and epidemiological methods (Table 4.1).

Incidence

The suggested incidence of dementia is about 0.5% up to the age of 75, increasing to about 1–3% aged 90. There is debate as to whether it levels off in the very old.

Gender

There is no gender difference in prevalence rates, but racial and community differences have been found, possibly due to the confounding effect of poorer education. Incidence studies have suggested that there is a higher incidence in women, and a higher incidence in New York compared with London.

Alzheimer's disease

The EURODEM prevalence rates for Alzheimer's disease are given in Table 4.2 (Rocca *et al*, 1991). Neuropathological studies have suggested that plaques and tangles affect 5% of all subjects aged 65 to 74 coming to post-mortem, 20% of those 75 to 84 and 45% of those over 85. There is a suggestion that Alzheimer's disease is more common in women than in men, while the reverse is true for vascular dementia. Alzheimer's disease is the most common dementing illness in clinical studies from Europe and North America, while vascular dementia is more common in reports from Russia, Japan and China. Neuropathologically,

Table 4.1 EURODEM prevalence rates for dementia (adapted from Rocca *et al*, 1991)

Age band	%
65–69	1
70–74	4
75–79	6
80–84	13
85–89	22
90–94	32
95–99	35

Table 4.2 EURODEM prevalence rates for Alzheimer's disease (adapted from Rocca *et al*, 1991)

Age band	%
60–69	0.3
70–79	3
0–89	20

however, Alzheimer's disease appears to be the most common throughout the world.

Clinical features

Symptoms usually start insidiously and relatives are characteristically unable to pin down their origin with any accuracy. Often, presentation is related to an identifiable life event (e.g. bereavement or retirement). The features may be observed by others. The patient misses an appointment or forgets an arrangement had ever been made. Sometimes the first manifestation is a lack of self-care and the family notice the home becoming dirtier, personal care deteriorating and eating habits neglected. Wandering can be an early sign and is particularly dangerous if the patient gets lost, especially during winter. By the time the patient comes to the psychiatric services (with the exception of a selected group of subjects who tend to refer themselves and make use of memory clinics) the degree of dementia is apparent and obvious cognitive deficits will be seen (see Box 4.1).

Amnesia

Amnesia is universal and characteristically said to be for recent memory. Not unusually, relatives say that the patient is able to remember events happening many years ago but not earlier that day. Disorientation is the rule, with disorientation for time usually being more obvious than for place.

Aphasia

Aphasia usually supervenes later, and is often a mixture of a receptive and expressive problem. Occasionally, an expressive aphasia is obvious during normal conversation, but usually it is apparent only on close questioning.

Apraxia

Apraxia is often tested for by asking the patient to copy a design, or demonstrate a simple task. From the history there may be evidence of an inability to put on clothes in the correct sequence or there may be a suggestion of an inability to eat correctly with a knife and fork.

Agnosia

Agnosia may be demonstrated as an inability to recognise parts of the body (not to be confused with an inability to name them). A particular form is finger agnosia, which in conjunction with right–left disorientation, acalculia and dysgraphia indicates the Gerstmann syndrome. Failure to recognise faces (prosopagnosia) may lead to the belief that a relative is not real, and occasionally this misidentification is combined with a duplication or replacement phenomenon (Capgras syndrome).

Psychiatric symptoms

Psychiatric symptoms are of three main types (Burns *et al*, 1990*a*):

Disorders of thought content

These occur in about 15% of patients and include delusions and paranoid ideation (persecutory beliefs not held with delusional intensity). Delusional ideas may take many forms. Simple uncomplicated beliefs may occur (e.g. that a handbag or other personal possession has been stolen, while in reality it has been misplaced). Generally, delusional ideas require relative preservation of cerebral structures.

Disorders of perception

These include visual and auditory hallucinations (affecting about 10–15% of patients over the course of their disease). Various forms of misidentification have been described, including misidentification of mirror image, of other people, of events on the television and also the belief that another person is living in the house (the 'phantom boarder' syndrome which may also be classified as a delusion). Hallucinations have been associated with a rapid cognitive decline. Misidentifications appear to be present in younger patients.

Disorders of affect

These are relatively common, depression occurring in up to half of patients but usually of a mild nature. Depressive symptomatology requiring treatment can occur in up to 20% of patients. By contrast, mania is rare.

There have been a number of instruments published for the assessment and quantification of neuropsychiatric features of dementia. The Manchester and Oxford University Scale Psycho-pathological Assessment of Dementia (MOUSEPAD; Allen *et al*, 1996), based on the work of Burns *et al* (1990*a*) is a structured interview with carers, and tracks the development and severity of neuro-psychiatric features over the evolution of the dementia. Other published instruments include the BEHAVE-AD (Reisberg *et al*, 1987), the Present Behavioural Examination (Hope & Fairbairn, 1992) on which the MOUSEPAD is based, the Columbia University Scale for Psychopathology in Alzheimer's Disease (CUSPAD; Devanand *et al*, 1992*b*) and the Neuropsychiatric Inventory (NPI; Cummings *et al*, 1994). Each has advantages and disadvantages, and the choice of instrument depends on the nature of the question being asked.

Behavioural disturbances

Behavioural disturbances are particularly important as they can affect a patient's ability to live in the community. Behavioural disturbances include: aggression, wandering, excessive eating, sexual disinhibition, explosive temper, incontinence and searching behaviour.

Personality changes

Personality changes are said to occur early in the course of dementia and changes often involve coarsening of affect and egocentricity. They are probably non-specific and so do not offer much in terms of diagnosis (see Chapter 11).

Subtypes

Subtypes of Alzheimer's disease have been described by a number of authors. Mayeux *et al* (1985) described four groups: (a) a benign group

---

Box 4.1 Clinical features of Alzheimer's disease

Insidious onset
Amnesia, aphasia, apraxia and agnosia
Disorders of thought content
Disorders of perception
Disorders of affect
Behavioural disturbances
Personality changes

which had little or no progression over a four-year follow-up; (b) a group with myoclonus, severe intellectual decline and a younger onset; (c) a group with extrapyramidal signs, severe intellectual and functional impairment and associated psychotic symptoms; and (d) a 'typical' group which had a gradually progressive decline without distinguishing features.

The early- and late-onset dichotomy has also received widespread attention. It is said that cases with an early onset (defined as 65 years or less) have more aphasia and apraxia, a more rapid course and a poor survival rate. It has also been suggested that more early-onset cases are left handed, perhaps indicating left hemisphere damage and a genetic component. The presence of agraphia may be associated with autosomal dominant transmission of disease. Certainly, apraxia and parietal lobe involvement have been associated with a poorer survival, even in groups of patients over the age of 65.

Differential diagnosis

When presented with a patient in whom dementia is suspected, two fundamental questions need to be answered:

(a) Does the patient has a confusional state (alone or in conjunction with an underlying dementia)?
(b) What is the cause of the dementia syndrome?

There are many causes of dementia, the most common being Alzheimer's disease and vascular dementia (see Chapter 5). For reviews of rare and potentially treatable dementias see Reichman & Cummings (1990) and Byrne (1987). There are a number of pointers in the history and investigations which are suggestive of one or other types of dementias. These are mentioned briefly, emphasising their importance in the differential diagnosis of Alzheimer's disease (Box 4.2).

Diagnostic criteria

ICD–10

Until recently, a diagnosis of Alzheimer's disease was essentially one of exclusion. A summary of the ICD–10 (World Health Organization, 1992) criteria for Alzheimer's disease is: presence of a dementia; insidious onset with slow deterioration; absence of evidence that the cause may be due to another condition such as hypothyroidism; and absence of sudden onset or focal neurological signs.

Box 4.2 Pointers suggestive of the type of dementia

Vascular dementia has a sudden onset, stepwise deterioration and risk factors for cardiovascular disease

Huntington's disease has prominent non-cognitive symptoms, choreiform movements and often a family history

Pick's disease starts with personality and mood changes, with relative preservation of memory. Age of onset is usually younger and the electroencephalogram is more often normal

Lewy body dementia is recognised by the presence of Lewy bodies in the cortex and is associated with features of parkinsonism, acute confusional episodes and hallucinations. A presentation of intermittent confusion with these other signs is suggestive of the disorder

Dementia of the frontal lobe type is being increasingly recognised, with personality changes and frontal lobe signs. It may be a variant of Pick's disease

Parkinson's disease shows mental slowing and cognitive changes, but an absence of cortical abnormalities. Other features of Parkinson's disease are usually present (up to one-third of patients with Parkinson's disease have a dementia syndrome and not uncommonly they have Alzheimer changes at post-mortem)

Progressive supranuclear palsy is indicated by paralysis of vertical gaze, rigidity and pseudobulbar palsy, and is the paradigm of subcortical dementia

Dementia pugilistica is suggested by a history of repeated head injury

Focal cerebral atrophy is suggested by isolated aphasia, apraxia or agnosia

Motor neurone disease has been described in association with dementia of frontal lobe type

Cerebral lesions are often suspected because of abnormal neurological signs and are usually diagnosed on a brain scan

Normal pressure hydrocephalus has the classical triad of dementia, gait disturbance and incontinence. Occasionally (not invariably) diverting cerebrospinal fluid may improve the dementia

Toxins such as alcohol, drugs and various metals are usually implicated by association, and a careful history is essential in these cases

Thyroid disease, hepatic and renal failure, vitamin deficiencies and endocrine disorders are uncovered on routine screening of blood

Whipple's disease is associated with malabsorption, a trial of antibiotics may be justified

Lymphoma and endocrine disorders are revealed on general medical examination

Further categories include early and late onset. While recognising that associated psychiatric symptoms occur, ICD–10 suggests that additional (functional) diagnoses are made in these cases.

National Institute of Neurological and Communicative Disorders and Stroke and the Alzheimer's Disease and Related Disorders Association

Research into Alzheimer's disease reached such a pitch in the 1970s and early 1980s that it was considered necessary to supplement existing diagnostic criteria with additional guidelines. In 1984, the National Institute of Neurological and Communicative Disorders and Stroke and the Alzheimer's Disease and Related Disorders Association (NINCDS–ADRDA) produced the criteria in Box 4.3 (McKhann *et al*, 1984).

These criteria have been validated neuropathologically and have a high positive predictive value, sensitivity and specificity rate (Tierney *et al*, 1989; Burns *et al*, 1990*b*). While some aspects are unsatisfactory (e.g. whether to place a patient who has hypertension or diabetes in the probable or possible groups), these criteria represent a significant

---

Box 4.3 NINCDS–ADRDA criteria for Alzheimer's disease

Probable Alzheimer's disease

Criteria include the presence of dementia, deficits in at least two areas of cognition, progressive deterioration, no clouding of consciousness, age between 40 and 90, absence of systemic disorders

Diagnosis is supported by: progressive deterioration of individual cognitive function, impaired activities of daily living, family history of dementia, normal lumbar puncture, electroencephalogram and evidence of atrophy (or progression) on CT scan

Features consistent with the diagnosis: plateaus in the course of the disease, associated psychiatric symptoms, neurological signs, seizures, normal CT scan

Diagnosis unlikely if: sudden onset, focal neurological signs, seizures or gait disturbance early in the disease

Possible Alzheimer's disease

Diagnosis can be made in the presence of atypical features, in the presence of a systemic disease (not considered to be the cause of dementia), in the presence of a single progressive cognitive deficit

Definite Alzheimer's disease

Criteria are the clinical criteria for probable Alzheimer's disease and histopathological evidence of the disorder

advance in diagnosis. Combined with standardised neuropathological criteria they represent a major step in the categorisation of dementia of the Alzheimer type.

Assessment

History

Any investigative procedure in the elderly begins with a thorough history (also from an informant) and examination. A sudden onset of disturbance of relatively recent origin, with variation in the clinical picture during 24 hours, is strongly suggestive of an acute confusional state.

Mental state examination

The mental state examination should detect clouding of consciousness, which is diagnostic of a confusional state, although its presence can be difficult to ascertain. It also assesses the presence of symptoms such as depression, delusions, paranoid ideations, hallucinations or misidentification phenomena (Burns *et al*, 1990*a*).

Cognitive testing

Cognitive testing is essential. It is useful (especially if the practitioner is not familiar with such tests) to conceptualise the domains to be assessed by being familiar with one of the standard neuro-psychological instruments. Examples are the Abbreviated Mental Test Score (AMTS; Hodkinson, 1972), the Mini-Mental State Examination (MMSE; Folstein *et al*, 1975) and the CAMCOG (part of the CAMDEX, Roth *et al*, 1986) (see Chapter 1).

It is particularly useful to test functions from each of the following areas: (a) orientation; (b) short-term memory (name and address after two minutes); (c) long-term memory (date of first World War); (d) knowledge of current events (e.g. name of the Queen or Prime Minister); (e) aphasia (receptive and express-ive); (f) apraxia; (g) concentration (e.g. counting from 20 down to one).

Physical examination

Examination of the central nervous system is important for the presence or absence of focal signs and primitive reflexes, abnormal plantar response, cranial nerve lesions, myoclonus, gait disturbance or signs of Parkinson's disease.

Blood tests

Blood tests should be routinely performed to assess general physical health and exclude other causes of dementia. These include a full blood count, erythrocyte sedimentation rate, urea and electrolytes, liver function tests, blood glucose, thyroid function tests, syphilis serology, serum B12 and folate. A urine culture is also important. In selected cases testing for HIV should be considered.

Electrocardiogram

An electrocardiogram may reveal signs of cardiovascular disease.

Imaging

A chest X-ray may show a malignancy. By far the most useful neuroimaging technique has been computer tomography (CT), which is acceptable to patients, and widely available (see Chapter 12). The main use of CT is to exclude intracranial lesions such as tumours (primary or secondary), brain abscess or subdural hematomas. Shrinkage of the brain (atrophy) (either cortical or subcortical) can be detected by sulcal widening or ventricular enlargement. In individual cases, the changes seen can be striking but are often unhelpful since, generally speaking, the degree of shrinkage corresponds to the degree of dementia (in other words, by the time obvious shrinkage occurs the degree of dementia is apparent). However, subtle changes of cerebral shrinkage support a clinical diagnosis of early Alzheimer's disease. Ventricular enlargement increases with normal ageing, accelerating in subjects over 60. Correlations have been found between ventricular enlargement and cortical atrophy, and the degree of dementia. Other changes such as cerebral infarctions, white matter changes and basal ganglia calcification can be detected and are helpful in the differential diagnosis. Serial changes in CT are also helpful in diagnosis (Burns *et al*, 1991).

Magnetic resonance imaging (MRI) has the advantage of showing cerebral structures in greater detail than CT and does not use radiation. However, the procedure is much more arduous for the individual and not really suitable for many patients with Alzheimer's disease.

Functional imaging is reviewed by Burns *et al* (1989*a*), Beats *et al* (1991) and Geaney & Abou-Saleh (1990). Single photon emission computed tomography uses gamma cameras, which are available in most nuclear medicine departments, whereas positron emission tomography (PET) requires specialist machinery (a cyclotron) to make radiotracers (see Chapter 12). Patterns of blood flow have been documented in Alzheimer's disease which appear quantitatively and qualitatively different to normal ageing, and deficits in the temporal, parietal and occipital lobes have been documented which correlate with neuropsychological changes (Burns *et al*, 1989*b*).

Electroencephalogram

The electroencephalogram (EEG) is an important additional investigation. In normal ageing there is a generalised slowing of the alpha rhythm, with an increase in theta, delta and beta activity. In acute confusional states the EEG is the most sensitive diagnostic procedure, and slowing of the tracing occurs. In Alzheimer's disease the tracing is usually normal in the early stages. Thereafter, a slowing in alpha and beta activity occurs, with increased delta and theta waves. As with all investigations there is overlap between the changes in normal ageing and in dementia. Soininen *et al* (1982) found abnormalities in 52% of Alzheimer's disease patients but in only one of 90 age-matched controls. The EEG is more often normal in Pick's disease than Alzheimer's disease (an observation of little practical benefit when dealing with an individual). In Creutzfeldt–Jakob disease, there are characteristic paroxysmal sharp waves with a slow background rhythm. The EEG can be used to make 'maps' of cerebral activity which can be of diagnostic use (Loeches *et al*, 1991).

Box 4.4 Investigations of suspected Alzheimer's disease

History: present illness, family history

Mental state examination: psychiatric symptoms, behavioural changes and personality changes

Cognitive function (including Abbreviated Mental Test Score, Mini-Mental State Examination, CAMCOG)

Full physical examination

Blood tests: full blood count, erythrocyte sedimentation rate, urea and electrolytes, liver function tests, glucose, syphilis serology, thyroid function tests, vitamin B12 and folate (red cell and serum), calcium, HIV

Urine culture

Chest X-ray, CT head

Electrocardiogram, electroencephalogram

Further investigations include a lumbar puncture, magnetic resonance imaging, single photon emission computerised tomography, positron emission tomography and brain electrical activity mapping

---

Prognosis

Survival

There is no doubt that Alzheimer's disease is a progressive condition and survival, compared with the general population, is greatly reduced. It was differential survival patterns which formed the basis for Roth's validation of clinical categories in old age psychiatry (Roth, 1955). Studies suggest elderly patients with Alzheimer's disease survive for about 30% of the normal age related life expectancy. Box 4.5 lists factors associated with a poorer survival. More recent papers have commented on the fact that survival for patients with Alzheimer's disease has improved over the past four decades (Burns & Lewis, 1993). There are probably several reasons for this including general improvement of care and the introduction of better medical treatment to control illnesses such as intercurrent infection. Age at diagnosis has been compared in several studies, and controlling for the degree of cognitive impairment, a young age is predictive of poorer survival. It has been shown that elderly patients, while surviving for at least 70% of their disease duration outside hospital, die more quickly once admitted.

Cognitive decline

It is part of the definition of Alzheimer's disease that progressive impairment in cognitive function occurs. A number of studies have attempted to document cognitive decline and identify features which predict cognitive deterioration. Cognition does not deteriorate significantly over a matter of weeks, and testing at least three months

---

Box 4.5 Factors associated with diminished survival

Parietal lobe damage (as evidenced by parietal lobe signs or decreased density on CT scan)
Being male
Age of onset of less than 65 years
Prominent behavioural abnormalities (such as irritability and wandering)
More severely impaired cognitive function (in particular evidence of apraxia)
Depression observed by a rater
The absence of misidentification phenomenon (i.e. misidentification appears to be protective despite its association with younger age)

apart is necessary to demonstrate statistically significant differences. There is large variation in the degree and rate of cognitive decline. Several studies have shown a subgroup of patients in whom progression in cognitive impairment is very slow (corresponding to the benign subgroup described by Mayeux *et al*, 1985).

Global ratings of dementia severity (including functional and cognitive measures) are better at demonstrating progressive impairment than either measure alone. Attempts at quantifying cognitive decline have shown remarkable consistency, despite wide variations in numbers of patients involved, diagnostic practices, selection criteria and placement. Deterioration occurs at a rate of about 10% per annum. However, the clinical observation that decline in the succeeding 12 months can be based on the last 12 months is not borne out by some studies (e.g. Salmon *et al*, 1990). It has been suggested that a shorter duration of illness is associated with an increased rate of further decline. There is also evidence that rate of cognitive decline correlates with the rate of ventricular enlargement (Burns *et al*, 1991).

Aetiology

Genetics

The existence of familial cases of Alzheimer's disease was demonstrated over 40 years ago (Sjogren *et al*, 1953). These familial cases, usually of early onset, were considered to be rare causes of Alzheimer's disease. Today, evidence suggests that familial genetic factors account for a considerable proportion of Alzheimer's disease in all age groups. This is difficult to verify in an elderly population with characteristically high drop-out rates, because the onset of Alzheimer's disease can vary over a wide age range. The estimated lifetime risk to develop Alzheimer's disease comes close to 50% for first-degree relatives, independent of their gender. This is consistent with an autosomal dominant inheritance. On the other hand, the observed concordance rate in monozygotic twins is less than 50%, indicating the importance of environmental factors (Nee *et al*, 1987).

At least four different genetic sites have been implicated in Alzheimer's disease, and this holds promise for future treatments of the disorder. Missense mutations have been found on chromosome 21 in the gene encoding for the beta amyloid precursor protein (Goate *et al*, 1991), emphasising the central place that amyloid formation has in the genesis of the disease. This seems to account for approximately a quarter of early-onset Alzheimer's disease cases, the remaining three-quarters being found on chromosome 14, the gene of which has been cloned (Sherrington *et al*, 1995). This has been referred to as

---

Box 4.6 The genetics of Alzheimer's disease

Presenilin 2 gene (chromosome 1)
Presenilin 1 gene (chromosome 14)
Beta amyloid precursor protein gene (chromosome 21)
Apolipoprotein E gene (chromosome 19)

---

presenilin 1. More recently, a presenilin 2 gene has been identified on chromosome 1 (Levy-Lahad *et al*, 1995), which also seems to be transmitted as an autosomal dominant condition.

Interest has also focused on chromosome 19 where the gene for apolipoprotein E is situated. Apo E is a plasma protein involved in the transport and metabolism of cholesterol. A number of studies have confirmed that the proportion of patients with Alzheimer's disease possessing one or more apolipoprotein E4 genes, is raised compared to the normal population (15% in normal people, up to 40% in patients with Alzheimer's disease) (Strittmater & Roses, 1995). Apolipoprotein E is produced by astrocytes in the brain, confirming the special role E4 may have in connection with neurodegeneration (for a summary see National Institute on Ageing, 1996). A recent study (Myers *et al*, 1996), showed that the risk ratio compared with persons without an E4 allele, was four times higher for those with E3/E4, and 30 times for those homozygous for E4. Fifty-five per cent of patients with E4/E3 developed Alzheimer's disease by age 80, compared to 27% who were E3/E4 and 9% for those without an E4 allele. The association between E4 and Alzheimer's disease is one of the most consistent biological findings in late-onset Alzheimer's disease and represents the first real biological risk factor identified for late-onset disease. With regard to studies on aetiology, it is likely that it will be useful in teasing out environmental and biological risk factors (Myers *et al*, 1996).

Other factors

Many other risk factors have been implicated in the genesis of Alzheimer's disease, which suggests no single aetiological factor is responsible. It is important not to confuse the finding of an association between Alzheimer's disease and a particular factor with a causal connection. The following summarises some of the better known associations (see also reviews by Henderson (1988) and Jorm (1990)).

Head injury

Head injury has been examined as a possible precipitating factor and is of particular interest as dementia pugilistica (caused by the repeated head injuries of boxing) is associated with the presence of neurofibrillary tangles in the neocortex, and the clinical syndrome of dementia. Often the head injury is many years prior to the onset of dementia. Despite some positive findings, several more studies have failed to find an association between dementia and head injury.

Aluminium

Aluminium received attention following a study (Martyn *et al*, 1989) which showed an association between dementia and the level of aluminium in drinking water. It suggested that the poisoning of a water supply in Cornwall was associated with cognitive impairment. Generally, there is no good evidence that excessive intake of aluminium in drinking water (or in antacid preparations) causes an increased risk of dementia. The bioavailability of aluminium, the effect of cooking acidic food in aluminium pans and a possible interaction between aluminium and calcium have all been investigated.

Smoking

Smoking has been found in several studies not to be associated with an increased rate of Alzheimer's disease, although the association has been reviewed.

Organic solvents

Exposure to various organic solvents has been associated with dementia, as has exposure to phenacetin.

Thyroid disease

Thyroid disease was suggested in one study to be associated with Alzheimer's disease. This was of particular interest in view of a previous association between Down's syndrome and thyroid dysfunction. However, this finding has not been confirmed.

Other conditions

Many associated medical conditions such as diabetes, infections and vascular dementia have been reported to have an increased risk of Alzheimer's disease, but the information is too sketchy to be conclusive. One of the earliest findings was an association between lymphomas and Alzheimer's disease, a search prompted by the association between these conditions and Down's syndrome. These findings have not been replicated, and the few positive results which were found, represented mainly an association with early-onset cases. The association of advanced paternal age and Down's syndrome has led to the search for a similar association in Alzheimer's disease. Both maternal and paternal age have been implicated in Alzheimer's disease, but the body of evidence is generally against such an association.

Neuropathology

Macroscopic changes

Brain atrophy is a frequent, but inconsistent, finding in Alzheimer's disease. Normal ageing is accompanied by minimal loss of brain weight and volume after the age of 50. The volume normally decreases by no more than 2% per decade. However, severe atrophy can occur in the absence of Alzheimer's disease, whereas severe Alzheimer pathology is not necessarily accompanied by corresponding macroscopic changes. The most severe cerebral atrophy (with weight loss of up to 300 g) is usually observed in early-onset Alzheimer's disease.

Sulcal widening in Alzheimer's disease is initially most pronounced over the temporal and parietal lobes, and in the later stages over the frontal lobes. These changes are mostly bilateral and symmetrical; in rare cases they can be unilateral or circumscribed. The most likely nature of this cortical atrophy is not a decrease of cortical thickness, but a reduction in length of the cortical ribbon due to a loss of perpendicularly organised columns of neurons and fibres. Ventricular enlargement has already been mentioned in the section on neuroimaging. Neuropathology studies are generally in agreement with CT findings (see Chapter 12).

Histological changes

Neurofibrillary tangles

Alzheimer (1907), described "the very peculiar neurofibrillary changes" of his famous first case, as the hallmark of this disease. Silver impregnation shows neurofibrillary tangles as flame-shaped or globose, intracellular inclusions in neural perikarya and dendritic processes. Sometimes, the neurofibrillary tangles can occur extracellularly in the neuropil of the dentate gyrus, or as resistant remnants of destroyed nerve cells in other areas of the brain (ghost tangles). Insolubility makes it difficult to isolate the neurofibrillary tangles and has precluded protein sequencing.

The neurofibrillary tangles consist of paired helical filaments twisted into a coil. High levels of hydroxyproline are probably responsible for the cross-linkage of the filaments. The presence of various constituents of neurofibrillary tangles has been demonstrated with neuroimmunological methods:

(a) Tau is a cytoskeletal protein which is abnormally phosphorylated in neurofibrillary tangles.
(b) Ubiquitin is a small, 'ubiquitous', phylogenetically old protein which is present in any eukaryotic cell. Ubiquitin is thought to label short-lived, or abnormal, proteins undergoing non-lysosomal enzymatic degradation.
(c) Immunostaining of the amino acid sequence A68 with the antibody Al$_z$SO is currently considered to have a high specificity for Alzheimer's disease typical neurofibrillary tangles.

Neurofibrillary tangles occur in normal ageing and in a number of diseases (Table 4.3). In Alzheimer's disease, neurofibrillary tangles are usually found in the pyramidal cells of the layers III and IV of the mediotemporal cortex and in the CA1 region of the hippocampus. In more advanced stages of illness, neurofibrillary tangles can occur with increasing density in all cortical lobes, and in the multipolar cells of numerous areas in the brainstem.

Plaques

Alzheimer (1907) recognised miliary plaques (i.e. spherical argyrophilic lesions in the neurophil of the upper cortical layers),

Table 4.3 Histological changes in ageing and disease

	Neurofibrillary tangles	Amyloid deposition	Inclusion bodies
Ageing	+	+	GV, Hirano bodies
Alzheimer's disease	++	++	GV, Hirano bodies
Down's syndrome	++	++	GV
Parkinson's disease	(+)	(+)	Lewy bodies (brainstem), GV
Lewy body dementia	(+)	(+)	Lewy bodies (diffuse), GV
Progressive supranuclear palsy	+	++	GV
Pick's disease	+	++	Pick bodies, Hirano bodies, GV
Amyotrophic lateral sclerosis	+	(+)	Hirano bodies, GV
Dementia pugilistica	++	++	

++, essential component; +, occurs in a large proportion of cases; (+) probably incidental finding. GV, granulovacuolar degeneration.

Box 4.7 Neuropathological criteria for the diagnosis of Alzheimer's disease (adapted from Khatchaturian, 1985)

Examination of the frontal, temporal, parietal lobes, amygdala, hippocampus, basal ganglia, substantia nigra, cerebellum and spinal cord to exclude other obvious forms of dementia
Any neocortical field of 1 mm^2 examined with magnification x200 has to show (in the presence of a positive clinical history these criteria should be revised downwards):

Age (years)	Plaques	Neurofibrillary tangles
<50	> 2	> 2
50–65	> 7	(+)
66–75	> 10	(+)
>75	> 15	(+)

---

but he did not pay great attention to the finding. Their presence in senile dementia and in old people with other illnesses had been known for a long time. Similarly to neurofibrillary tangles, plaques are found in a large number of diseases (Table 4.3). Therefore diagnostic neuropathological standards have to take account of their numbers, and not only of their presence (Glenner & Wong, 1984) (Box 4.7). To date, the diagnostic significance of plaques is valued higher than neurofibrillary tangles because the number of plaques seems to be linked more closely to the degree of cognitive impairment.

At least three forms of plaques can be distinguished. They may reflect different developmental stages:

(a) The early immature plaque consists primarily of argyrophilic fibres. Closer scrutiny with more advanced techniques reveals swollen neurites staining for acetylcholinesterase and neuropeptide transmitters, indicating that neurotransmitter alterations can occur early in the course of illness.
(b) The classical mature plaque consists of an amyloid centre surrounded by neuritic debris, reactive astrocytes and neuroglia.
(c) Isolated amyloid cores were considered as burnt-out, hypermature plaques. Advances in molecular biology have led to the discovery of a very early preplaque of diffuse amyloid protein. There is increasing evidence that morphologically similar plaques in normal ageing, and in Alzheimer's disease, may be immunologically distinct.

Other microscopic features

Amyloid protein

Amyloid protein can be found around arteries, capillaries and venules of the hippocampus and occipital lobe in most Alzheimer's disease cases (Lantos, 1990). This amyloid angiopathy, and the observation of capillaries in the centre of amyloid plaques raise the question of whether the amyloid protein can be imported from the periphery across the blood–brain barrier. Milder forms of such amyloid changes can also be seen in clinically normal elderly people. Severe isolated forms can cause infarction, or lethal bleeds in hereditary cerebral haemorrhage with amyloidosis Dutch type (see Chapter 5).

Granulovacuolar degeneration

The pyramidal cells of the hippocampus often contain vacuoles which are filled with argentophilic or eosinophilic granules. This granulovacuolar degeneration can also occur in Pick's disease, Down's syndrome and other illnesses (Table 4.3).

Lewy bodies

Lewy bodies (i.e. globoid, rod- or serpent-shaped eosinophilic inclusions) surrounded by blue halo (haematoxylin-eosin stain), found frequently in the substantia nigra of patients with Parkinson's disease, have been reported with increasing frequency in the cortex of patients with concomitant Alzheimer pathology. It is unclear whether this is a coincidence, or whether it represents a variant of Alzheimer's disease.

Hirano bodies

Hirano bodies, short eosinophilic rod-shaped structures, can be found in the CA1 area of the hippocampus.

Astrocytes

Hypertrophic and proliferating activated astrocytes, intensely staining with glial fibrillary acidic protein, are seen in the upper-cortical layers and in the white matter of patients with Alzheimer's disease.

White matter changes

Cranial CT and MRI have led to increased awareness of white matter changes in the elderly. Such alterations, leuko-araiosis, are a common finding in Alzheimer's disease. Their nature is currently under debate. These changes could be due to subacute incomplete white matter infarctions or, in the absence of risk factors, to Wallerian 'dying back' neuropathy. They seem to have a weak relationship with more severe cognitive impairment and poor prognosis.

Neurochemistry

Neurotransmitter changes

The widespread nature of the histological changes in Alzheimer's disease suggests that multiple neurotransmitter systems can be involved secondarily (Rossor, 1987). Table 4.4 gives a brief outline of some of the cell groups affected by underlying pathological changes, consecutive neurotransmitter alterations and reported changes of receptor density and sensitivity.

Acetylcholine

It has been suggested that impaired cholinergic function could cause the cognitive impairment in Alzheimer's disease. A number of findings support this hypothesis:

(a) Ninety per cent of the large multipolar neurons in the basal nucleus of Meynert are cholinergic and responsible for the cholinergic innervation of the cerebral cortex. These neurons are subject to severe changes in the course of Alzheimer's disease: tangle formation, reduction in cell size and eventually cell death (Whitehouse *et al*, 1982).

(b) The activity of cholineacetyltransferase and consequently acetylcholine, is reduced in cortical and subcortical structures.

(c) A subclass of muscarinic receptors, the presynaptic M2 receptors, appear to be reduced in density.

All these changes can be explained by the degeneration of cholinergic neurons in the basal nucleus of Meynert. The alterations correlate with clinical measurements of cognitive impairment.

Other neurotransmitters

Aminergic deficits in Alzheimer's disease are caused by the degeneration of noradrenergic cells in the locus coeruleus and by the loss of serotonergic neurons in the raphe nuclei. Dopamine was reported to be normal in the cerebral cortex, but low in amygdala and striatum. Gamma-aminobutyric acid from inhibitory cortical interneurons and glutamate, probably from pyramidal cells of layer

Table 4.4 Neurotransmitter changes in Alzheimer's disease

Origin	Neurotransmitter	Receptor
Basal nucleus of Meynert	D choline-acetyltransferase	N nicotinergic
	D acetylcholine	D muscarinergic (M2)
Locus coeruleus	D dopamine-beta-hydroxylase	N alpha
	D noradrenaline	N beta
Dorsal raphex nucleus	D serotonin D	5-HT$_2$
Striatum/amygdala	D dopamine	
Cortical neurones	?D GABA	
	?D glutamate	
	?D somatostatin	D STH
	?D CRF	? supersensitivity

D, decrease; N, no consistent change.

III, was reduced, but this change could be due to post-mortem decay. Neuropeptides, which can coexist in cholinergic, monoaminergic and gamma-aminobutyric acid neurons, are affected by the disease process to a variable extent. Decreases of cortical somatostatin and corticotrophin releasing factor have been observed. Nucleolar volume and cytoplasmatic ribonucleic acid are reduced in the basal nucleus of Meynert, hippocampus and locus coeruleus, indicating impaired intracellular signalling and protein formation.

Conclusion

Alzheimer's disease is a significant cause of morbidity and mortality in the elderly. Its onset is usually insidious, and primarily affects memory, although there are a number of associated clinical features. It is important to differentiate Alzheimer's disease from other causes of dementia. This process is being refined with the development of more precise clinical, imaging, genetic and pathological criteria. The aetiology of Alzheimer's disease is better understood than ever before, and advances in genetic research offer the hope of new treatments.

References

Allen, N., Gordon, S., Hope, T., *et al* (1996) Manchester and Oxford University Scale for the Psychopathological Assessment of Dementia (MOUSEPAD). *British Journal of Psychiatry*, 169, 293–307.

Alzheimer, A. (1907) Tiber eine eigenartige Erkrankung der Hirnrinde. *Allgemeine Zeitschrift fur Psychiatrie und Psychisch-Gerichtliche Medizin*, 64, 146–148.

Beats, B., Burns, A. & Levy, R. (1991) Single photon emission tomography in dementia. *International Journal of Geriatric Psychiatry*, 6, 57–62.

Burns, A., Tune, L., Steele, C., *et al* (1989*a*) Positron emission tomography in dementia – a clinical review. *International Journal of Geriatric Psychiatry*, 4, 67–72.

——, Philpot, M., Costa, D., *et al* (1989*b*) Investigation of dementia of the Alzheimer type with single photon emission tomography. *Journal of Neurology, Neurosurgery and Psychiatry*, 52, 248–253.

——, Jacoby, R. & Levy, R. (1990*a*) Psychiatric phenomena in Alzheimer's disease. *British Journal of Psychiatry*, 157, 72–94.

——, Luthert, P., Jacoby, R., *et al* (1990*b*) Accuracy of clinical diagnosis of Alzheimer's disease. *British Medical Journal*, 301, 1026.

——, Jacoby, R. & Levy, R. (1991) Computed tomography in Alzheimer's disease – a longitudinal study. *Biological Psychiatry*, 29, 383–390.

—— & Lewis, G. (1993) Survival in dementia. In *Ageing and Dementia: A Methodological Approach*, pp. 125–143. London: Edward Arnold.

Byrne, J. (1987) Reversible dementias. *International Journal of Geriatric Psychiatry*, 2, 72–81.

Cummings, J., Mega, M., Dray, K., *et al* (1994) The Neuropsychiatric Inventory. *Neurology*, 44, 2308–2314.

Devanand, D., Miller, L., Richards, M., *et al* (1992) The Columbia University Scale for Psychopathology in Alzheimer's Disease. *Archives of Neurology*, 49, 371–376.

Folstein, M. F., Folstein, S. E. & McHugh, P. R. (1975) Mini-Mental State: a practical method for grading the cognitive state of patients for clinicians. *Journal of Psychiatric Research*, 12, 189–198.

Geaney, D. & Abou-Saleh, M. (1990) The use and applications of single photon emission computerised tomography in dementia. *British Journal of Psychiatry*, 157 (suppl. 9), 66–75.

Glenner, G. G. & Wong, C. W. (1984) Alzheimer's disease and Down's syndrome: sharing of a unique cerebrovascular amyloid vascular protein. *Biochemical and Biophysical Research Communications*, 122, 1131–1135.

Goate, A., Chartier-Harlin, M.-C., Mullen, M., *et al* (1991) Segregation of a missense mutation in the amyloid precursor protein gene with familial Alzheimer's disease. *Nature*, 349, 704–706.

Henderson, A. (1988) The risk factors for Alzheimer's disease: a review and a hypothesis. *Acta Psychiatrica Scandinavica*, 78, 257–275.

Hodkinson, H. (1972) Evaluation of a mental test score for assessment of mental impairment in the elderly. *Age and Aging*, 1, 233–238.

Hofman, A., Rocca, A., Brayne, C., *et al* (1991) The prevalence of dementia in Europe. *International Journal of Epidemiology*, 20, 736–748.

Hope, R. & Fairbairn, C. (1992) The Present Behavioural Examination. *Psychological Medicine*, 22, 223–230.

Ineichen, B. (1987) Measuring the rising tide. *British Journal of Psychiatry*, 150, 193–200.

Jorm, A. (1990) *The Epidemiology of Alzheimer's Disease and Related Disorders*. London: Chapman and Hall.

Khatchaturian, Z. (1985) Diagnosis of Alzheimer's disease (Conference report). *Archives of Neurology*, 42, 1097–1105.

Lantos, P. (1990) Ageing and dementias. In *Systematic Pathology* (3rd edn), Vol. 4: *Nervous System, Muscle and Eyes* (ed. R. O. Weller), pp. 361–396. Edinburgh: Churchill-Livingstone.

Levy-Lahad, E., Wasco, W., Poorkaj, P., *et al* (1995) Candidate gene for the chromosome 1 familial Aizheimer's disease locus. *Science,* 269, 973–977.

Loeches, M., Gil, P., Jimenez, F., *et al* (1991) Topographic maps of brain electrical activity in primary degenerative dementia of the Alzheimer type and multi-infarct dementia. *Biological Psychiatry,* 29, 211–223.

Martyn, C., Barker, D., Osmand, C., *et al* (1989) Geographical relation between Alzheimer's disease and aluminium in drinking water. *Lancet, i,* 59–62.

Mayeux, R., Stern, Y. & Spanton, S. (1985) Heterogeneity in dementia of the Alzheimer type: evidence of subgroups. *Neurology,* 35, 453–461.

McKhann, G., Drachman, D., Folstein, M., *et al* (1984) Clinical diagnosis of Alzheimer's disease. *Neurology,* 34, 939–944.

Myers, R., Schaefer, E., Wilson, P., *et al* (1996) Apolipoprotein E4 association with dementia in a population-based study. *Neurology,* 46, 673–677.

National Institute on Ageing/Alzheimer's Association Working Group (1996) Consensus Statement: Apolipoprotein E genotyping in Alzheimer's disease. *Lancet,* 347, 1091–1095.

Nee, L. E., Eldridge, R, Sunderland, T., *et al* (1987) Dementia of the Alzheimer type: clinical and family study of 22 twin pairs. *Neurology,* 37, 359–363.

Reichman, W. & Cummings, J. (1990) Diagnosis of rare dementia syndromes: an algorhythmic approach. *Journal of Geriatric Psychiatry and Neurology,* 3, 73–84.

Reisberg, B., Borenstein, J., Franssen, E., *et al* (1987) BEHAVE-AD. In *Alzheimer's disease – Problems, Prospects and Perspectives* (ed. H. Aitman), pp. 1–16. New York: Plenum Press.

Rocca, A., Hofman, A., Brayne, C., *et al* (1991) Frequency and distribution of Alzheimer's disease in Europe. *Annals of Neurology,* 30, 381–390.

Rossor, M. (1987) Alzheimer's disease: neurobiochemistry. In *Dementia* (ed. B. Pitt). Edinburgh: Churchill-Livingstone.

Roth, M. (1955) The natural history of mental disorder in old age. *Journal of Mental Science,* 101, 281–301.

—, Tym, E., Mountjoy, C. Q., *et al* (1986) CAMDEX. A standardised instrument for the diagnosis of mental disorder in the elderly with special reference to the early detection of dementia. *British Journal of Psychiatry,* 149, 698–709.

Salmon, D., Thal, L., Butters, N., *et al* (1990) Longitudinal evaluation of dementia of the Alzheimer type. *Neurology,* 40, 1225–1230.

Sherrington, R., Rogaev, E. & Liang, Y. (1995) Cloning of a gene bearing missense mutations in early onset familial Alzheimer's disease. *Nature,* 375, 754–760.

Sjogren, T., Sjogren, H. & Lundgren, A. G. H. (1953) Morbus Alzheimer and morbus Pick: a genetic, clinical and pathoanatomical study. *Acta Psychiatric Scandinavica Supplementum,* 82, 9–152.

Soininen, H., Partanen, V., Halkala, E., *et al* (1982) EEG findings in senile dementia in normal aging. *Acta Neurologica Scandinavica,* 65, 59–70.

Strittmatter, W. & Roses, A. (1995) Apolipoprotein E in Alzheimer's disease. *Proceedings of the National Academy of Science of the United States of America,* 92, 4725–4727.

Tierney, M., Fisher, R., Lewis, A., *et al* (1988) The NINCDS/ADRDA workgroup criteria for the clinical diagnosis of probable Alzheimer's disease: a clinico-pathologic study of 57 cases. *Neurology*, 38, 359–364.

Whitehouse, P. J., Price, D. L., Struble, R. G., *et al* (1982) Alzheimer's disease and senile dementia: loss of neurons in the basal forebrain. *Science*, 215, 1237–1239.

World Health Organization (1993) *The ICD–10 Classification of Mental and Behavioural Disorders. Diagnostic Criteria for Research*. Geneva: WHO.

5 Vascular and other dementias

Jeremy Brown and Martin Rossor

Vascular dementia ● *Rare causes of vascular dementia* ● *Non-Alzheimer degenerative dementias* ● *Treatable dementias* ● *Conclusion*

The non-Alzheimer dementias are a heterogeneous group of disorders, accounting for approximately a third of all dementias. Many dementias have familial forms and molecular techniques have identified the gene mutations responsible for Alzheimer's disease, Huntington's disease, familial Creutzfeldt–Jakob disease and a form of vascular dementia. These genetic defects lie at the start of pathological cascades which lead to disease, and they provide a powerful means of classification. This will hopefully extend to the other dementias with familial forms, such as vascular, and frontal lobe dementias.

Vascular dementia

Presentation

Vascular disease is the second most common cause of dementia after Alzheimer's disease. In addition to those individuals with a 'pure' vascular dementia, many individuals have clinical and pathological evidence of both Alzheimer's disease and vascular disease. The presentation of vascular dementia is variable and the clinical spectrum is wide. Patients may present with an insidious onset of cognitive problems, suggestive of a degenerative dementia, or with a series of strokes and widespread physical abnormalities.

Vascular dementia can be divided on clinical features into three major subtypes, although individuals may have features of more than one subtype: cognitive deficits following a single stroke, multi-infarct dementia and progressive small vessel disease (Binswanger's disease). There are also rare causes of vascular dementia (Box 5.3).

Cognitive deficits following a single stroke

The major causes of stroke (haemorrhage, infarct and embolism) can all produce dementia, although many single strokes leave little apparent cognitive deficit. When there are cognitive problems following a stroke, the site of the lesion usually determines the clinical

---

Box 5.1 Key features of the ICD–10 classification of vascular dementia (World Health Organization, 1992)

Vascular dementia
A dementia resulting from vascular disease
Uneven impairment of cognitive function
Abrupt onset or stepwise deterioration
Focal neurological signs and symptoms
May coexist with Alzheimer's dementia

Multi-infarct dementia
More gradual onset
Follows a number of minor ischaemic episodes

Subcortical vascular dementia
A history of hypertension
Deep white matter ischaemia
Cerebral cortex is well preserved

---

picture. For example, a dominant middle cerebral artery infarct results in dysphasia, dyscalculia and dysgraphia. The dementia tends to be particularly severe in certain midbrain or thalamic strokes. Few patients have formal neuropsychological assessment following a single stroke and it is likely that many mild cognitive deficits are not detected. As with physical disability, the cognitive problems may remain fixed or recover, partially or totally.

Multi-infarct dementia

In a classical case of multi-infarct dementia there is a history of successive strokes, each leading to greater cognitive deficits. These strokes produce a step-like deterioration, with intervening periods when patients remain stable (or may improve). Multi-infarct dementia can be produced through similar mechanisms to a single stroke. The recurrent nature of multi-infarct dementia suggests that there is underlying disease predisposing to stroke, such as hypertension or valvular heart disease. Multi-infarct dementia can be produced by large vessel disease, small vessel disease or a combination of the two.

Progressive small vessel disease (Binswanger's disease)

In Binswanger's disease the diagnosis may initially be less clear. The course is of a slow intellectual decline, either gradual or step-like.

The clinical picture may be dominated by the dementia, or there may be concomitant physical problems, such as gait disorders or dysarthria. Brain imaging reveals periventricular lucencies and extensive white matter changes. The changes are often particularly marked on magnetic resonance imaging. There may be small distinct infarcts (lacunae), or more generalised white matter changes (leukoariosis). This distribution of the radiological and pathological changes suggests that the disease is affecting the small perforating vessels. This subtype of vascular dementia has had a number of names, including Binswanger's disease and subcortical arteriosclerotic encephalopathy. The cognitive profile of progressive small vessel disease is suggestive of a subcortical dementia, with slowing of intellectual processes, rather than the specific deficits such as dysphasia and dyscalculia, produced by large cortical strokes.

Epidemiology

Vascular disease contributes to about a quarter of all cases of dementia in published series. Vascular dementia shows marked geographical and racial variation and, not surprisingly, is common in countries such as Japan which have a high incidence of vascular disease. The prevalence of vascular dementia is higher with increasing age and in males. Patients often have a family history of vascular disease. There are many medical associations of vascular dementia, including hypertension, diabetes, hyperlipidaemia, polycythaemia, homocystinuria, sickle cell anaemia, coagulopathies and valvular heart disease. Vascular disease is more common in smokers. In a few families there is an autosomal dominant pattern of inheritance, with onset around the age of 45. This syndrome has been termed cerebral autosomal dominant arteriopathy with subcortical infarcts and leukoencephalopathy (CADASIL).

Clinical features

The variety of presentations of stroke are legion, and so are the features of vascular dementia. The differential diagnosis is usually between vascular dementia and a degenerative dementia, although treatable causes of dementia must not be forgotten. There are certain clinical features, such as the sudden onset of a deficit, which are highly suggestive of vascular dementia. A scoring system was developed by Hachinski and colleagues (1975) which allows the clinician to quantify the likelihood of a patient having a vascular, rather than degenerative dementia (Box 5.2). A score above six suggests vascular dementia.

On examination there may be clues to the aetiology of the dementia: physical signs such as a hemiparesis, hemianopia or

---

Box 5.2 The Hachinski ischaemia score (adapted from Hachinski *et al*, 1975)

Abrupt onset	2
Stepwise deterioration	1
Fluctuating course	2
Nocturnal confusion	1
Relative preservation of personality	1
Depression	1
Somatic complaints	1
Emotional incontinence	1
History of hypertension	1
History of strokes	2
Atherosclerosis	2
Focal neurological symptoms	2
Focal neurological signs	2

---

pseudobulbar palsy are typical features of a vascular dementia and unusual in degenerative dementias. As well as performing a neurological examination, it is important to record the blood pressure and look for evidence suggestive of extracranial vascular disease. The presence of significant cardiac murmurs or atrial fibrillation should prompt further investigations. The presence of carotid bruits or absence foot pulses signifies clinical vascular disease.

Investigations

Investigations need to be tailored to the individual patient. Blood tests include a full blood count, erythrocyte sedimentation rate, biochemical screen, syphilis serology, lipids, B12 levels and thyroid function tests. An electrocardiogram and chest X-ray should be done. In young-onset patients and patients in whom embolic disease seems likely (patients with large discrete infarcts affecting several vascular territories), an echocardiogram is appropriate to look for a cardiac source of emboli. Trans-sternal echocardiography is often used as a screening test for cardiac defects, but transoesophageal echocardiography is a more sensitive investigation. If there is history of an event in a carotid territory and the patient is suitable for surgery, a Doppler ultrasound of the carotid vessels should be performed to look for a surgically treatable stenosis. Brain imaging is often appropriate to exclude treatable forms of dementia and to confirm the presence of macroscopic infarcts or periventricular lucencies.

In unusual cases many more investigations may be done, including a prothrombotic screen, autoantibody screen and tests aimed at looking for rare neurological diseases such as mitochondrial disease,

Fabry's disease and homocystinuria. There are several causes of strokes which typically occur in young people without obvious vascular risk factors. These include the lupus anticoagulant syndrome, arterial dissections and paradoxical embolism from a deep venous thrombosis through a patent foramen ovale. These diagnoses are important because medical treatment may reduce the risk of future strokes, however they are extremely rare causes of vascular dementia.

Management

The most important initial step in the management of vascular dementia is to search for the treatable causes of stroke. If there is a cardiac source of emboli, such as an enlarged, fibrillating atrium or valvular heart disease, many patients will benefit from anticoagulation. If there is a history of a vascular event within a carotid territory and a significant stenosis of that artery, carotid endarterectomy or angioplasty may be indicated. Medical diseases such as hypertension, hyperlipidaemia and diabetes should be treated by diet or drugs. Aspirin may be prescribed in cases of vascular dementia, in whom there is no contraindication, although there are no trials to suggest it slows the progression of the disease. It is important also to manage problems produced by the dementia, such as disinhibited behaviour and depression (see Chapter 6).

Preventive measures in the population offer the best means of reducing the incidence of vascular dementia. Initiatives such as the UK Government's *Health of the Nation* targets (Department of Health, 1992) seek to do this by promoting dietary changes and regular exercise. Treatment of hypertension is important as relatively small decreases in mean diastolic blood pressure can substantially reduce the risk of stroke.

Prognosis

The prognosis of vascular dementia is poor, and may be worse than Alzheimer's disease. Most patients die within a few years of the onset of the dementia. Clearly, if there is a treatable cause such as a valvular heart lesion, then the disease progression can be halted, however often the cognitive decline continues despite treatment of risk factors. The poor prognosis emphasises the importance of preventative measures.

Rare causes of vascular dementia

Cerebral autosomal dominant arteriopathy with subcortical infarcts and leukoencephalopathy

CADASIL is a familial form of vascular dementia (Tournier-Lasserve *et al*, 1993). The term CADASIL for this disease was adopted by the French group and is now widely accepted; although there are several reports of a similar disease in the earlier literature. Patients with CADASIL usually present with recurrent stroke, at an average age of 43 years. There is often a history of migraine, and many patients later develop a subcortical dementia and pseudobulbar palsy. Magnetic resonance imaging shows widespread white matter changes and is often abnormal in presymptomatic relatives at risk of developing the disease. The disease is transmitted as an autosomal dominant trait with high penetrance. Several pedigrees have been described, mainly from continental Europe. Molecular genetic linkage studies have assigned the disease gene to the long arm of chromosome 19. Recent work has associated mutations in the Notch 3 gene on chromosome 19 with CADASIL in several families.

Vasculitis

Patients with a cerebral vasculitis may develop cognitive problems and dementia, as a result of repeated infarcts. The history of dementia may be steadily progressive or step-like, but is usually of rapid progression compared with the degenerative dementias. There are often marked systemic features with the vasculitis involving several different organs, but the clinical features may be limited to the central nervous system. The more common causes of cerebral vasculitis include systemic lupus erythematosus, giant cell arteritis, isolated cerebral vasculitis and polyarteritis nodosa. The diagnosis can sometimes be made through a series of autoantibody tests including: double stranded DNA and ANCA (antineutrophil cytoplasmic antibody); looking at inflammatory markers; brain imaging; examination of the cerebrospinal fluid; and the search for evidence of vasculitis in other affected organs. In many cases the diagnosis is less clear, and cerebral angiography and cerebral or meningeal biopsy may be needed.

Cerebral haemorrhage

In acute cerebral haemorrhage and extracerebral haemorrhage, dementia is not usually the presenting problem but patients are often left with residual cognitive problems. Large arteriovenous malformations can cause cognitive problems through pressure and steal effects, or through cerebral haemorrhage. There are also two autosomal dominant forms of vascular dementia associated with repeated lobar haemorrhages:

  (a) Hereditary cerebral haemorrhage with amyloidosis, Dutch type. This condition is caused by mutations in the amyloid precursor protein gene and is associated with the deposition of beta amyloid.

(b) Hereditary cerebral haemorrhage with amyloidosis, Icelandic type. This is caused by mutations in the cystatin C gene and is associated with cystatin C deposition.

Chronic subdural haematoma

Chronic subdural haematoma is one of the more common treatable causes of dementia. The patient is usually elderly and there may be no history of previous trauma. If the haematoma is unilateral, the patient presents with features of a lateralised space occupying lesion. If the subdurals are bilateral, then the diagnosis may be more difficult. Examination often reveals clues to the diagnosis, such as papilloedema or bilateral extensor plantar responses.

Other vascular dementias

Dementia can also be produced by multiple infarcts occurring during hypotensive crises. Such infarcts typically affect the watershed areas of the brain, which lie between two vascular territories. These infarcts may occur in the survivors of cardiac arrest. Cognitive problems can also follow myocardial infarction and cardiac surgery.

Non-Alzheimer degenerative dementias

Dementia with Lewy bodies

Patients who present with Parkinson's disease may develop a progressive dementia. A subgroup of Alzheimer's disease type patients develop marked extrapyramidal problems. Pathological examination of patients dying with these two clinical pictures often reveals the presence of cortical Lewy bodies (Kosaka *et al*, 1988). These are seen particularly well with anti-ubiquitin staining. Such patients are described as having dementia with Lewy bodies (formally called cortical Lewy body disease, and diffuse Lewy body disease, among other names). Dementia with Lewy

---

Box 5.3 Types of vascular dementia

Cognitive deficits following a single stroke
Multi-infarct dementia
Progressive small vessel disease (Binswanger's disease)
CADASIL
Vasculitis
Cerebral haemorrhage
Chronic subdural haematoma

bodies is one of the more common degenerative dementias. However, there is clinical and pathological overlap in these patients with Alzheimer's disease and idiopathic Parkinson's disease. Clinical features strongly suggestive of dementia with Lewy bodies include rapid fluctuations in cognitive ability and visual hallucinations (Box 5.4). Treatment with l-dopa and the standard anti-parkinsonian drugs often improves the motor symptoms, but can lead to confusion and hallucinations. Patients are very sensitive to neuroleptics, which can considerably worsen the Parkinsonian symptoms.

Frontotemporal dementia

A significant minority of patients with a degenerative dementia present with symptoms such as personality change and behavioural problems, suggestive of frontal lobe dysfunction. In some series, up to 20% of cases of degenerative presenile dementia present with this anterior cortical picture rather than the typical temporoparietal deficits seen in Alzheimer's disease (Gustafson *et al*, 1992). The disease progresses and patients tend to develop a non-fluent aphasia. Patients often develop features suggestive of temporal lobe dysfunction, such as hyperorality. In contrast to Alzheimer's disease, memory is affected later and less severely. Spatial orientation is well-preserved, even late in the illness. Insight is characteristically lost early.

On post-mortem examination the pathological features are variable. In the majority of cases there is mild frontal and temporal lobe atrophy, without the distinctive histopathological features such as plaques, tangles and intraneuronal inclusion bodies seen in other degenerative dementias. This syndrome has been described under many names, including frontal lobe degeneration of non-Alzheimer type. Following a consensus statement it is now called frontotemporal dementia (Brun *et al*, 1994).

There is a high proportion of familial cases, about 50% of presenile cases having a positive family history for dementia. Recently, one of the mutations responsible for this form of dementia has been mapped to chromosome 3 (Brown *et al*, 1995). The dementia in other families is linked to a locus on chromosome 17 (Wilhelmsen *et al*, 1994). The disease is steadily progressive and there is no specific treatment. Patients with clinical frontotemporal dementia may have a variety of other pathological features, including those of motor neuron disease in the absence of the typical clinical signs of these diseases (Cooper *et al*, 1995).

Pick's disease

Pick's disease is currently regarded by most authorities as a form of frontotemporal dementia. It is differentiated from the other forms of

---

Box 5.4 Features of frontotemporal dementia

Personality change
Early loss of insight
Non-fluent aphasia
Hyperorality
Well-preserved spatial orientation

---

frontotemporal dementia by pathological features, such as severe 'knife-edge' atrophy of the frontal and temporal lobes and the presence of argyrophilic inclusion bodies (Pick bodies) in neurones. Swollen, achromatic neurones (also called ballooned neurones or Pick cells) are present in other neurodegenerative diseases and do not reliably identify Pick's disease. The clinical features do not distinguish it from other forms of frontotemporal dementia; it may present with the features of a frontal lobe dementia, or less frequently, with features of selective temporal lobe disease. Classical Pick's disease is the cause of a small minority of cases of frontotemporal dementia. There are rare published reports of familial classical Pick's disease (many of the reported familial cases have clinical frontotemporal dementia without the pathological features of Pick's disease) (Brown, 1992).

Dementia associated with other neurological diseases

Many neurological diseases, including motor neuron disease, progressive supranuclear palsy and multiple sclerosis, are associated with dementia. Often the dementia occurs in patients who have had these diseases for many years, but occasionally dementia can be an early or presenting feature. The cognitive assessment of these patients is often complicated by their physical problems.

Huntington's disease

There are many genetic causes of dementia, the best known of which is probably Huntington's disease. This condition may present with cognitive problems, or a movement disorder. It is inherited as an autosomal dominant trait. The mutation producing the disease has been identified (Huntington's Disease Collaborative Research Group, 1993). The disease arises as a result of an abnormal expansion of a trinucleotide repeat sequence within the gene. This is one of a group of so called 'triplet repeat disorders', which can produce neurological disease. The gene product has been named Huntingtin. The disease can now be diagnosed using molecular genetic techniques.

Prion dementia

These are a clearly defined group of disorders characterised by an accumulation of an abnormal form of a normal human protein, prion protein (Prusiner, 1991). The first human form, Kuru, was described in the cannibal Fore people in New Guinea. Gadjusek and colleagues showed that Kuru was transmissible to chimpanzees by intracerebral inoculation of a brain extract (Lampert *et al*, 1969). Neuropathological morphological similarities were noted between Kuru and Creutzfeldt–Jakob disease, a rare disease first described in Europe. Gadjusek and colleagues showed that Creutzfeldt–Jakob disease was also transmissible.

Creutzfeldt–Jakob disease is a rare disease, affecting about one person per million per year. Affected individuals develop a rapidly progressive dementia with cerebellar ataxia and myoclonus. Typical cases die within a few months of onset of the disease. Neuropathological examination reveals spongiform degeneration. Immunocytochemistry shows the deposition of prion protein. Familial forms of prion disease account for about 15% of all cases. Some patients have clinical features very similar to sporadic cases. Two variants have been described:

(a) Gerstmann–Straussler syndrome, which has a more chronic course and prominent cerebellar ataxia.
(b) Fatal familial insomnia, which presents with insomnia and a thalamic dementia.

A series of mutations in the prion protein gene on chromosome 20 have been shown to cause the familial forms. Iatrogenic cases of Creutzfeldt–Jakob disease have been reported following neurosurgery and injection of growth hormone obtained from pooled human cadavers. Recent evidence suggests that a new form of Creutzfeldt–Jakob disease may have appeared in the UK, as a result of people eating offal from cows suffering from a bovine prion disease (bovine spongiform encephalopathy, BSE).

Box 5.5 ICD–10 other diseases causing dementia (World Health Organization, 1992)

Pick's disease
Creutzfeldt–Jakob disease
Huntington's disease
Parkinson's disease
Human immunodeficiency virus disease

Treatable dementias

Metabolic and endocrine

Dementia is such a devastating disease that it is important to consider a treatable cause in all patients (Box 5.6). Virtually any metabolic or endocrine derangement can cause cognitive problems, and simple blood tests should be performed to exclude metabolic causes for cognitive problems, including renal disease, liver disease and hypothyroidism.

Infective

Neurosyphilis is now a very rare cause of dementia, but should be considered in all cases of dementia since it is treatable. Patients with positive serology require further investigation, usually including a cerebrospinal fluid examination and a full course of antibiotic treatment. Problems in diagnosis may arise with patients who have been exposed to other treponemal diseases, such as yaws.

The acquired immune deficiency syndrome (AIDS) can produce dementia through direct invasion of the brain by the virus, or as a result of a number of associated central nervous system infections and neoplasms. In neurological practice it is a very rare cause of dementia in patients not previously known to have human immunodeficiency virus (HIV) infection.

Whipple's disease is almost certainly an infective disease which produces a dementia. There are often clues to the diagnosis, with a history of intestinal problems and systemic symptoms. The physical examination may reveal typical signs, such as a supranuclear gaze palsy. Magnetic resonance image scanning typically shows both grey and white matter lesions. Treatment is with long-term antibiotics.

Vitamin deficiencies

Several vitamin deficiencies can cause cognitive decline. It is important to screen for B12 deficiency in all patients with dementia,

---

Box 5.6 Treatable dementias

Metabolic and endocrine: renal disease, liver disease, hypothyroidism
Infections: neurosyphilis, HIV, Whipple's disease
Vitamin deficiencies: B12, folate, nicotinic acid, thiamine
Toxins and drugs: anticonvulsants, alcohol
Neoplastic
Normal pressure hydrocephalous

and to be aware that not all have the characteristic haematological abnormalities. Folate deficiency and nicotinic acid deficiency, among other vitamin deficiencies, may also produce cognitive problems.

Thiamine deficiency can produce an acute encephalopathy, Wernicke's encephalopathy, which is preventable. Furthermore, it can be an iatrogenic disease precipitated by infusion of glucose into patients at risk of thiamine deficiency. The most common cause of thiamine deficiency is alcohol misuse, but it can occur in patients with malabsorption syndromes or malignancy. Wernicke's encephalopathy is characterised by: ophthalmoplegia (typically bilateral lateral rectus palsies), nystagmus, ataxia and disturbed consciousness.

Wernicke's encephalopathy needs immediate treatment with intravenous thiamine. Chronically the condition is termed Korsakoff's psychosis and is characterised by loss of short-term memory. Patients often confabulate; psychometry usually reveals widespread deficits, including problems in remote memory.

Toxins and drugs

Toxins and drugs should be excluded as causes. Alcohol has been suggested as a cause of dementia, but people with chronic alcohol dependency often have other associated conditions such as vitamin deficiencies, head injuries and subdural haematomas. Many drugs have been found to cause cognitive problems, common examples include the anticonvulsants. Most drug-induced cognitive changes are reversible on withdrawal of the drug, although the recovery may be slow.

Neoplastic

Neoplasms can produce dementia in three main ways:

(a) Through local effects of the primary growth. There may be few associated neurological symptoms and signs, particularly with frontal tumours. Many such tumours are intrinsic gliomas and the long-term prognosis is poor, but dementia can be produced by meningiomas, which are curable.
(b) Through secondary spread.
(c) Through para-neoplastic mechanisms such as brainstem encephalitis or progressive multifocal leukoencephalopathy.

Normal pressure hydrocephalus

Normal pressure hydrocephalus produces a clinical triad of: progressive dementia, urinary incontinence and gait disturbance

The dementia is of the subcortical type, with marked cognitive slowing, in the absence of focal cortical deficits. There may be a history of subarachnoid haemorrhage or meningitis. It can be very difficult to distinguish normal pressure hydrocephalus (where the hydrocephalus causes the symptoms) from patients with degenerative or vascular dementia with periventricular atrophy (where the hydrocephalus is secondary to cerebral atrophy). In the past, normal pressure hydrocephalus was overdiagnosed, it is probably a very rare cause of dementia. It is possible to make a definite diagnosis with intraventricular pressure monitoring, but this is invasive and not always conclusive. Some patients show a temporary improvement following lumbar puncture to remove 20–50 ml of cerebrospinal fluid, to lower the cerebrospinal fluid pressure. Treatment is difficult. A few patients improve dramatically following insertion of a permanent shunt. However, others are left worse off as a result of the complications of shunting, such as shunt infections and subdurals.

Conclusion

There are many causes of dementia, some of which are treatable. Advances are being made into the genetic basis of these disorders and this should help diagnosis, prevention and treatment. Good practice demands the thorough assessment of all patients presenting with dementia.

References

Brown, J. (1992) Pick's disease. *Balliere's Clinical Neurology*, 1, 535–557.
——, Ashworth, A., Gydesen, S., *et al* (1995) Familial non specific dementia maps to chromosome 3. *Human Molecular Genetics*, 4, 1625–1628.
Brun, A., Englund, B., Gustafson, L., *et al* (1994) Clinical and neuropathological criteria for frontotemporal dementia. *Journal of Neurology, Neurosurgery and Psychiatry*, 57, 416–418.
Cooper, P. N., Jaken, M., Lennox, G., *et al* (1995) Tau, ubiquitin and alpha beta crystallin immunohistochemistry define the principal causes of frontotemporal dementia. *Archives of Neurology*, 52, 1011–1015.
Department of Health (1992) *The Health of the Nation: A Strategy for Health in England*. London: HMSO.
Gustafson, L., Brun, A. & Passant, U. (1992) Frontal lobe degeneration of non-Alzheimer type. In *Unusual Dementias* (ed. M. N. Rossor), pp. 559–582. London: Ballèire Tindall.
Hachinski, V. C., Lliff, L. D., Kilhka, M. *et al*, (1975) Cerebral blood flow in dementia. *Archives of Neurology,* 32, 632–637.
Huntington's Disease Collaborative Research Group (1993) A novel gene containing a trinucleotide repeat that is expanded and unstable on the "Huntington's disease chromosome". *Cell*, 72, 971–983.

Kosaka, K., Tsuchiya, K. & Yoshimurra, M. (1988) Lewy body disease with and without dementia: a clinicopathological study of 35 cases. *Acta Neuropathologica,* 7, 299–305.

Lampert, P. W., Earle, K. M., Gibbs, C. J., *et al* (1969) Experimental Kuru encephalopathy in chimpanzees and spider monkeys. *Journal of Neuropathology and Experimental Neurology,* 28, 353–370.

Prusiner, S. B. (1991) Molecular biology of prion diseases. *Science,* 252, 1515–1522.

Tournier-Lasserve, E., Joutel, A., Melki, J., *et al* (1993) Cerebral autosomal dominant arteriopathy with subcortical infarcts and leukoencephalopathy maps to chromosome 19q12. *Nature Genetics,* 3, 256–259.

Wilhelmsen, K. C., Lynch, T., Pavlov, E., *et al* (1994) Localization of disinhibition-dementia-parkinsonism-amyotrophy complex to 17q 21-22. *American Journal of Human Genetics,* 55, 1159–1165.

World Health Organization (1992) *The Tenth Revision of the International Classification of Diseases and Related Health Problems* (ICD–10). Geneva: WHO.

6 Management of dementia

Tony Hope & Brice Pitt

Historical context ● *Structured approach* ● *Treatable causes of dementia*
● *Concurrent illness* ● *Troublesome behaviours* ● *Medication* ●
Psychological interventions ● *Social interventions* ● *Carers* ● *Primary
health care* ● *Multi-disciplinary team* ● *Care Programme Approach* ●
Problem-orientated approach ● *Conclusion*

There are no simple recipes for managing dementia. Imagination is required to find solutions to the various problems. However, imagination needs structure, and ideas with which to play. It is the purpose of this chapter to offer these.

Historical context

The 'mere oblivion' of Shakespeare's seventh age, to which dementia as well as sensory impairment must have contributed, has always been a fate threatening those few men and women who survived into their eighth decade. Until the present century they were so scarce as to present little or no problem to society as a whole, though they may have been a burden on some families. Extended families, where three generations lived within a mile or so of each other, coped with their frailer elders, if they were not too disabled or deranged. Otherwise there were, for the poor, workhouses and asylums. The former were gradually replaced by local authority homes under Part III of the National Assistance Act, while the latter were used for those with 'senile dementia' unable to give informed consent to institutional care, who were compulsorily admitted (a procedure involving a magistrate) under the Lunacy Act.

The 20th century has seen the remarkable ageing of populations in the developed countries, so that those over 65 years of age in the UK have grown from 5 to 17% of the population. The burden of ageing and dementia has vastly increased, and resources have changed. Families continue to offer most support, but health services (including the specialities of geriatrics and the psychiatry of old age), social services and voluntary organisations have developed. Recent genetic and pharmacological advances in Alzheimer's disease may herald more resources and better care for those with dementia and their carers.

Structured approach

Box 6.1 gives a simple, four-point check-list as an initial approach to management, using the mnemonic DIPS (Burns & Hope, 1997). In practice, treatable causes of dementia are uncommon, and treating concurrent illnesses usually leaves several problems unsolved. Constructing a list of problems is often the most valuable part of the assessment. These problems are prioritised; it is unlikely that all problems can be tackled at once. An overall perspective should be maintained. For example, one patient displayed a large number of behavioural difficulties; but the key problem was her daughter's guilt at the thought of her moving to an old people's home. Once the problem list is made, solutions to the most pressing problems are generated. It is important to support the carer and involve them in the management plans as far as possible.

Treatable causes of dementia

The management of dementia starts with a full assessment of the patient. This includes a history, mental state examination, physical examination and investigations (see Chapter 1). It is helpful to speak to an informant such as a carer, as well as gathering information from other services including the general practitioner (GP) and social services. The assessment aims initially at excluding other conditions such as delirium or depression, and arriving at the type of dementia syndrome. It is particularly important to exclude the treatable causes of dementia (see Chapter 5). These are reviewed in Lishman (1998).

Concurrent illness

People with dementia are not immune from other illness and disability. However, dementia may mask the symptoms and interfere with eliciting signs. Any alteration in behaviour in someone suffering from dementia may be the result of concurrent illness (Granacher, 1982; Moss *et al*, 1987; O'Connor, 1987). Box 6.2 lists important conditions and disabilities.

Box 6.1 DIPS: a structured approach to management of dementia

Dementia: treat the cause where possible
Illness: treat concurrent illness
Problem list: tackle each major problem
Support the supporters: care for the carers

Box 6.2 Concurrent illness and disability

Physical illness and symptoms
Infection (e.g. chest, urine)
Metabolic disturbance (e.g. dehydration, diabetes, renal failure,
    liver failure)
Cardiac failure or anaemia
Drug toxicity
Hypothermia
Malnutrition
Constipation
Pain

Symptoms of mental illness
Depression
Delusions or hallucinations
Anxiety

Disabilities
Poor hearing or vision
Dental problems
Foot problems
Incontinence

Depression

Depression commonly accompanies dementia, and may benefit from treatment in its own right. Assessment can be difficult if the dementia is too severe for patients to give a good account of their mood and thoughts. In these circumstances, fearfulness and the appearance of sadness may be useful indicators of depression. It may be possible to gain some access to the thoughts of people with moderate dementia, by paying attention to the content of spontaneous speech. The Depressive Signs Scale (Katona & Aldridge, 1985) rates depression in people with dementia (Box 6.3). The nine items are useful indicators of depression in patients with dementia. A history of depressive illness increases suspicion of a present depression.

Two principles should be followed in prescribing antidepressant medication: proceed cautiously using relatively safe drugs with few side-effects (e.g. fluoxetine, lofepramine or trazodone) and define clearly the criteria for success or failure. For further discussion of antidepressant medication and dementia see Satlin & Cole (1988).

Delusions and hallucinations

Delusions and hallucinations commonly occur in the course of dementia (Table 6.1). Often delusions take the form of paranoia where the patient

---

Box 6.3 Items associated with depression in dementia (Katona & Aldridge, 1985)

A sad appearance
Alleviation of sad appearance by external circumstances
Agitation
Slowness of movement
Slowness of speech
Early wakening
Loss of appetite
Diurnal variation in mood
Loss of interest in surroundings

---

accuses people of stealing something they have mislaid. A gentle approach usually proves helpful in these circumstances. Visual hallucinations should raise suspicion of an added delirium or dementia with Lewy bodies. For psychotic symptoms which are persistent, and disturbing for the patient, antipsychotic medication may help (see Chapter 16). Particular care should be taken to prescribe the lowest effective dose of neuroleptic, and to closely monitor for side-effects.

Troublesome behaviours

There are a range of troublesome behaviours which may be identified from the history (Table 6.1). These should be listed, and strategies generated to deal with them. Carers often find these behaviours particularly difficult to deal with and stressful (see Chapter 18).

Table 6.1 The frequency of troublesome behaviours found in a sample of patients with dementia (Swearer *et al*, 1988)

	%
Angry outbursts	51
Dietary change	46
Sleep disturbance	45
Paranoia	32
Phobia	25
Delusions and hallucinations	22
Assaultative/violent behaviour	21
Bizarre behaviour	21
Incontinence	17

Aggression

Overt, directed aggression is rare in dementia. What is far more common is irritability or anger at being disturbed at times of washing, dressing or eating. At home this anger is usually directed at carers, while in institutions, staff or other residents may be on the receiving end. Aggression needs a considered response:

(a) Maintain an unhurried, friendly and respectful manner.
(b) Exclude obvious causes of anger such as pain, depression, psychosis or nicotine withdrawal.
(c) Use a behavioural approach like ABC (see below)
(d) Distraction may be helpful.
(e) A short period of 'time out' is justified as part of a behavioural programme.
(f) A very small dose of a neuroleptic can be effective, but avoid sedation.

Wandering

Wandering may result from many causes and the management depends on the cause (Box 6.4). Often a more structured and fuller day is required and the person may require more interaction. The design of the environment can have an important effect. Sometimes it may be necessary to lock doors. Physical restraint should be avoided if possible. Medication may be helpful for anxiety, depression or psychosis but its use as a 'chemical straitjacket' should also be avoided. It needs to be closely monitored and stopped if failing or harmful.

Restlessness at night

Patients with dementia often become more agitated and confused at night (sundowning). Their sleep cycle may become so disturbed that they are up all night and sleep during the day. They may find the quietness and darkness of night threatening. Delirium should be excluded. Efforts should

---

Box 6.4 Causes of wandering

Boredom and lack of stimulation
Lack of exercise
Habit
Anxiety, agitation, depression or psychosis
Seeking out somewhere such as the shops or home
Pain or discomfort

be directed at ensuring rewarding activities (and little sleep) during the day. This is often easier said than done. Other advice is to establish a routine with a fixed bedtime late in the evening, avoid stimulants such as tea and coffee, encourage a reasonable sized meal a few hours before bedtime, and to make sure the bed is warm and comfortable. If these measures fail then medication may help. This could be a neuro-leptic such as thioridazine, a sedating antidepressant such as trazodone, or a hypnotic such as temazepam or chlormethiazole (see Chapter 16).

Incontinence

Incontinence has many causes (Box 6.5). Those associated with dementia include poor planning, disorientation, being unable to recognise the toilet, not caring, and less cortical control of bladder or bowel. Management depends upon the cause. Measures include:

(a) regular visits to the toilet especially before travelling;
(b) clear labelling of a convenient toilet;
(c) avoiding drinks before bedtime;
(d) treating constipation or urinary tract infections;
(e) incontinence pads; and
(f) an anticholinergic for an unstable bladder (be wary of hastening cognitive decline).

Sexual disinhibition

This is often stressful for carers (see Chapter 18). Behaviour includes exposing self, extreme sexual language, masturbation and propositioning others. It is important not to reinforce the behaviour, and a behavioural approach may be helpful. Rarely it can be necessary to use a libido suppressant such as benperidol, as an alternative to secure or single gender institutionalised care (see also Chapter 11).

Box 6.5 Causes of incontinence

Stress incontinence
Immobility
Urgency associated with prostatism
Urinary tract infection
Over sedation
Diabetes
Diuretics
Epilepsy

Uncooperativeness

Ideally all management plans, including attending day centres or hospital admission, should be discussed with the patient and agreement reached. However, services are sometimes rejected by patients who may refuse any help, or expect their carer to offer all the support. At other times, patients with dementia may refuse medication or hospital admission. In these circumstances, it is best to explain the situation clearly and calmly to the patient, and try not to be too confrontational. Gentle persuasion or leaving the discussion for a little while can be effective. Some ideas sound more acceptable from doctors than carers, and vice versa. A visit to a day centre may relieve fears for the patient and carer. Medication, such as a small dose of neuroleptic, may relieve some of the anxiety associated with change.

Use of legislation is usually reserved for those situations where it is felt the patient is putting themselves at risk. The Mental Health Act (1983) can be used in order to assess and treat someone in hospital compulsorily. Similarly, guardianship is sometimes used to require someone to live at a specific place such as a residential home (see Chapter 19). In practice, many people with dementia are admitted to hospital or residential care without real consent.

Medication

There are two broad categories of medication used in dementia: drugs aimed at improving cognitive function; and drugs aimed at reducing problematic behaviour. These approaches are considered separately in Chapter 16.

Psychological interventions

Psychological treatments have emphasised the importance of a structured approach to solving specific problems, and have provided a much needed reminder that a person with dementia has experiences and wishes which should be respected. Treatments can be broadly divided into therapies for dementia and therapies aimed at specific problems. The general therapies of reality orientation, reminiscence, validation therapy, memory therapy and resolution therapy are covered in Chapter 17. Therapies aimed at specific problems are described in the following section. Garland (1997) provides a good review of the applications of psychological treatments to elderly people, including those with dementia.

Behavioural analysis

One of the most important contributions of psychology to the management of dementia has been the development of a structured approach to tackling behavioural problems. It involves three stages:

(a) Observing what events and situations *activate* (or are *antecedent* to) the behaviour.
(b) The *behaviour* itself is precisely described.
(c) Identify the *consequences* of the behaviour (for example, how carers respond).

This approach is usefully known as the ABC analysis of behaviour. Stokes (1990) gave an example of aggressive behaviour. The first step involves finding out when and where the behaviour takes place, what the person was doing immediately before the aggression and what else was happening around this time. The second step means describing exactly what the person did. The third step identifies how the victim, and other people reacted, and how the aggressor responded.

Usually a period of at least several days' structured observation is required before any therapeutic interventions are introduced. The effectiveness of these is then assessed through further observations. The interventions may involve reducing the likelihood of the person being in the provoking situations, they may be aimed at altering the responses of other people or they may involve a combination of the two.

Strengths-based approach

A focus on solving problems needs to be tempered by a strengths-based approach which emphasises the importance, in therapy, of capitalising on what the individual patient can do and enjoy.

Social interventions

Social treatments involve changing the environment of the person and helping those who are principally involved in the care. Good reviews of these treatment strategies are provided by Moriarty & Levin (1993), Morris & Morris (1993), Bradshaw (1997), Levin (1997) and Moore & Buckland (1997).

Restructuring the environment

This looks at how the environment can be: made more safe; altered to enable the person to cope better; and be pleasant and stimulating.

Safety

Box 6.6 is a check-list of some of the ways in which people with dementia might be unsafe and come to harm. A patient's safety needs to be kept under regular review, particularly in the light of increasing impairment. Maintaining a balance between safety and the restriction of a patient's

---

Box 6.6 Ways in which people with dementia can come to harm

Falling on slippery floors
Falling down stairs
Falling from bed onto hard floor or against furniture
Starting fire with matches, candles or cooker
Scalding with hot tap water or kettle
Wandering away and spending night outside or hit by traffic
Choking
Unsuitable ingestion of medication
Abuse from carer

---

freedom is one of the most difficult aspects of caring for people with dementia. For example, people who wander off from their home are often at some risk of being hit by traffic. However, the degree of restriction which would prevent this behaviour may interfere greatly with the freedom enjoyed by both patient and carer.

Coping better

The environment should be reviewed to help the patient cope with problems. Some simple examples of environmental manipulations are summarised in Box 6.7. More sophisticated measures include radio-tagging devices to ensure that someone cannot get lost if they wander off (McShane *et al*, 1994), and floor designs in front of exit doorways, which are thought to decrease the chance of confused people leaving the ward (Hussian & Brown, 1987).

Pleasant and stimulating

A discussion of the environment should not concentrate exclusively on solving problems. It is also important to design an environment which is

---

Box 6.7 Environmental manipulations to help patients to cope

Clear labelling of toilet rooms
Maintain consistent furniture arrangement
Enable carers to develop one-to-one relationships with patient
Maintain adequate lighting in all areas used by patients
Use identification necklace for those who wander off and become lost
Remove inedible objects which patient attempts to eat

likely to be pleasant and stimulating. Care must be taken, however, to take the patients' perspective. There is a danger that in trying to make the surroundings stimulating they become confusing. The Domus philosophy of residential care is one recent attempt to improve the quality of those in long-term residential care (Lindsay *et al*, 1995). It is based on four assumptions:

(a) That the residence (domus) is the person's home for life.
(b) That the needs of the staff are as important as those of the residents.
(c) That the domus should aim to correct the avoidable consequences of dementia and accommodate those that are unavoidable.
(d) That the residents' individual psychological and emotional needs may take precedence over the physical aspects of their care.

Carers

Those intimately concerned with looking after people with dementia need two kinds of support: practical and emotional (see Chapter 18 for a fuller account).

Practical support

Financial

Many carers are not receiving all the financial support to which they are entitled. It is important to ensure that they are properly informed and helped with making financial claims.

Respite

Many carers want to continue to look after the person with dementia, but their ability to cope is undermined by the lack of any respite. Day care can allow carers to carry out necessary tasks, such as shopping. It may enable them to continue in paid work with both financial and social advantages, and it can give them some much needed time to enjoy themselves. 'Holiday admissions' in which the person with dementia is admitted for residential or hospital care for several days at a time, are another way in which carers can be given time to recreate themselves. It is sometimes possible for a sitter to look after the patient for several hours, in their own home, either during the day or at night, in order to allow the principal carer some respite.

Tasks

Help with providing food (e.g. meals on wheels), cleaning, washing and dressing (e.g. a home help) can also relieve some of the burden from the principal carer.

Education

The importance of education for the carer must not be underestimated (Pollitt, 1994). This includes information about the disease, its prognosis and likely consequences. It may include training in carrying out a programme of behaviour modification and information about giving medication. It can include information about the various means of obtaining practical support.

Emotional support

It is important that the carer is also cared for. Opportunities are needed for carers to talk about the problems they are having, and about their feelings, including the negative feelings about the person with dementia. Carers' support groups as well as experienced counsellors (such as community psychiatric nurses) can be of great benefit.

One carer, whose wife had Alzheimer's disease, writing about his own experience (Reveley, 1988) offered these pieces of advice: do not hide the disease from those around you; take care of yourself; enlist help in all areas; and take calculated risks.

Professional carers such as nurses, residential home staff, doctors and social workers, also need support and care. A professional team needs to build into it a mechanism to enable such support to be given. Hospital-based professionals can help the staff of residential homes to think about and to achieve their goals (see Garland, 1991).

Primary health care

The early diagnosis of dementia is important, not only to exclude treatable conditions, but because it is often the trigger for health and community

---

Box 6.8 Support the supporters; care for the carers

Financial: ensure financial entitlements
Respite: day care, holiday admissions, day sitting service, night sitting service
Practical: meals on wheels, home help
Education: about disease process, about medication, about behaviour modification programme, about support services
Care: individual counselling (e.g. community psychiatric nurses), carers groups (e.g. through Alzheimer's Disease Society), family and friends

services. In particular, a person with dementia is entitled to an assessment of needs under the 1990 Community Care Act. GPs act as gatekeepers to specialist services, but there is evidence that they tend to underdiagnose dementia (Ilffe *et al*, 1991). All people over 75 should now be offered an annual check by their GP and this may improve detection. After referral, it is important that community health teams and hospital-based teams liaise with the primary health care team. It is easy for hospital doctors to forget that GPs provide the major medical support for most people with dementia.

The multi-disciplinary team

The management of people with dementia requires many different tasks to be undertaken. It is not usually appropriate for one person to carry out all of these tasks and effective teamwork is vital. Box 6.9 lists some of the professions who contribute to the team. For management to be effective, good and frequent communication between the team members is needed.

Care Programme Approach

The Care Programme Approach requires that all patients accepted by specialist mental health services must have a keyworker who is

---

Box 6.9 Professional groups and some of their roles

Doctors: evaluation of concurrent illness; prescription of medication; facilitating provision of hospital and community services

Nurses: general care of in-patients and nursing home residents; carrying out behaviour modification regimes; education and counselling of relatives; coordination of community services

Clinical psychologists: initiating behaviour modification programmes, offering advice and support to staff in a caring role

Social workers: facilitating provision of local authority services such as residential care, respite care, home care; counselling of carers

Occupational therapists: design of environment; education of carers; identification of strengths and abilities of patient

responsible for making sure that their health and social needs are fully assessed. The keyworker is responsible for a care plan that is negotiated with the patient and their carers. Depending upon the local services, many people with dementia will be assessed by the old age psychiatric services, management suggestions made, and their care discharged back to their GP. Other patients will be followed up by the community team and require regular Care Programme Approach reviews.

Problem-orientated approach

The main steps in a problem-oriented approach to management need to be planned, if possible, with the whole team. Involve the patient, carers and the primary health care team in these processes as far as is possible. The steps are summarised in Box 6.10.

Conclusion

The management of dementia is sometimes thought to be an unrewarding area, of little intellectual interest. This is far from the case. Certainly there are no cures for the disease. For this reason, management requires the ability to think widely and imaginatively. This chapter has emphasised a structured approach to management. Of equal importance is attitude. Above all, management must be centred on respect for the individual.

Box 6.10 Steps taken in a problem-oriented approach to the management of dementia

Identify problems which might need addressing
Identify strengths of patient and the support system
Establish priorities for problems list
Set clear goals for management – these should be realistic
For each aspect of management decide who should be involved
Ensure patient and carers are well informed of plans
Set time for review
Carry out review: assess effectiveness of management plan and reassess problems and priorities

References

Bradshaw, M. (1997) Social work with older persons. In *Psychiatry in the Elderly* (eds R. Jacoby & C. Oppenheimer), 2nd edn, pp. 217–231. Oxford: Oxford University Press.

Burns, A. & Hope, T. (1997) Clinical aspects of the dementias of old age. In *Psychiatry in the Elderly* (eds R. Jacoby & C. Oppenheimer), 2nd edn, pp. 456–493. Oxford: Oxford University Press.

Garland, J. (1991) *Making Residential Care Feel Like Home: Enhancing Quality of Life for Older People.* Bicester: Winslow Press.

—— (1997) Psychological assessment and treatment. In *Psychiatry in the Elderly* (eds. R. Jacoby & C. Oppenheimer), 2nd edn, pp. 246–256. Oxford: Oxford University Press.

Granacher, R. P. (1982) Agitation in the elderly. An often-treatable manifestation of acute brain syndrome. *Postgraduate Medicine*, 72, 83–96.

Hussian, R. A. & Brown, D. C. (1987) Use of two-dimensional grid patterns to limit hazardous ambulation in demented patients. *Journal of Gerontology*, 42, 558–560.

Illife, S., Haines, A., Gallivan, S., *et al* (1991) Assessment of elderly patients in general practice. 1. Social circumstances and mental state. *British Journal of General Practice*, 41, 9–12.

Katona, C. & Aldridge, D. (1985) The DST and depression signs in dementia. *Journal of Affective Disorders*, 8, 83–89.

Levin, E. (1997) Carers – problems, strains and services. In *Psychiatry in the Elderly* (eds R. Jacoby & C. Oppenheimer), 2nd edn, pp. 392–402. Oxford: Oxford University Press.

Lindesay, J., Briggs, K., Lawes, M., *et al* (1995) The Domus Philosophy: a comparative evaluation of residential care for the demented elderly. In *Geriatric Psychiatry: Key Research Topics for Clinicians* (eds E. Murphy & G. Alexopoulos), pp. 259–273. Chichester: John Wiley and Sons.

Lishman, W. A. (1998) *Organic Psychiatry.* Oxford: Blackwell Scientific.

McShane, R., Wilkinson, J. & Hope, T. (1994) Tracking patients who wander: ethics and technology. *Lancet*, 343, 1274.

Moore, S. & Buckland, A. (1997) Nursing in old age psychiatry. In *Psychiatry in the Elderly* (eds R. Jacoby & C. Oppenheimer), 2nd edn, pp. 303–317. Oxford: Oxford University Press.

Moriarty, J. & Levin, E. (1993) Services to people with dementia and their carers. In *Ageing and Dementia: A Methodological Approach* (ed. A. Burns), pp. 237–250. London: Edward Arnold.

Morris, R. G. & Morris, L. W. (1993) Psychological aspects of caring for people with dementia: conceptual and methodological issues. In *Ageing and Dementia: A Methodological Approach* (ed. A Burns), pp. 251–274. London: Edward Arnold.

Moss, R., D'Amico, S. & Maletta, G. (1987) Mental dysfunction as a sign of organic illness in the elderly. *Geriatrics*, 42, 35–42.

O'Connor, M. (1987) Disturbed behaviour in dementia: psychiatric or medical problem. *Medical Journal of Australia*, 147, 481–485.

Pollitt, P. A. (1994) The meaning of dementia to those involved as carers. In *Dementia and Normal Ageing* (eds F. A. Huppert, C. Brayne & D. W. O'Connor), p. 257. Cambridge: Cambridge University Press.

Reveley, J. B. (1988) One caregiver's view. In *Treatments for the Alzheimer Patient* (eds L. F. Jarvik & C. H. Winograd), pp. 137–144. New York: Springer Publishing.

Satlin, A. & Cole, J. O. (1988) Psychopharmacologic interventions. In *Treatments for the Alzheimer Patient* (eds L. F. Jarvik & C. H. Winograd), pp. 59–79. New York: Springer Publishing.

Stokes, G. (1990) Behavioural analysis. In *Working with Dementia* (eds G. Stokes & F. Goudie), pp. 181–190. Bicester: Winslow Press.

Swearer, J. M., Drachmann, D. A., O'Donnell, B. F., *et al* (1988) Troublesome and disruptive behaviours in dementia – relationships to diagnosis and disease severity. *Journal of the American Geriatrics Society*, 76, 784–790.

Additional reading

Jarvik, L. F. & Winograd, C. H. (eds) (1998) *Treatments for the Alzheimer Patient*. New York: Springer Publishing.

Woods, R. T. & Britton, P. G. (1985) *Clinical Psychology with the Elderly*. London: Croom Helm.

Stokes, G. & Goudie, F. (eds) (1990) *Working with Dementia*. Bicester: Winslow Press.

Garland, J. (1991) *Making Residential Care Look Like Home: Enhancing Quality of Life for Older People*. Bicester: Winslow Press.

Pitt, B. (ed.) (1987) *Dementia*. Edinburgh: Churchill Livingstone.

Jacoby, R. & Oppenheimer, C. (1997) *Psychiatry in the Elderly,* 2nd edn. Oxford: Oxford University Press.

7 Depression

Robert Baldwin

Classification • *Epidemiology* • *Clinical presentation* • *Assessment* •
Differential diagnosis • *Aetiology* • *Management* • *Prognosis* •
Conclusion

Functional disorders are nowadays seen almost as often, in many old age
psychiatric services, as dementia. Depression is a common, sometimes
the most common, reason for referral.

Classification

'Depressive illness' is synonymous with depressive episode in ICD–10
(World Health Organization, 1993) (Box 7.1) and major depressive episode
in DSM–IV (American Psychiatric Association, 1994).

Epidemiology

The prevalence of depressive symptoms far exceeds that of depressive
illness. Classic research from Newcastle (Kay *et al*, 1964) found a
prevalence of 10% for depression in community residents, although less
than 2% met criteria for what would now correspond to depressive illness.
In a cross-national comparison, Gurland *et al* (1983) found levels of
'pervasive depression' in 13% of New York elderly residents and 12% of
Londoners. Point (past month) prevalence of manic depressive or
depressive disorder, akin to depressive illness, was found to be 1.3 and
2.5%, respectively. The rates are double this in general practice attenders,
and considerably higher in hospital settings (Jackson & Baldwin, 1993).

Clinical presentation

Clinical features normally regarded as more common in elderly depressed
patients include: neuro-vegetative symptomatology, somatic preoccupation,
agitation, forgetfulness and delusions. However, these stereotypic descriptions
of depression in later life derive, in the main, from the study of in-patients
and may reflect illness severity. Blazer *et al* (1986), using an approach which
controlled for symptoms that may increase fortuitously with age, found:

Box 7.1 ICD–10 classification of depression (World Health Organization, 1993)

Mild depressive episode (at least two from (b) and at least four from (c)). Moderate depressive episode: at least six of the symptoms under (c). Severe depressive episode: all three from section (b) and at least five from section (c) (at least eight symptoms in total)

(a) The syndrome of depression must be present for at least two weeks, no history of mania, and not attributable to organic disease or psychoactive substance
(b) At least two of the following three symptoms must be present:
  (i) Depressed mood to a degree that is definitely abnormal for the individual, present for most of the day and almost every day, largely uninfluenced by circumstances, and sustained for at least two weeks
  (ii) Loss of interest or pleasure in activities that are normally pleasurable
  (iii) Decreased energy or increased fatiguability
(c) An additional symptom or symptoms from the following (at least four):
  (i) Loss of confidence or self-esteem
  (ii) Unreasonable feelings of self-reproach or excessive and inappropriate guilt
  (iii) Recurrent thoughts of death or suicide; suicidal behaviour.
  (iv) Complaints or evidence of diminished ability to think or concentrate, such as indecisiveness or vacillation;
  (v) Change in psychomotor activity, with agitation or retardation (either subjective or objective)
  (vi) Sleep disturbance of any type
  (vii) Change in appetite (decrease or increase) with corresponding weight change

---

(a) Older depressed subjects reported more somatic symptoms.
(b) Older people had more thoughts about death and had a greater preoccupation with the wish to die than younger people, although not significantly so.
(c) Surprisingly, it was the younger rather than the older people with depression who reported more memory problems.
(d) There was no support for the notion of masked depression in the elderly.

More recently, Musetti *et al* (1989) could find no symptoms which reliably differentiated older community dwelling patients with major depression from younger ones. Against expectations, the group over 65 years, exhibited more retardation than agitation. In terms of clinical presentation, the adage 'depression is depression at any age' has some truth to it. However, the pathoplastic influences of age and ageing alter the presentation of depression among the elderly. The main influences are shown in Box 7.2.

Coexistence with physical illness

A common difficulty arises from the coexistence of lowered mood and physical illness. For example, symptoms such as weight loss, fatigue and insomnia may overlap in someone with rheumatoid arthritis. Diagnostic sensitivity is increased if attention is paid to the following.

   (a) The history may indicate a change in symptoms at a time of static physical health.
   (b) Appropriate questions must be asked, e.g. 'Do you feel tired even when at rest?', not 'Have you no energy?'.
   (c) Particular care must be directed towards uncovering anhedonia and depressive ideation (self-deprecation, guilt, etc.).

Complaining of depression

In the elderly a complaint of depression may be denied or minimised (Georgotas, 1983). In fact, DSM–IV recognises this and allows anhedonia, instead of low mood, for a diagnosis of major depression. Depression has only recently been an acceptable reason for consulting a doctor. Instead, elderly people more frequently develop excessive physical preoccupation in the form of hypochondriasis (Gurland, 1976). There may be an actual pain for which no organic cause can be uncovered or, more commonly, disproportionate complaining about known organic pathology.

Box 7.2 Factors which may alter or obscure presentation

Overlap of physical and somatic psychiatric symptoms
Reduced expression of sadness
Somatisation or disproportionate complaints associated with physical disorder
Neurotic symptoms of recent onset
Medically 'trivial' deliberate self-harm
Pseudodementia
Depression superimposed upon dementia
Behavioural disorder
Accentuation of abnormal personality traits
Late-onset alcohol dependency syndrome

Other neuroses

Neuroses such as obsessive–compulsive disorder, hypochondriasis and hysteria are rare as primary disorders among the elderly. When neurotic symptoms occur for the first time in an older person they are usually secondary (sometimes referred to as 'symptomatic') with depression being the most common underlying cause. Likewise, anxiety symptoms may dominate the clinical picture with the danger that an underlying depression is missed.

Deliberate self-harm

Perhaps the most serious error is to dismiss an act of deliberate self-harm in an older person because in medical terms it was 'trivial'. Likewise, depressive illness is a very frequent accompaniment of any act of deliberate self-harm. Any older individual who deliberately harms themselves should always have a full psychiatric assessment.

Other behaviours

These behaviours may indicate an underlying depressive illness:

(a) Behavioural disorder: the sudden occurrence of food refusal, aggression or inappropriate micturition, usually in a residential facility and within a context of resented dependency.
(b) Shoplifting.
(c) Alcohol dependence arising for the first time in later life.
(d) An accentuation of premorbid personality traits: such individuals are often theatrical and importuning, and a depressive illness may easily be overlooked.

In these instances a thorough history from the patient and an informant often clears up uncertainty. Evidence of recent change is crucial and a comprehensive past personal and family psychiatric history must be obtained, along with a full drug and alcohol history. Depressive cognition may have been noticed by relatives, e.g. 'I wish the Lord would take me'.

Pseudodementia

Another important, if controversial, presentation is depressive pseudodementia. The term is unsatisfactory. Other terminology such as 'the dementia of depression' (Pearlson *et al*, 1989) has been proposed, but pseudodementia seems here to stay. Perhaps it is best used as a reminder that severe depression can mimic dementia. The term has been used in at least three ways:

(a) Depressed patients who perform poorly on a bedside screening test for dementia. Since dementia is defined clinically and not on the basis of a test result, this use should be discouraged.

(b) Depressed, usually elderly patients who have cognitive impairment which does not meet the diagnostic criteria for dementia. These patients have a general impairment in effortful tasks, especially those concerned with memory, rather than an impairment in cortical function (language, praxis, construction) (Weingartner *et al*, 1981). After reviewing the literature, Reynolds *et al* (1988*a*) suggest a prevalence of between 10 and 20% of depressed patients. There is evidence that these cognitive deficits arise from subcortical dysfunction, suggesting that depressive illness may cause a subcortical dementia. However, since most elderly patients with depressive illness have some degree of cognitive impairment the term pseudodementia used this way may be rather meaningless.

(c) To define a characteristic, if dramatic, presentation of dementia. Post (1982) provides a vivid account. The patient appears perplexed and may be inaccessible at interview, although non-verbally may convey considerable distress. The history is months at most and poor memory can often be dated accurately, unlike the insidious onset and course of dementia. Patients with dementia try their best but are inaccurate and are often unaware of their errors when asked questions concerning cognitive function. Pseudodementia patients become irritable and complain vociferously of bad memory. Such patients are usually described as giving 'don't know' answers. Post makes the point that the term 'pseudodementia' should really be reserved for those patients who can be tested, rather than those who are inaccessible and not really testable.

Assessment

History

A detailed history is required from the patient and an informant. Evidence suggesting recent change is very important and areas such as a family and personal history of depression, and a full drug and alcohol history must be covered. Treatments and responses in previous depressive episodes should be clarified. Information about major adverse life events, for example bereavement and other losses such as ill-health, should be documented, along with previous capacity to cope with stressful situations and difficulties. This covers aspects of personality. Personality traits may be difficult to assess but they are important in setting a realistic target to therapy. For example, an individual with long-standing dysthymia may become severely depressed and require treatment, but restitution to a former state of relative gloom may be more realistic than attempting to help the patient attain perfect happiness. Availability and the quality of support from family, friends, neighbours, and statutory and voluntary sectors are important, as they may influence prognosis.

Mental state examination

Care must be taken not to overlook suicidal ideation and delusional phenomena. Evidence of cognitive impairment should be carefully documented so that comparisons can be made after recovery. Routine neuropsychological testing is not usually warranted unless dementia is suspected, and even then the findings are likely to be equivocal. However, it is useful to include a screening measure such as the Mini-Mental State Examination (Folstein *et al*, 1975) (see Chapter 1).

Physical examination

A physical examination is important because of the close association between physical illness and depression (Box 7.3). As well as possibly causing depression, physical illness is a poor prognostic factor. Cases of diagnostic difficulty usually need admission to hospital for skilled psychiatric nursing observation.

Investigations

Laboratory investigations include haemoglobin and red blood cell indices which may indicate B12 deficiency or excessive alcohol intake. B12 estimation should be undertaken in a first episode. Folate should be measured if severe depression has been present for some weeks, as a state of under-nutrition may have developed. For similar reasons urea and electrolytes are important. A low serum potassium may delay electroconvulsive therapy (ECT). An elevated calcium is occasionally associated with depression, in primary hyperparathyroidism and metastatic

---

Box 7.3 Causes of organic ('symptomatic' or 'secondary') depression

Occult carcinoma: lung, pancreas
Metabolic or endocrine: hypothyroidism, hypercalcaemia, Cushing's disease
Drugs: steroids, beta-blockers, methyldopa, clonidine, nifedipine, digoxin, L-dopa, tetrabenazine
Infections: post-viral, myalgic encephalomyelitis, brucellosis, neurosyphilis
Organic brain disease: space occupying lesion, dementia

cancer. Thyroid function tests may reveal hypothyroidism or an 'apathetic hyperthyroidism', both of which can be mistaken for depression. The main clinical use of an electroencephalogram (EEG) is to help differentiate depression from an organic brain syndrome. Abnormal investigations may be responsible for depression, or the result of depression (Table 7.1).

Imaging

Imaging is not routinely carried out in depression in the elderly, but only if indicated by other factors such as a rapid onset or the presence of neurological symptoms or signs. However researchers are looking at ways in which the newer imaging techniques may be clinically useful in diagnosis or treatment. For example, O'Brien *et al* (1994) have found that measures of temporal lobe atrophy on magnetic resonance imaging discriminate between depression and Alzheimer's disease (see Chapter 12).

Biological markers

More contentious is the role of markers of depressive illness. The best known of these is the dexamethasone suppression test (DST). The rationale is that there is hyperactivity of the hypothalamic-pituitary-adrenal axis in depression, which leads to a failure to suppress cortisol after ingestion of dexamethasone. Following initial encouraging reports (Carroll *et al*, 1981) a deluge of publications ensued, all enthusiastically supporting the DST as a 'diagnostic tool' for major depression, only to be followed by doubt

Table 7.1 Investigations

	First episode	Recurrence
Full blood count	Yes	Yes
Urea and electrolytes	Yes	Yes
Calcium	Yes	If symptoms indicate
Thyroid function	Yes	If symptoms indicate, or > 12 months previously
B12	Yes	If symptoms indicate, or > 2 years previously
Folate	Yes	If indicated by nutritional state
Liver function	Yes	If indicated (e.g. alcohol intake)
Syphilitic serology	Yes; if atypical presentation	If not already done
CT (brain)	If clinically indicated	If neurologically indicated
Electroencephalogram	If clinically indicated	If neurologically indicated

and uncertainty. Clearly the DST is less specific for depressive illness than was first thought. For old age psychiatry the situation is even less promising, as a consensus seems to be emerging that DST non-suppression gradually increases with age, particularly after 75 years. Furthermore the DST does not appear to differentiate between dementia and depression (Spar & Gerner, 1982).

Assessment schedules

Another approach to diagnosis concerns schedules. These are useful in improving detection in areas such as residential and nursing home facilities, where the prevalence of depression is known to be high. The Geriatric Depression Scale (GDS) which is available in either a 30-item and a 15-item version (Yesavage, 1988) is probably the most widely used.

Differential diagnosis

ICD–10

The main differential diagnoses in ICD–10 are:

(a) organic depressive disorder, the aetiology of which may be systemic or cerebral;
(b) dysthymia, a form of chronic 'low grade' depression;
(c) delusional disorder, in which the judgement is whether delusional symptoms are mood-congruent, in which case psychotic depression is most likely; and
(d) adjustment disorder, with either a brief (one to six months) or prolonged (more than six months) depressive reaction, adjustment disorder is sometimes secondary to a bereavement in older people.

Bereavement

Some of the symptoms of bereavement overlap with those of depressive illness. Certain features point more clearly towards depressive illness and to a consideration of antidepressants:

(a) progress over the first few months only to slip back for no apparent reason;
(b) suicidal thoughts;
(c) pervasive guilt (not merely remorse over what more might have been done to prevent death);
(d) disability; and
(e) 'mummification', maintaining grief by keeping everything unchanged.

Aetiology

Predisposing factors

Genetic

The genetic contribution to depressive illness decreases with age. Hopkinson (1964) reported that the risk to first degree relatives of probands with depressive illness was 20% in early onset but only 8% in late onset. Others have confirmed this difference (Mendelwicz, 1976).

Gender

Depression in all age groups is more common in women and this is true in later life. The ratio is approximately seven to three, female to male. Some studies have reported higher rates of depression in those widowed or divorced.

Neurobiology

Amine changes may predispose to depression, or be altered as a consequence of it. Perhaps not surprisingly, no clear consensus has emerged in respect of the amine theory in later life depression. However, some biological changes associated with ageing are similar to those seen in depression. Both ageing and depression are associated with decreased brain concentrations of serotonin, dopamine, noradrenaline and their metabolites, and increased MAO-B activity (Veith & Raskind, 1988).

Neuroendocrinology

A variety of neuroendocrine changes are associated with ageing (Veith & Raskind, 1988). However, the site of action is not clear and may involve changes at cortical, limbic, hypothalamic or pituitary level. Depression in all age groups is associated with hyperactivity and dysregulation of the hypothalamic-pituitary-adrenal axis. The TSH response to thyroid-releasing hormone is less age dependent than cortisol non-suppression, but is not specific for depression, and there has been very little research on depressed subjects in later life. Schneider (1992) concluded that none of the neurochemical markers or neuroendocrine challenge tests is sufficiently sensitive or specific to be of clinical use in depression of old age.

Electroencephalogram

Variables measured during sleep show similar changes in depression and ageing (Veith & Raskind, 1988). These include night time wakefulness and decreases in slow wave sleep, total rapid eye movement sleep and rapid eye movement latency. Using discriminant function analysis,

Reynolds *et al* (1988*b*) found that four EEG sleep variables correctly differentiated depressed elderly patients from those with dementia in 80% of cases.

Structural brain changes

Over a quarter of a century ago, Felix Post (1968) wrote "subtle cerebral changes may make ageing persons increasingly liable to affective disturbance". Recently several factors have renewed interest in this hypothesis:

(a) The attenuation of genetic risk, an important factor in 'younger' depression, ought to lead to a reduced prevalence of depression in later life. Since this has not been demonstrated, other factors such as subtle brain damage may be active.

(b) Biological and clinical markers have been described which may distinguish early from late-onset depressions. These include a lower sedation threshold to barbiturates, both before and after treatment; latency in auditory cortical evoked responses, midway between patients with dementia and controls; and a higher than expected rate of death from vascular causes (Murphy *et al*, 1988).

(c) There is growing evidence that structural and functional brain changes occur in depression in old age. Findings include (see Chapter 12): ventricular enlargement on computerised tomography (Jacoby & Levy, 1980); magnetic resonance imaging changes (white matter change of possible vascular aetiology) (reviewed by Baldwin, 1993); single photon emission tomography changes in blood flow (Sackheim *et al*, 1990); and focal abnormalities in cerebral blood flow with positron emission tomography (Bench *et al*, 1992).

Physical health

Diseases, some with occult presentation, may predispose to severe depression (Box 7.3). Some neurological illnesses, such as stroke and idiopathic Parkinson's disease, may have specific organic links with depressive illness.

Personality

Surprisingly little has been written about this (see Chapter 11). Roth (1955) believed that those with late-onset depressive illness had more robust personalities than those with depression arising earlier in life. Post (1972) noted that severe depression was associated with less premorbid personality dysfunction than milder depression. However, differentiating current illness from premorbid personality is very difficult, and even informants often provide biased accounts. Even so, Bergmann (1978) and Post (1972) note that patients with predominantly neurotic symptom profiles of depression have often been categorised anxiety-prone individuals. Bergmann (1978), basing his argument on the influential work of Bowlby, suggested that satisfactory attachment behaviour in early life was necessary to adaptively cope with the real threats of old age. Post (1972) noted that obsessional traits were over-represented in his in-patient group. Abrams *et al* (1987) found an association of 'avoidant' and 'dependent' types with late-life depression. Murphy (1982) found that a life-long lack of a capacity for intimacy, a personality variable, seemed to be a risk factor for depression in later life.

Social supports and intimacy

Most of the vulnerability factors for depression, identified by Brown & Harris (1978), are not relevant to the elderly. One potentially relevant one, loss of mother before aged 11, was not confirmed by Murphy (1982) in her study of depressed elderly patients. Murphy's research suggested that a confidant may buffer social losses. The increased realisation in recent years that childhood sexual abuse often has severe and long-lasting damaging effects, including depression, should not be overlooked when treating elderly patients. One woman in her seventies who presented to me with a late-onset depressive illness after a difficult orthopaedic procedure, revealed for the first time (to the female nurses) that she had been sexually abused by her father many years earlier.

Precipitating factors

Life events

As with depression in younger age groups, a recent adverse life event is an important precipitant. Post (1962) reported these in two-thirds of severely depressed in-patients. Murphy (1982) found that 48% of depressed in- and out-patients had experienced threatening or loss events in the preceding year, compared to 23% of controls. In addition, major chronic

---

Box 7.4 Aetiology

Genetic (reduced)
Gender (female)
Neurobiology
Neuroendocrinology
Structural brain changes
Physical health
Personality
Social supports

social difficulties (as distinct from abrupt events) lasting at least two years were associated with depression. These findings are comparable to the life event studies of Brown & Harris (1978), except for one difference: in the elderly a recent grave physical illness or a chronically disabling disorder assumed a far more conspicuous role (Murphy, 1982).

Perpetuating factors

Social factors

There is evidence that, on the whole, social factors exert less influence on the course of depressive illness in later life. Nevertheless, it is important to examine the social factors which may influence outcome for the better. Oxman *et al* (1992) examined the effect of social networks and supports on depressive symptoms, in people seen three years apart. Using multiple regression analysis, most variance was explained by disability, but there were important social variables such as loss of spouse, adequacy of emotional support, presence of 'tangible' support and the role of family and confidantes. Although the evidence is meagre and at times contradictory, poor support is likely to be a maintenance factor for depression.

Carers

Hinrichsen & Hernandez (1993) found three factors which associated with poorer outcome at one year from major depression in a cohort of patients with a mean age of just over 70 (see Chapter 18): psychiatric symptoms in the carer, reported difficulties and poorer carer health.

Management

Biological treatments

Antidepressants

How antidepressants are prescribed is perhaps as important as knowing what to give. Some elderly people are somewhat in awe of their doctors. Rather than causing offence, because they do not consider tablets to be the answer to depression, they will discreetly bin their antidepressants or retain them in their bottles or sealed packages. Start with an explanation that depression which warrants treatment with tablets is an illness, and that it is common, treatable and not a sign of moral weakness. Many patients need reassurance that the tablets are not addictive and that depression is not 'senility' or a harbinger of dementia. Involve the patient in an agreed treatment plan. They need to be told, in layman's terms, why they should not expect immediate results. A keyworker from the old age psychiatric team should coordinate the care and act as a point of contact for the patient and family (for a fuller account see Chapter 18).

Electroconvulsive therapy

ECT remains the most effective treatment for depressive illness at any age, with recovery rates of around 80%. It is the treatment of choice for patients exhibiting profound disability, food or fluid refusal and suicidal behaviour. It is often considered the treatment of choice in delusional depression. It is tolerated well by elderly people (Benbow, 1989). The factors which predict a good response to ECT are the same at all ages and, in general, encompass the symptomatology of severe depression. The elderly, unlike younger patients seem to respond well when anxiety dominates the clinical picture (Benbow, 1989). Memory impairment is measurably worse in older patients given ECT, which is why clinicians often prescribe unilateral electrode placement. However, this may be counterbalanced by arguments that this memory effect may be of negligible clinical relevance, and that bilateral placement may be more effective therapeutically (Benbow, 1989).

All the contraindications to ECT are relative (Box 7.5). It may be given to a patient who is desperately ill with depression, even though their physical health is also poor. A careful physical examination is the most important way to screen for problems (Abramczuk & Rose, 1979), with subsequent investigations (ECG, chest radiograph, pulmonary function testing, etc.) and referral to specialists as appropriate. ECT can be given to patients with a pacemaker provided the patient is insulated and no-one touches him or her during the passage of electricity.

Patients detained under Section 3 of the 1983 Mental Health Act can be given ECT without consent, but a doctor appointed by the Mental Health Act Commission must agree with the decision. Under such circumstances it is worth remembering that the 'standard' six treatments given to younger depressives is probably insufficient for elderly patients (Baldwin & Jolley, 1986). It is reasonable to specify a course of up to 12 treatments when giving ECT under Section 3.

Treatment-resistant depression

When faced with a patient whose depression has not shown worthwhile improvement after six weeks treatment with an adequate dose of antidepressant, the options are as follows (see review, Baldwin, 1996):

(a) Extend the trial beyond the 'traditional' six-week period, ensuring the dose is optimal, for between three and six more weeks. There is some evidence that this helps up to 50% of patients (Georgotas & McCue, 1989).

```
┌─────────────────────────────────────────────────────────────┐
│         Table 7.5 Contraindications to ECT (all relative)     │
│                                                               │
│  Myocardial infarct within three months                       │
│  Stroke within three months                                   │
│  Markedly compromised respiratory reserve                     │
│  Uncontrolled hypertension                                    │
│  Uncontrolled heart failure                                   │
│  Predisposition to dysrhythmia                                │
│  Aortic or carotid aneurysm                                   │
│  Traditional monoamine oxidase inhibitor within 10 days       │
└─────────────────────────────────────────────────────────────┘
```

(b) Change to an antidepressant of another class, a popular strategy for which there is remarkably little convincing evidence.
(c) Use an augmentation strategy such as lithium.

Lithium augmentation

Flint (1995) reviewed the literature on lithium augmentation and was unable to draw firm conclusions. There have only been four prospective studies of lithium augmentation in elderly patients. Zimmer *et al* (1988) and Flint & Rifat (1994) found response rates of around 20%, much lower than open studies of younger adults. Parker *et al* (1994) compared a group treated with a single antidepressant with a lithium augmented group, in a prospective study. The lithium augmentation group were significantly less depressed at follow-up. However, this study did not use random allocation, or blinded measures, so the results are encouraging but preliminary. There have been no double-blind, placebo-controlled trials of augmentation therapy in elderly patients, to date.

Psychological treatments

Psychotherapy

This has not been as extensively evaluated as drug treatment in the elderly. Jarvik *et al* (1982) treated elderly depressives in either a psychodynamic group, or with group cognitive–behavioural therapy. Both did better than a third placebo group. Thompson *et al* (1987) reported similar results in elderly depressives, who were randomly allocated to behavioural, cognitive or psychodynamic individual therapy (see Chapter 17).

Cognitive–behavioural therapy

Interest in this therapy has accelerated in recent years. Yost *et al* (1986) provide a comprehensive guide for those wishing to work with the elderly.

However, the major role of cognitive–behavioural therapy may be as an adjunct to pharmacotherapy, especially in the acute and continuation phases of depression (Reynolds *et al*, 1992, 1994).

Family therapy

Old age psychiatrists are well aware of the potency of the family to promote or disrupt recovery of an elderly depressed member. Attention to communication, explanation and a consistent approach to management, which excludes no relevant family member, are clearly important. Interventions with families vary in complexity. Blazer (1982) has summarised some of the important roles adopted by family members: others are beginning to modify systems theory in order to give formal family therapy to elderly depressed patients and their families (Benbow *et al*, 1990). The effectiveness of such interventions have yet to be evaluated over usual practice with a multi-disciplinary team.

Marital therapy and bereavement counselling

These are further skills which may be offered with benefit to selected depressed patients, after resolution of the more severe symptoms.

Social interventions

Social aspects of treatments should not be overlooked. For example, poor housing, poverty, high local crime rates and other indices of deprivation are important in the prognosis of depression in old age (Murphy, 1983). Also, evidence that elderly depressed people report a lack of diffuse (as opposed to intimate) contacts in the community (Henderson *et al*, 1986) suggests possible treatment strategies, such as the imaginative use of a day centre.

Prognosis

Although the recovery rate for an individual episode of depression with energetic treatment is good (around 75–80% (Flint & Rifat, 1996)), the longer-term prognosis is poorer. Murphy (1983) applied modern investigational techniques to a cohort of depressed patients and found that only 35% had good outcomes. The short follow-up period (one year) and possible under-treatment (judged by the ECT data offered) might partially explain these gloomy findings. More recent studies have been less pessimistic (Baldwin & Jolley, 1986; Burvill *et al*, 1991). In a review of 10 studies, Cole (1990) calculated that 60% of patients (with a mean follow-up time of 32 months) had either remained well, or had suffered relapses which had been successfully treated. Of the remaining 40%, between 7 and 10% remain unremittingly depressed, and around a third have been characterised as having 'depressive invalidism'; in other words, some recovery but residual symptoms, such as anxiety and hypochondriasis.

Outcome compared to younger patients

Depressive illness is prone to relapse, recurrence and chronicity irrespective of age. However, several studies have shown a better outcome in elderly depressed patients than younger ones (Murphy, 1983; Baldwin & Jolley, 1986; Meats *et al*, 1991). Other studies have found outcome to be at least as good (Hinrichsen, 1993; Hughes *et al*, 1993; Reynolds *et al*, 1994; Alexopoulos *et al*, 1996). This impressive weight of evidence is clearly contrary to the received wisdom, still evident in some textbooks.

Mortality

Another outcome is death. A number of studies point to a higher than expected death rate, in the short term, for elderly depressives (Murphy, 1983; Rabins *et al*, 1985; Burvill *et al*, 1991; Kivela *et al*, 1991). However, in the longer term the death rate for older depressives may not be significantly higher than the base population (Robinson, 1989). Whereas Ciompi (1969) reported an excess of deaths due to suicide, recent studies have not confirmed this, either in the medium term (Murphy *et al*, 1988) or the long term (Robinson, 1989). The obvious answer, that the excess is accounted for by greater physical morbidity in the depressed group, is also probably incorrect. Murphy *et al* (1988) controlled for physical illness severity but still found an excess of deaths in the depressed group compared to non-depressed controls, especially from cardiovascular causes.

Cognitive impairment

It is uncertain whether depression predisposes to dementia. Sometimes depression is a harbinger of what, with the passage of time, is clearly dementia. Several other neurodegenerative disorders may present in this way. There is evidence that depressed patients who present with pseudodementia have an increased risk of developing true dementia. For example, an often quoted study is Kral & Emery (1989), who reported that 89% of patients previously diagnosed as having pseudodementia went on to develop unequivocal dementia. Alexopoulos *et al* (1993) found the same. Abas *et al* (1990) noted that despite successful treatment of mood, the cognitive impairment that they had detected (which did not amount to dementia) persisted in around a third of those patients who had it at the outset. On the other hand, long-term naturalistic studies have not confirmed these findings. It seems that when a depressed patient presents with marked confusion, this may herald dementia, so careful follow-up is required. In general, however, depression in old age is not a risk factor for dementia.

Suicide

Elderly people are over-represented in the suicide statistics and the relationship between depression and suicide is particularly strong. Barraclough (1971) found that nearly 90% of successful suicides had clear-cut evidence of depression. Worryingly, 90% had been seen by their general practitioners within the previous three months, half within the preceding week. Furthermore, unlike parasuicide in young people, approximately two-thirds of elderly attempters have a psychiatric disorder. Manipulative overdoses are uncommon in elderly attempters.

There are three interrelated risk factors for suicide:

(a) Psychiatric disorder – most closely associated with severe depression. The clinical picture is of agitation, guilt, hopelessness, hypochondriasis and insomnia and, contrary to expectation, the illness is often a first-onset, non-psychotic depression of only moderate severity.

(b) Chronic – often painful, physical health problems.

(c) Social isolation – however, many more elderly people live alone than ever attempt suicide. It may be then that better social conditions serve to reduce a vulnerability to suicide rather than removing a cause of it (Lindesay, 1986).

Predictors of poor outcome

General factors associated with poorer outcomes (Box 7.6) are:

(a) Initial and supervening serious physical illness, presenting acutely or chronically disabling (Murphy, 1983; Baldwin & Jolley, 1986).

(b) Cerebral pathology, either coarse (Post, 1962) or subtle (Jacoby *et al*, 1981). Baldwin *et al* (1993) failed to replicate Post's findings, suggesting that modern antidepressants may be more effective in depression associated with cerebral organic disorder.

Predictors of good outcome

Adequate treatment

Late-life depression is undertreated in primary care settings (McDonald, 1986), and the more sparing use of physical treatments in specialist settings is associated with poorer prognoses (Baldwin, 1991). There is a large

---

Box 7.6 Factors associated with a poor prognosis

Presence of cerebral organic pathology
Preceding severe physical health problems
Supervening health events
Slower recovery
More severe initial depression
Duration of symptoms of more than two years
Two or more previous episodes in the last two years or three
in five years

---

variation in the use of antidepressant drugs, lithium and ECT in naturalistic studies (Baldwin, 1991).

Planned after-care

Relapse is most likely in the first 18 months to two years after an initial episode (Godber *et al*, 1987; Flint, 1992). Since relapses are often undetected without planned after-care (Sadavoy & Reiman-Sheldon, 1983) it makes sense to have a clear plan of follow-up for at least 18 months. After-care can be by a member of a multi-disciplinary old age psychiatric team or the primary care team.

Prophylaxis

The Old Age Depression Interest Group (1993) found that of 219 patients with major depression, 69 recovered sufficiently to enter a two-year, double-blind, placebo-controlled trial of dothiepin. Dothiepin (75 mg daily) reduced their relative risk of relapse by a factor of two and a half.

Prevention

There is a case for indefinite prophylactic treatment of any new episode of major depression in an older patient. An elderly person in his or her 70s may have an expected life span of five years. Preventing six months morbidity due to the recurrence of a depressive illness is an important gain. However, blanket prophylaxis risks over-treatment. Furthermore there are difficulties with the long-term use of tricyclics, notably weight gain and dental decay. Clearly studies are needed which look at the efficacy of selective serotonin reuptake inhibitors, and other new antidepressants, in the prevention of relapse and recurrence of depression in older patients. Lithium carbonate should be considered for those who have had either two episodes of depression in the last two years, or three in the past five years (Abou-Saleh & Coppen, 1983). To date there are no controlled evaluations of maintenance ECT in the prevention of relapse.

Drugs are not the only form of prophylaxis. Ong *et al* (1987) demonstrated that a simple weekly support group for recovered depressives significantly reduced both relapses and readmissions. The emphasis in prevention is increasingly on the combined use of antidepressant drugs and psychological interventions such as inter-personal psychotherapy. The early evidence is that this approach is as effective in older patients as younger ones (Reynolds *et al*, 1994).

Conclusion

Advances have been made in the aetiology and management of depression in the elderly. In spite of this, most depression remains undetected and untreated. Health professionals tend to see the older people who are most susceptible to depression, including the physically unwell or those living in residential accommodation. In these circumstances it may become tempting to consider depression as an inevitable part of ageing, and that little can be done. This is not the case.

References

Abas, M. A., Sahakian, B. J. & Levy, R. (1990) Neuropsychological deficits and CT scan changes in elderly depressives. *Psychological Medicine*, 20, 507–520.

Abou-Saleh, M. T. & Coppen, A. (1983) The prognosis of depression in old age: the case for lithium therapy. *British Journal of Psychiatry*, 143, 527–528.

Abramczuk, J. A. & Rose, N. M. (1979) Pre-anaesthetic assessment and the prevention of post-ECT morbidity. *British Journal of Psychiatry*, 134, 582–587.

Abrams, R. C., Alexopoulos, G. S. & Young, R. C. (1987) Geriatric depression and DSM–III–R personality disorder criteria. *Journal of American Geriatric Society*, 35, 383–386.

Alexopoulos, G. S., Meyers, B. S., Young, R. C., *et al* (1993) The course of geriatric depression with 'reversible dementia': a controlled study. *American Journal of Psychiatry*, 150, 1693–1699.

Alexopoulos, G. S., Meyers, B. S., Young, R. C., *et al* (1996) Recovery in geriatric depression. *Archives of General Psychiatry*, 53, 305–312.

American Psychiatric Association (1994) *Diagnostic and Statistical Manual of Mental Disorders* (4th edn) (DSM–IV). Washington, DC: APA.

Baldwin, B. (1991) The outcome of depression in old age. *International Journal of Geriatric Psychiatry*, 6, 395–400.

Baldwin, R. C. (1988) Delusional and non-delusional depression in late life: evidence for distinct subtypes. *British Journal of Psychiatry*, 152, 39–44.

—— (1993) Late life depression and structural brain changes: a review of recent magnetic resonance imaging research. *International Journal of Geriatric Psychiatry*, 8, 115–123.

—— (1996) Refractory depression in late life: a review of treatment options. *Reviews in Clinical Gerontology,* 6, 343–348.

—— & Jolley, D. J. (1986) The prognosis of depression in old age. *British Journal of Psychiatry,* 149, 574–583.

——, Benbow, S. M., Marriott, A., *et al* (1993) The prognosis of depression in later-life: a reconsideration of cerebral organic factors in relation to outcome. *British Journal of Psychiatry,* 163, 82–90.

Barraclough, B. M. (1971) Suicide in the elderly. In *Recent Developments in Psychogeriatrics* (eds D. W. K. Kay & A. Walk), pp. 87–97. Ashford: Headley Bros.

Benbow, S. B. (1989) The role of electroconvulsive therapy in the treatment of depressive illness in old age. *British Journal of Psychiatry,* 155, 147–152.

——, Egan, D., Marriott, A., *et al* (1990) Using the family life cycle with later life families. *Journal of Family Therapy,* 12, 321–340.

Bergmann, K. (1978) Neurosis and personality disorder in old age. In *Studies in Geriatric Psychiatry* (eds A. D. Isaacs & F. Post), pp. 41–75. Chichester: John Wiley and Sons.

Bench, C. J., Friston, K. J., Brown, R. G., *et al* (1992) The anatomy of depression – focal abnormalities of cerebral blood flow in major depression. *Psychological Medicine,* 22, 607–615.

Blazer, D. G. (1982) *Depression in Later Life,* pp. 221–235. St Louis, CV: Mosby.

——, George, L. & Landerman, R. (1986) The phenomenology of late life depression. In *Psychiatric Disorders in the Elderly* (eds P. E. Bebbington & R. Jacoby), pp. 143–152. London: Mental Health Foundation.

Brown, G. W. & Harris, T. O. (1978) *The Social Origins of Depression.* London: Tavistock.

Burvill, P. W., Hall, W. D., Stampfer, H. G., *et al* (1991) The prognosis of depression in old age. *British Journal of Psychiatry,* 158, 64–71.

Carroll, B. J., Feinberg, M., Greden, J. F., *et al* (1981) A specific laboratory test for the diagnosis of melancholia. *Archives of General Psychiatry,* 38, 15–22.

Ciompi, L. (1969) Follow-up studies on the evolution of former neurotic and depressive states in old age. *Journal of Geriatric Psychiatry,* 3, 90–106.

Cole, M. G. (1990) The prognosis of depression in the elderly. *Canadian Medical Association Journal,* 143, 633–639.

Flint, A. J. (1992) The optimum duration of antidepressant treatment in the elderly. *International Journal of Geriatric Psychiatry,* 7, 617–619.

—— (1995) Augmentation strategies in geriatric depression. *International Journal of Geriatric Psychiatry,* 10, 137–146.

—— & Rifat, S. L. (1994) A prospective study of lithium augmentation in antidepressant-resistant geriatric depression. *Journal of Clinical Psychopharmacology,* 14, 353–356.

—— & —— (1996) The effect of sequential antidepressant treatment on geriatric depression. *Journal of Affective Disorders,* 36, 95–105.

Folstein, M. F., Folstein, S. E. & McHugh, P. R. (1975) Mini-Mental State: a practical method for grading the cognitive state of patients for the clinician. *Journal of Psychiatric Research,* 12, 185–198.

Georgotas, A. (1983) Affective disorders in the elderly: diagnostic and research considerations. *Age and Ageing,* 12, 1–10.

—— & McCue, R. (1989) The additional benefit of extending an antidepressant trial past seven weeks in the depressed elderly. *International Journal of Geriatric Psychiatry*, 4, 191–195.

Godber, C., Rosenvinge, H., Wilkinson, D., *et al* (1987) Depression in old age: prognosis after ECT. *International Journal of Geriatric Psychiatry*, 2, 19–24.

Gurland, B. J. (1976) The comparative frequency of depression in various adult age groups. *Journal of Gerontology*, 31, 283–292.

——, Copeland, J., Kuriansky, J., *et al* (1983) *The Mind and Mood of Aging*. New York: Haworth Press.

Henderson, A. S., Grayson, D. A., Scott, R., *et al* (1986) Social support, dementia and depression among the elderly living in the Hobart community. *Psychological Medicine*, 16, 379–390.

Hinrichsen, G. A. (1993) Recovery and relapse from major depressive disorder in the elderly. *American Journal of Psychiatry*, 149, 1574–1579.

—— & Hernandez, N. A. (1993) Factors associated with recovery from and relapse into major depressive disorder in the elderly. *American Journal of Psychiatry*, 150, 1820–1825.

Hopkinson, G. (1964) A genetic study of affective illness in patients over 50. *British Journal of Psychiatry*, 110, 244–254.

Hughes, D. C., DeMalie, D. & Blazer, D. G. (1993) Does age make a difference in the effects of physical health and social support on the outcome of the major depressive episode. *American Journal of Psychiatry*, 150, 728–733.

Jacoby, R. J. & Levy, R. (1980) Computed tomography in the elderly. 3: Affective disorder. *British Journal of Psychiatry*, 136, 270–275.

——, —— & Bird, J. M. (1981) Computed tomography and the outcome of affective disorder: a follow-up study of elderly patients. *British Journal of Psychiatry*, 139, 288–292.

Jackson, R. & Baldwin, B. (1993) Detecting depression in elderly medically ill patients: the use of the Geriatric Depression Scale compared with medical and nursing observations. *Age and Ageing*, 22, 349–353.

Jarvik, L. S., Mintz, J., Steuer, J., *et al* (1982). Treating geriatric depression: a 26 week interim analysis. *Journal of American Geriatric Society*, 30, 713–717.

Kay, D. W., Beamish, P. & Roth, M. (1964) Old age mental disorders in Newcastle-Upon-Tyne. Part I: a study of prevalence. *British Journal of Psychiatry*, 110, 146–158.

Kivela, S. -L., Pahkala, K. & Laippala, P. (1991) A one year prognosis of dysthymic disorder and major depression in old age. *International Journal of Geriatric Psychiatry*, 6, 81–87.

Kral, V. A. & Emery, O. B. (1989) Long-term follow-up of depressive pseudodementia of the aged. *Canadian Journal of Psychiatry*, 34, 445–446.

Lindesay, J. (1986) Suicide and attempted suicide in old age. In *Affective Disorders in the Elderly* (ed. E. Murphy), pp. 187–202. Edinburgh: Churchill Livingstone.

MacDonald, A. J. D. (1986) Do general practitioners 'miss' depression in elderly patients? *British Medical Journal*, 292, 1365–1367.

Meats, P., Timol, M. & Jolley, D. (1991) Prognosis of depression in the elderly. *British Journal of Psychiatry*, 159, 659–663.

Mendelwicz, J. (1976) The age factor in depressive illness: some genetic considerations. *Journal of Gerontology*, 31, 300–303.

Murphy, E. (1982) Social origins of depression in old age. *British Journal of Psychiatry*, 141, 135–142.

—— (1983) The prognosis of depression in old age. *British Journal of Psychiatry*, 142, 111–119.

——, Smith, R., Lindesay, J., *et al* (1988) Increased mortality rates in late-life depression. *British Journal of Psychiatry*, 152, 347–353.

Musetti, L., Perugi, G., Soriani, A., *et al* (1989) Depression before and after age 65: a re-examination. *British Journal of Psychiatry*, 155, 330–336.

O'Brien, J. T., Desmond, P., Ames, D., *et al* (1994) The differentiation of depression from dementia by temporal lobe magnetic resonance imaging. *Psychological Medicine*, 24, 633–640.

Old Age Depression Interest Group (1993) How long should the elderly take antidepressants? A double blind placebo-controlled study of continuation/ prophylaxis therapy with dothiepin. *British Journal of Psychiatry*, 162, 175–182.

Ong, Y. -L., Martineau, F., Lloyd, C., *et al* (1987) Support group for the depressed elderly. *International Journal of Geriatric Psychiatry*, 2, 119–123.

Oxman, T. E. , Berkman, L. F., Kasl, S., *et al* (1992) Social support and depressive symptoms in the elderly. *American Journal of Epidemiology*, 135, 356–368.

Parker, K. L., Mittmann, N., Shear, N. H., *et al* (1994) Lithium augmentation in geriatric depressed outpatients: a clinical report. *International Journal of Geriatric Psychiatry*, 9, 995–1002.

Pearlson, G. D., Rabins, P. V., Kim, W. S., *et al* (1989) Structural brain CT changes and cognitive deficits with and without reversible dementia ('pseudodementia'). *Psychological Medicine*, 19, 573–584.

Post, F. (1962) *The Significance of Affective Symptoms in Old Age,* Maudsley Monographs 10. London: Oxford University Press.

—— (1968) The factor of ageing in affective disorder. In *Recent Developments in Affective Disorders*, Royal Medico-Psychological Association Publication No. 2 (eds A. Coppen & A. Walk). Ashford: Headley Bros.

—— (1972) The management and nature of depressive illnesses in late life: a follow-through study. *British Journal of Psychiatry*, 121, 393–404.

—— (1982) Functional disorders. In *The Psychiatry of Late Life* (eds R. Levy & F. Post), pp. 190–191. Oxford: Blackwell Scientific Publishers.

Rabins, P. V., Harvis, K. & Koven, S. (1985) High fatality rates of late-life depression associated with cardiovascular disease. *Journal of Affective Disorders*, 9, 165–167.

Reynolds, C. F., Hoch, C. C., Kupfer, D. J., *et al* (1988*a*) Bedside differentiation of depressive pseudodementia from dementia. *American Journal of Psychiatry*, 145, 1099–1103.

——, Kupfer, D. J., Houck, P. R., *et al* (1988*b*) Reliable discrimination of elderly depressed and demented patients by electroencephalographic sleep data. *Archives of General Psychiatry*, 45, 258–264.

——. Frank, E., Perel, J. M., *et al* (1992) Combined pharmacotherapy psychotherapy in the acute and continuation treatment of elderly patients with recurrent major depression. *American Journal of Psychiatry*, 149, 1687–1692.

——, ——, ——, *et al* (1994) Treatment of consecutive episodes of major depression in the elderly. *American Journal of Psychiatry*, 151, 1740–1743.

Robinson, J. R. (1989) The natural history of mental disorder in old age – a long term study. *British Journal of Psychiatry*, 154, 783–789.

Roth, M. (1955) The natural history of mental disorder in old age. *Journal of Mental Science*, 101, 281–301.

Sackeim, H. A., Prohovnik, I., Moeller, J. R., *et al* (1990) Regional cerebral blood flow in mood disorders. 1. Comparison of major depressives and normal controls at rest. *Archives of General Psychiatry*, 47, 60–70.

Sadavoy, J. & Reimaan-Sheldon, E. (1983) General hospital geriatric psychiatric treatment: a follow-up study. *Journal of the American Geriatric Society*, 31, 200–205.

Schneider, L. S. (1992) Psychobiologic features of geriatric affective disorders. *Clinics in Geriatric Medicine*, 8, 253–265.

Spar, J. E. & Gerner, R. (1982) Does the dexamethasone suppression test distinguish dementia from depression? *American Journal of Psychiatry*, 139, 238–240.

Thompson, L., Gallagher, D. & Breckenbridge, J. (1987) Comparative effectiveness of psychotherapies for depressed elders. *Journal of Consulting and Clinical Psychology*, 55, 385–390.

Veith, R. C. & Raskind, M. A. (1988) The neurobiology of aging: does it predispose to depression? *Neurobiology of Aging*, 9, 101–117.

Weingartner, H., Cowan, R. M., Murphy, D. L., *et al* (1981) Cognitive processes in depression. *Archives of General Psychiatry*, 38, 42–47.

World Health Organization (1993) *The ICD–10 Classification of Mental and Behavioural Disorders. Diagnostic Criteria for Research*. Geneva: WHO.

Yesavage, J. A. (1988) Shortened Geriatric Depression Scale. *Psychopharmacology Bulletin*, 24, 709–710.

Yost, E. B., Beutler, L. E., Corbishley, M. A., *et al* (1986) *Group Cognitive Therapy: A Treatment Approach for Depressed Older Adults*. New York: Pergamon Press.

Zimmer, B., Rosen, J., Thornton, J. E., *et al* (1988) Adjunctive low dose lithium carbonate in treatment resistant depression: a placebo-controlled study. *Journal of Clinical Psychopharmacology*, 8, 120–124.

8 Mania

Ken Shulman

Classification ● *Epidemiology* ● *Aetiology* ● *Age of onset and clinical course* ● *Clinical presentation* ● *Management* ● *Prognosis* ● *Conclusion*

Mania occurring in later life has come under closer scrutiny in recent years. As a result, important issues related to the classification and the neurobiological basis of affective illness have become clearer.

Classification

Historical context

Kraepelin (1921) established the separateness of affective disorders from other major psychoses by developing the concept of manic–depressive illness. This was a unitary concept combining mania and depression. It was not until the 1960s that the bipolar–unipolar dichotomy was postulated (Perris, 1966). Despite preliminary evidence of support, recent thinking has shifted away from the notion that manic disorders are fundamentally different from unipolar depression. Indeed, the study of elderly bipolars reveals that many of them 'convert' from a unipolar depressive pattern after many years and multiple depressive episodes (Shulman & Post, 1980; Snowdon, 1991).

Spectrum of affective disorders

Akiskal *et al* (1983), noted that young people with depression, followed prospectively for 3–6 years, developed mania in about 20% of cases. Moreover, it is difficult clinically to determine when a picture of mild pressure of speech or disinhibition, following treatment of major depression, represents a 'true' hypomania. Therefore, the idea of a spectrum of affective disorders was developed in which a hierarchy of different patterns of illness is described (Akiskal, 1983). These range from milder expressions, such as cyclothymia and dysthymia, to unipolar major depression, bipolar II (with mild hypomania) and bipolar I (full-blown manic episodes). Tsuang *et al* (1985) suggest a "threshold hypothesis" in which mania is a more severe form of affective disorder, requiring lower levels of stress to precipitate a decompensation.

125

Mixed affective states

To emphasise the blurring of manic and depressive phases, Clothier *et al* (1992) described the condition of 'dysphoric mania', a mixed affective state. Kraepelin (1921) has already provided a classification of six sub-types of 'mixed' affective states. These are: depressive/anxious mania, excited depression, mania with poverty of thought, manic stupor, depression with flight of ideas and inhibited mania. Careful and systematic clinical observations in young and old patients force us to reconsider our fundamental view of mania and its relationship to depression.

ICD–10

ICD–10 (World Health Organization, 1992) considers mood disorders as a spectrum, with mania and severe depression at opposite ends. Mood disorders are divided into: manic episode, bipolar affective disorder, depressive episode, recurrent depressive disorder and persistent mood disorders. Bipolar affective disorder is characterised by repeated episodes of mood disturbance, at least one of which is mania or hypomania, and one of which is depression. Manic episodes are divided into hypomania, mania without psychotic symptoms, and mania with psychotic symptoms (Box 8.1).

Epidemiology

Data regarding the incidence and prevalence of mania in old age show opposite trends. The incidence, as measured by first admission rates to

---

Box 8.1 Summary of the ICD–10 criteria for a manic episode (World Health Organization, 1992)

Without psychotic symptoms:
Elevated mood or irritability
Increased energy and overactivity
Pressure of speech
Decreased sleep
Social disinhibition
Poor attention and marked distractibility
Grandiose or over-optimistic ideas
Extravagant schemes and over spending
Aggressive or amorous episodes

With psychotic symptoms; as above and:
Severe and sustained excitement
Flight of ideas
Mood congruent delusions or hallucinations

hospital, increases with age even in the extremes of old age (Eagles & Whalley, 1985). However, the community prevalence decreases with age (Weissman *et al*, 1988). One-year prevalence rates are 0.1% in over 65s (Box 8.2) and 1.4% in the 18- to 44-year-old age group. This prompts the question 'where have all the young bipolars gone?'. This is addressed later in this chapter.

The prevalence of mania on psychogeriatric in-patient units has been reviewed by Yassa *et al* (1988) and Shulman *et al* (1992). Over the course of a year, an average unit can expect to treat eight patients suffering from mania severe enough to require hospitalisation. This represents 12% of all affective disorders treated on specialised geriatric psychiatry units. The gender ratio of elderly manic patients shows a female preponderance, with a ratio of about two to one.

Aetiology

Genetics

Affective disorders are known to have a marked genetic predisposition (Goodwin & Jamison, 1984). Bipolar disorders have usually been considered to have a stronger genetic component than depression (Gershon *et al*, 1975). However, Tsuang *et al* (1985) could find no difference in risk for affective disorder between the relatives of younger bipolar and unipolar probands. This led to the conclusion that both phenotypes share a common aetiological pool including environmental, psychological, biological and genetic factors.

Studies of first degree relatives of elderly manic probands have found a quarter to a half are affected (Glasser & Rabins, 1984; Stone, 1989; Broadhead & Jacoby, 1990; Snowdon, 1991; Shulman *et al*, 1992). The relatively high yield of positive family history may reflect the longer periods of exposure in the parents, siblings and children of elderly probands who present with mania. Earlier age of onset is associated with a positive family history (Stone, 1989), while the presence of coarse neurological disorders has a lower genetic predisposition (Snowdon, 1991; Shulman *et al*, 1992). In the Shulman *et al* (1992) study, the elderly people with mania with neurological disorders had a significantly lower family history than those without. None the less, the prevalence of affective illness in first degree relatives was still 32%.

Box 8.2 Epidemiology of mania in older patients

Average age at onset 55 years
Female to male ratio 2:1
One year community prevalence 0.1%
Proportion of in-patient affective patients 12%

Brain disease

All studies that have systematically assessed the prevalence of cerebral-organic disorders in elderly people with mania have found a significant association between brain disease and mania (Table 8.1). Depending on the rigorousness of the search (i.e. whether by case notes, neurological examination, imaging or cognitive testing), the prevalence of organic brain disorders in patients with mania ranges from 20–40%. In the two studies where a consistent methodology was applied, the proportion of neurological disorders was closer to 40% (Broadhead & Jacoby, 1990; Shulman *et al*, 1992). Broadhead & Jacoby (1990) used computerised tomography scans, a Kendrick battery and a clinical assessment. They found a significant increase in cortical atrophy and an increase in cognitive impairment on the Kendrick. However, clinical assessment did not confirm the presence of dementia, a finding similar to other studies (Shulman & Post, 1980; Shulman *et al*, 1992). Consistent with the concept of secondary mania as defined by Krauthammer & Klerman (1978), 20% of the elderly people with mania had their first manic attack in close temporal proximity to a cerebral disorder, while this was not evident in any of the young people with mania.

There appears to be a trend for the secondary mania subgroup to have mania as the first affective episode (Broadhead & Jacoby, 1990; Shulman *et al*, 1992). As noted earlier, there is also a trend for the secondary manias to have a lower genetic predisposition. However, many of these patients do have a positive family history for affective disorder.

The brain diseases are heterogeneous in nature, without any consistent localising pattern according to the available data. Cerebrovascular disorders, chronic alcoholism and head injury appear most common (Shulman *et al*, 1992). Secondary mania has been systematically reviewed by Strakowski *et al* (1994), who concluded that lesions tend to involve right-sided brain structures. Similarly, Robinson *et al* (1988) found an association between right-sided stroke and mania. Silent cerebral infarctions have been noted more often in late-onset mania than matched elderly depressives (Fujikawa *et al*, 1995). Similarly, Kobayashi *et al* (1991)

Table 8.1 Aetiology

	Associations
Genetic	Earlier age of onset
	Absence of neurological damage
Brain disease	Cerebrovascular disease
	Chronic alcohol misuse
	Head injury
	Right-sided lesions

showed an increased incidence of silent cerebral infarctions with age among patients with mania.

Anecdotal case reports of cerebrovascular disease associated with mania have accumulated in recent years (Shulman, 1993). Neuroimaging studies have confirmed an increase in subcortical hyperintensities, presumably reflecting cerebrovascular pathology in old age (McDonald *et al*, 1991). Alzheimer's disease does not seem to be associated with mania in late-life. No more than the expected proportion in the population seem to progress to a full-blown dementia following a manic episode.

Summary of aetiology

Evidence suggests that there is a significant neurological substrate for mania in old age. In some elderly patients that vulnerability is manifested by earlier depressions that 'switch' to mania after a prolonged latency. In a second subgroup, coarse neurological disorders play a prominent role in producing a syndrome of 'secondary mania', and genetic factors are less important. None the less, it is uncertain why this relatively small group of patients present a different clinical picture to the vast majority of elderly patients who suffer neurological insults. New neuroimaging techniques such as the positron emission tomography, single photon emission tomography and magnetic resonance imaging scanners (see Chapter 12) may offer further insights into the nature of the cerebral changes associated with mania.

Age of onset and clinical course

On average, elderly people with mania have an onset of affective disorder in their late 40s. The onset of mania is later, at a mean age of about 55 years. However, the incidence figures reveal manic cases occurring for the first time, well into their 80s. For about half of elderly people with mania their first affective episode is depression (Shulman & Post, 1980; Broadhead & Jacoby, 1990; Snowdon, 1991). In this subgroup, an average of 16 years elapsed before mania became manifest, often preceded by repeated episodes of depression. This group tends not to suffer from coarse neurological disorders, which suggests that an 'ageing factor' may 'convert' affectively predisposed individuals to a manic presentation.

General adult studies of hospitalised patients with mania find an age of onset of about 30 years (Goodwin & Jamison, 1984; Tohen *et al*, 1990). The Epidemiologic Catchment Area (ECA) study using a community sample showed a very early onset, at a mean of 21 years (Weissman *et al*, 1988). In marked contrast, very few elderly people with mania have become manic before the age of 40 years (Shulman & Post, 1980; Snowdon, 1991). Available evidence points to two possible explanations.

The first is that the disorder beginning early in life eventually burns out after an initial clustering of affective episodes (Winokur, 1975).

The second explanation, supported by Snowdon (1991), suggests that premature death may be partly responsible. Goodwin & Jamison (1984) found a mortality among bipolars more than twice that of the general population, and half of these patients died before the age of 70. Long-term follow-up of bipolars shows higher suicide rates (Tsuang, 1978) and excess mortality (Weeke & Vaeth, 1986). Because prospective follow-up studies of 40–50 years are impractical, the best approach may be to prospectively study a large cohort of early-onset, middle-aged people with mania.

Clinical presentation

Earlier anecdotal observations suggested that mixed affective disorders were more common in elderly people with mania, as described in Kraepelin's "mixed states", such as dysphoric mania (Shulman & Post, 1980). Systematic analyses of the clinical features of elderly patients with mania, however, show no significant differences from younger bipolars (Broadhead & Jacoby, 1990), except that young people with mania have a more severe form of the disorder, as measured by a standardised rating scale. Therefore, one should expect the usual range of symptoms as described by Glasser & Rabins (1984) including: decreased sleep, physical hyperactivity, flight of ideas, thought disorder, overspending, grandiose delusions, irritability and hypersexuality (Box 8.1).

Management

Unfortunately, little systematic data are available regarding the treatment of mania in old age. Clinical reports suggest that lithium retains an important role but is associated with an increased incidence of neurotoxicity (Himmelhoch *et al*, 1980; Stone, 1989) (Table 8.2). Altered renal excretion and distribution, result in a prolonged half-life (Hardy *et al*, 1987) and require much lower doses, in the range of 150–600 mg per day. A mean dose of 300–450 mg per day should achieve blood levels of about 0.5 mmol/l (Shulman *et al*, 1987). More work is needed to confirm these reports and establish the range of dosage and blood levels necessary for effective and safe treatment in old age.

The anticonvulsants carbamazepine and valproate are now widely used in the management of mania (McElroy *et al*, 1992) but little is known of their use in old age. McFarland *et al* (1990) provide an anecdotal series of cases, suggesting that valproate is a useful adjunct to lithium in the management of refractory, elderly patients with mania. Kando *et al* (1996) found valproate to be well tolerated and efficacious in a retrospective

Table 8.2 Drug treatment of mania

	Treatment
Lithium	Plasma levels approximately 0.5 mmol/l
	Be aware of risk of toxicity
Carbamazepine	Risk of neurotoxicity
Valproate	Possible adjunct to lithium
	Risk of neurotoxicity

chart review of elderly patients suffering from an affective disorder. Concerns regarding neurotoxicity, however, suggest a cautious approach to the addition of these medications.

Prognosis

Studies have examined the outcome of mania in old age. Shulman *et al* (1992) used a retrospective cohort method to determine survival in elderly people with mania and an age- and gender-matched group of elderly people with depression. After an average follow-up period of six years (range 3–10 years), 50% of the patients with mania had died compared with only 20% of the unipolar patients with depression. This suggests that mania may have a poorer prognosis and represent a more severe disruption of central nervous system function. Interestingly, only one patient in the cohort of 100 was known to have committed suicide.

Dhingra & Rabins (1991) followed up elderly people with mania for 5–7 years (Table 8.3) and found that 34% had died. At follow-up, 32% of the patients with mania had experienced significant cognitive decline, as measured by a score of less than 24 on the Mini-Mental State Examination. However of those alive, 72% were symptom free and 80% were living independently. They concluded that the prognosis for mania in old age has improved considerably compared to that of the previous generation, reported by Roth (1955).

Table 8.3 Outcome after 5–7 year follow-up (adapted from Dhingra & Rabins, 1991)

	(*n*=38)
Symptom free	72%[1]
Living independently	80%[1]
Cognitive decline	32%[1]
Died	34%

1. Per cent of those surviving

Conclusion

Late-onset mania appears to be fundamentally different from early-onset mania in terms of clinical course, outcome and its association with coarse cerebral disorders. However, the clinical presentation is similar. The high mortality of patients with mania is of concern, and may mean that mania results from a more severe disruption of central nervous system. However, newer technologies and treatments offer hope for improved understanding and management of this important syndrome.

References

Akiskal, H. (1983) Diagnosis and classification of affective disorders: new insights from clinical and laboratory approaches. *Psychiatric Developments*, 2, 123–160.
——, Walker, P., Puzantian, V. R., *et al* (1983) Bipolar outcome in the course of depressive illness. *Journal of Affective Disorders*, 5, 115–128.
Broadhead, J. & Jacoby, R. (1990) Mania in old age: A first prospective study. *International Journal of Geriatric Psychiatry*, 5, 215–222.
Clothier, J., Swann, A. C. & Freeman, T. (1992) Dysphoric mania. *Journal of Clinical Psychopharmacology*, 12 (suppl.), 13S–16S.
Dhingra, U. & Rabins, P. V. (1991) Mania in the elderly: A 5–7 year follow-up. *Journal of the American Geriatrics Society*, 39, 581–583.
Eagles, J. M. & Whalley, L. J. (1985) Ageing and affective disorders: The age at first onset of affective disorders in Scotland, 1969–1978. *British Journal of Psychiatry*, 147, 180–187.
Fujikawa, T., Yamawaki, S. & Touhouda, Y. (1995) Incidence of silent cerebral infarction in patients with major depression. *Stroke*, 24, 1631–1634.
Gershon, E. S., Baron, M. & Leckman, J. F. (1975) Genetic models of the transmission of affective disorders. *Journal of Psychiatric Research*, 12, 301–317.
Glasser, M. & Rabins, P. (1984) Mania in the elderly. *Age and Ageing*, 13, 210–213.
Goodwin, F. K. & Jamison, K. R. (1984) The natural course of manic-depressive illness. In *Neurobiology of Mood Disorders* (eds R. M. Post & J. C. Ballenger). Edinburgh: Williams and Wilkins.
Hardy, B., Shulman, K., MacKenzie, S., *et al* (1987) Pharmacokinetics of lithium in the elderly. *Journal of Clinical Psychopharmacology*, 7, 153–158.
Himmelhoch, J. M., Neil, M. F., May, S. J., *et al* (1980) Age, dementia, dyskinesias and lithium response. *American Journal of Psychiatry*, 137, 941–945.
Kando, J. C., Tohen, M., Castillo, J., *et al* (1996) The use of valproate in an elderly population with affective symptoms. *Journal of Clinical Psychiatry*, 57, 238–240.
Kobayashi, S., Okada, K. & Yamashita, K. (1991) Incidence of silent lacunar lesions in normal adults and its relation to cerebral blood flow and risk factors. *Stroke*, 22, 1379–1383.
Kraepelin, E. (1921) *Manic Depressive, Insanity and Paranoia*. Edinburgh: Livingston. (Reprinted 1976, New York: Ages Company Publishers.)
Krauthammer, C. & Klerman, G. L. (1978) Secondary mania. Manic syndromes associated with antecedent physical illness or drugs. *Archives of General Psychiatry*, 35, 1333–1339.

McDonald, W. M., Krishnan, K. R. R., Doraiswamy, P. M., *et al* (1991) Occurrence of subcortical hyperintensities in elderly subjects with mania. *Psychiatry Research: Neuroimaging*, 40, 211–220.

McElroy, S., Keck, P., Pope, H., *et al* (1992) Valproate in the treatment of bipolar disorder: literature review and clinical guidelines. *Journal of Clinical Psychopharmacology*, 12 (suppl. 1), 42S–52S.

McFarland, B. H., Miller, M. R. & Straumfjord, A. A. (1990) Valproate use in the older manic patient. *Journal of Clinical Psychiatry*, 51, 479–481.

Perris, C. (1966) A study of bipolar (manic-depressive) and unipolar recurrent psychoses (I-X). *Acta Psychiatrica Scandinavica Supplementum*, 194, 1–189.

Robinson, R. G., Starstein, S. E. & Price, T. R. (1988) Post-stroke depression and lesion location. *Stroke*, 19, 125.

Roth, M. (1955) The natural history of mental disorder in old age. *Journal of Mental Science*, 101, 281–301.

Shulman, K. (1993) Mania in the elderly. *International Review of Psychiatry*, 5, 445–453.

—— & Post, F. (1980) Bipolar affective disorder in old age. *British Journal of Psychiatry*, 136, 26–32.

——, MacKenzie, S. & Hardy, B. (1987) The clinical use of lithium carbonate in old age: A review. *Progress in Neuro-Psychopharmacology*, 11, 159–164.

——, Tohen, M., Satlin, A., *et al* (1992) Mania compared with unipolar depression in old age. *American Journal of Psychiatry*, 149, 341–345.

Snowdon, J. (1991) A retrospective case-note study of bipolar disorder in old age. *British Journal of Psychiatry*, 158, 485–490.

Stone, K. (1989) Mania in the elderly. *British Journal of Psychiatry*, 155, 220–224.

Strakowski, S., McElroy, S. L., Keck, P. W., *et al* (1994) The co-occurrence of mania with medical and other psychiatric disorders. *International Journal of Psychiatry in Medicine*, 24, 305–328.

Tohen, M., Waternaux, C. M. & Tsuang, M. T. (1990) Outcome in mania: A four year prospective follow-up study utilizing survival analysis. *Archives of General Psychiatry*, 47, 1106–1111.

Tsuang, M. T. (1978) Suicide in schizophrenics, manics, depressives and surgical controls. *Archives of General Psychiatry*, 35, 153–155.

——, Farrone, S. V. & Fleming, J. A. (1985) Familial transmission of major affective disorders: is there evidence supporting the distinction between unipolar and bipolar disorders? *British Journal of Psychiatry*, 146, 268–271.

Weeke, A. & Vaeth, M. (1986) Excess mortality of bipolar and unipolar manic-depressive patients. *Journal of Affective Disorders*, 11, 227–234.

Weissman, M. M., Leaf, P. J., Tichler, G. L., *et al* (1988) Affective disorders in five United States communities. *Psychological Medicine*, 18, 141–153.

Winokur, G. (1975) The Iowa 500: heterogeneity and course in manic depressive illness (bipolar). *Comprehensive Psychiatry*, 16, 125–131.

Yassa, R., Nair, V., Nastase, C., *et al* (1988) Prevalence of bipolar disorder in a psychogeriatric population. *Journal of Affective Disorders*, 14, 197–201.

World Health Organization (1992) *The Tenth Revision of the International Classification of Diseases and Related Health Problems* (ICD–10). Geneva: WHO.

9 Anxiety disorders and other neuroses

James Lindesay

Classification ● *Epidemiology* ● *Aetiology* ● *Specific neurotic disorders* ●
Management ● *Conclusion*

Neurotic disorders are relatively neglected in the elderly. However, there is accumulating evidence that these conditions are clinically important in terms of their prevalence, the distress they cause, the cost to services and the potential for treatment and prevention (Lindesay, 1995). At all ages, neurotic disorders complicate and aggravate other psychiatric and physical disorders, and doctors should be able to recognise and manage these conditions.

Classification

The concept of 'neurosis' is going through troubled times. It was originally coined in the 18th century to describe a category of disorders of the peripheral nervous system (Knoff, 1970). As the central and psychological origin of many of these conditions came to be recognised, the meaning of the term was revised and reviewed. In the 20th century, it has usually been applied to emotional and behavioural disorders arising from the impact of stress factors on particularities of character. In recent years, this concept has been challenged by the growth of biological psychiatry. Researchers have dissected out specific conditions from the body of neurosis, on the basis of particular physiological characteristics, responses to drugs, genetic heritability and even neuropathology. In the US, the triumph of biology is complete, and words such as 'neurosis' and 'neurotic' no longer form any part of DSM–IV nosology (American Psychiatric Association, 1994). ICD–10 (World Health Organization, 1992) has also rejected the traditional division between neuroses and psychoses. Instead, it has placed many of the conditions previously associated with the neuroses in the group 'neurotic, stress-related and somatoform disorders' (Box 9.1).

The unifying concept of neurosis is not, however, obsolete. Advances in medical understanding come from lumping, as well as splitting clinical phenomena. The biological evidence for discrete disorders needs to be interpreted in the light of clinical and epidemiological evidence that within

---

Box 9.1 Summary of ICD–10 classification of neurotic, stress-related and somatoform disorders (World Health Organization, 1992)

Agoraphobia
Social phobias
Specific (isolated) phobias
Panic disorder
Generalised anxiety disorder
Obsessive–compulsive disorder
Post-traumatic stress disorder
Adjustment disorders
Dissociative disorders
Somatisation disorders

---

individuals, and over time, there is considerable comorbidity and interchangability between these disorders. Tyrer (1985) has argued that labelling episodes of illness purely in terms of current symptomatology is misleading, and that such cases are better understood, both clinically and nosologically, as a general neurotic syndrome with a prolonged course and varying presentations over time. This is most apparent in community and primary care populations, where dimensions of depression and anxiety underlie the manifest psychological symptoms in both younger and older adults (Goldberg *et al*, 1987; Mackinnon *et al*, 1994). The unitary model of neurotic disorders is also supported by evidence from genetic studies which suggest that it is not specific disorders that are inherited, so much as a general predisposing trait of neuroticism (Kendler *et al*, 1987; Andrews *et al*, 1990). In the elderly, where chronicity and multiple pathology are the norm, the concept of a general neurotic syndrome is useful in making sense of changing clinical pictures, in understanding the causes and outcome of neurotic presentations and in guiding their treatment.

Epidemiology

The prevalence rates of neurotic disorders in the elderly depend on the population studied. They are uncommon primary diagnoses in hospital populations, and while there is a steady accumulation of chronic cases in primary care settings, there is a decline, with age, in the rate of new consultations. As with younger adults, the highest rates of neurotic disorders, particularly anxiety, are found in the community. To some extent the discrepancy between clinical and community populations is due to a proportion of the community cases being mild and non-problematic.

However, there are clinically significant cases of neurotic disorder that either do not present to the health services or are not identified or treated (Macdonald, 1986; Thompson *et al*, 1988; Lindesay, 1991).

Table 9.1 summarises prevalence rates for specific DSM–III disorders in community samples of the over 65-year-olds, reported by the US Epidemiologic Catchment Area (ECA) study. Studies have tended to report different rates, due mainly to differences in the operation of hierarchical rules for diagnosis and in the level of severity required for caseness. In most neurotic disorders there is a fall in prevalence with age, in both genders, but the differences are not large compared with clinical populations. At all ages, prevalence rates for neurotic disorders are higher in women than in men, but this difference is least pronounced in the elderly. Community studies of neurotic disorders in the elderly confirm that the majority of cases are long-standing, with onset in young adulthood and middle age. However, a significant minority has an onset after the age of 65 years (Bergmann, 1972; Lindesay, 1991).

Aetiology

Physical illness

Epidemiological studies of community populations provide the least biased information about factors associated with neurotic disorder in the elderly (Box 9.3). As noted above, there is at all ages extensive comorbidity between specific neurotic disorders and depression (Boyd *et al*, 1984; Weissman & Merikangas, 1986). In the community elderly, neurotic disorders are also associated with increased mortality and physical

Table 9.1 Epidemiologic Catchment Area study: prevalence of neurotic disorders in the elderly (%)

	Male	Female	Total
One-year prevalence (Robins & Regier, 1991)			
Phobic disorder	4.9	7.8	–
Panic disorder	0.04	0.08	–
Generalised anxiety	–	–	2.2
Obsessive–compulsive disorder	0.8	0.9	1.7
One-month prevalence (Regier et al, 1988)			
Phobic disorder	2.9	6.1	4.8
Panic disorder	0.0	0.2	0.1
Obsessive–compulsive disorder	0.7	0.9	0.8
Somatisation disorder	0.0	0.2	0.1
Dysthymia	1.0	2.3	1.8

morbidity, notably cardiovascular, respiratory and gastrointestinal complaints (Kay & Bergmann, 1966; Bergmann, 1972; Lindesay, 1990). The relationship between physical and psychiatric disorders in the elderly is even more marked in clinical populations, and emphasises the importance of careful history taking and physical examination, particularly in late-onset cases.

To some extent, this association between neurotic and physical disorder may be due to increased bodily concern leading to presentation with physical, rather than psychological complaints; or to somatic anxiety symptoms being wrongly attributed, by patient and doctor, to physical illness. However, many important physical disorders may present with neurotic symptoms, particularly anxiety, and should be suspected if: the patient is male; there is no history of neurotic disorder; nothing in the patient's circumstances accounts for the episode. Box 9.2 sets out some of the physical conditions that may present as neurotic disorder in this age group. For most elderly people an episode of physical illness, with its associated investigations and treatments, is a threatening and frightening experience. In vulnerable individuals this may result in persistent neurotic disturbance, such as phobic withdrawal and generalised anxiety, as well as more transient adjustment reactions.

Psychosocial factors

Psychosocial factors are important in the aetiology of neurotic disorders in the elderly, particularly at the symptom level, where high scores are associated

---

Box 9.2 Physical causes of neurotic symptoms in the elderly (adapted from Pitt, 1995)

Cardiovascular: myocardial infarction, cardiac arrhythmias, orthostatic hypotension, mitral valve prolapse

Respiratory: pneumonia, pulmonary embolism, emphysema, asthma, left-ventricular failure, hypoxia, chronic obstructive airways disease, bronchial carcinoma

Endocrine and metabolic: hypo- and hyperthyroidism, hypo- and hypercalcaemia, Cushing's disease, carcinoid syndrome, hypoglycaemia, insulinoma, phaeochromocytoma, hyperkalaemia, hypokalaemia, hypothermia

Neurological: head injury, cerebral tumour, dementia, delirium, epilepsy, migraine, cerebral lupus erythematosus, demyelinating disease, vestibular disturbance, subarachnoid haemorrhage, central nervous system infections

Dietary and drug related: caffeine, vitamin deficiencies, anaemia, sympathomimetics, dopamine agonists, corticosteroids, withdrawal syndromes, akathisia, digoxin toxicity, fluoxetine

with low socio-economic status (Himmelfarb & Murrell, 1984; Kennedy *et al*, 1989). Studies of established cases of neurotic disorders have not found a substantive relationship with socio-economic indicators, such as occupational class or household tenure (Lindesay, 1991). However, generalised anxiety was associated with low household income in the ECA study.

Adverse life events can provoke the onset of some psychiatric disorders in vulnerable individuals; it is the meaning of the event for the individual that is important, rather than the severity. Loss events generally lead to depression, while threatening events may lead to anxiety (Brown *et al*, 1987; Brown, 1993). Age-related experiences such as retirement, bereavement and institutionalisation may cause acute psychological disturbance, but they do not appear to be a major cause of persistent disorders in the elderly.

In common with younger adults, early experience, such as parental loss, may be important in determining personal vulnerability to neurotic disorder (Zahner & Murphy, 1989; Lindesay, 1991). Perhaps, early experiences such as these lead to the development of particular cognitive habits and personality traits, which render the individual vulnerable to developing neurotic disorders in response to challenging experiences later in life (see Chapter 11). According to Andrews *et al* (1990) it is the lack of mastery over self and environment, and an inability to make use of effective coping strategies, that results in neurotic symptomatology. Unlike late-life depression, phobic disorders in the elderly are not associated with absence of confiding relationships (Lindesay, 1991); indeed, in some cases, the presence of close relationships may maintain phobic avoidance.

Biological factors

There has been very little research into possible biological factors involved in the development of neurotic disorders in old age (Philpot, 1995). Computerised tomography studies of elderly depressed patients have found that the milder, more 'neurotic' cases, and those with higher anxiety scores, tend to have normal scans. Studies of patients with post-stroke anxiety disorders suggest that the distribution of lesions is different from that seen in post-stroke depression, but there is no consistent location. Functional neuroimaging with younger patients with anxiety disorders is beginning to identify changes in regional cerebral blood flow associated with the provocation of symptoms, and with treatment.

There is no association between neurotic disorders and dementia in surveys of community populations, but clinical studies have found significant levels of anxiety in patients with dementia, particularly those in the early stages (Wands *et al*, 1990; Ballard *et al*, 1996). This anxiety may be associated with depression, psychotic symptoms or with the implications of the dementia and its impact on social functioning.

Box 9.3 Factors associated with neuroses in the elderly

Physical illness notably cardiovascular, respiratory and
    gastrointestinal complaints
Low income
Adverse life events
Early adverse experiences such as parental loss
Other psychiatric illness, including dementia

Specific neurotic disorders

Phobic disorder

The irrational fears reported by elderly people are similar to those in younger age groups: animals, heights, public transport, going out of doors, and so on (Lindesay, 1991). Unfortunately, much is made of the 'reasonableness' of some of these fears in the elderly, particularly those who live in run-down areas of inner cities, and clinically important fears may be dismissed as rational. In fact, the evidence from fear of crime surveys indicates that an individual's perception of vulnerability is determined principally by factors such as physical disability and the availability of social support (Fattah & Sacco, 1989). It is these, rather than age, that should be taken into consideration when judging the reasonableness, or otherwise, of fears.

Long-standing disorder

These are usually specific in nature, and associated with little in the way of distress or social impairment. These individuals have organised their lives so that they do not need to confront their fears, and it is only occasionally that the onset of old age makes such a confrontation unavoidable; for example, a needle phobic may have to contend with the onset of insulin-dependent diabetes or an agoraphobic may need to shop after the death of their spouse.

Late-onset disorder

These are often agoraphobic in nature and associated with clinically significant levels of distress and disability. They usually develop following a traumatic event such as an episode of physical illness, a fall or a mugging. The resulting impairment usually persists long after the physical consequences of the event have resolved. Unfortunately, the psychological effects of traumatic physical health events in old age are still poorly appreciated, with the result that the statutory services and the family may unwittingly collude with phobic avoidance by providing well-meaning but misguided domiciliary support. Very few elderly people with disabling phobic disorders receive any appropriate treatment for their problem (Lindesay, 1991).

Panic disorder

Panic attacks and panic disorder are rare in epidemiological studies of elderly community populations (Table 9.1), although cross-sectional surveys may underestimate the true rates. The evidence from case reports, and non-psychiatric patient and volunteer samples, suggests that panic in old age is less common than in early adulthood, is more common in women and widows and is symptomatically less severe than in early-onset cases (Sheikh *et al*, 1991). Elderly panic patients tend not to present to psychiatric services, but the prominent physical symptoms may result in their being referred instead to cardiologists, neurologists and gastroenterologists. In one study of cardiology patients with chest pain and no coronary artery disease, one-third of those aged over 65 years met diagnostic criteria for panic disorder (Beitman *et al*, 1991).

Generalised anxiety disorder

One result of the recognition of specific anxiety disorders, such as phobic disorders and panic disorder, by the new psychiatric classifications has been the relative eclipse of the concept of generalised anxiety as a diagnostic entity. Indeed in ICD–10, generalised anxiety disorder may only be diagnosed in the absence of any other mood disorder. The current unpopularity of generalised anxiety is probably due in part to the lack of specific treatments (Tyrer, 1985), and in part to the current emphasis on the organic as opposed to psychosocial causes of anxiety disorders (Blazer *et al*, 1991). In particular, the role of chronic stress in the aetiology of conditions such as generalised anxiety has been neglected in recent years.

Concern has been expressed that the diagnosis of generalised anxiety disorder may be inappropriately applied to elderly people because of their vulnerability and physical frailty (Shamoian, 1991). In fact, the epidemiological evidence indicates that only a small percentage of the elderly population meet diagnostic criteria for this disorder (Copeland *et al*, 1987a,b; Lindesay *et al*, 1989; Blazer *et al*, 1991; Manela *et al*, 1996).

Whatever the nosological status of generalised anxiety, the condition appears to be associated with an increased use of both physical and mental health services (Blazer *et al*, 1991). If service use is regarded as a criterion of clinical importance then generalised anxiety remains a useful concept, particularly at the primary care level.

'Neurotic' depression

Although ICD–10 has retained the concept of neurotic disorders (Box 9.1), no depressive condition appears in this group. As a diagnostic category, neurotic depression has always been unsatisfactory; the criteria are vague, and it is defined more by the absence of psychotic symptoms than by the presence of anything specific. Nevertheless, as Snaith (1991) points out, "consideration of aspects of depression is integral to the understanding of many neurotic disorders" because:

(a) Conditions such as phobic disorder, generalised anxiety disorder, agoraphobia, obsessive–compulsive disorder (OCD) and somatisation are often accompanied by depressive symptoms, and these often come to dominate the clinical picture over time, particularly if the neurotic symptoms are severe and disabling. This depressive element of the clinical picture may well require treatment in its own right.

(b) At all ages, the most common psychiatric disorder seen in primary care settings is a mild to moderate mixture of depressive and anxiety symptoms, arising in response to a specific stressor, often in the context of particular maladaptive personality traits.

(c) Depression in the elderly sometimes presents with apparently 'neurotic' behaviour, such as hypochondriasis, anorexia, importuning and screaming, that can mislead the unwary diagnostician.

Obsessive–compulsive disorder

Of all the specific neurotic disorders OCD is the most persistent and stable diagnosis. It has a chronic, fluctuating course (Rasmussen & Tsuang, 1986), and the clinical features of OCD in elderly patients are similar to those seen in younger adults. Although a proportion of patients with OCD also develop significant depressive symptoms, other evidence suggests that OCD is a distinct disorder involving the orbitofrontal cortex, basal ganglia, substantia nigra and ventrolateral pallidum (Montgomery, 1980; Goodman *et al*, 1989; Insel, 1992).

While the onset of OCD in old age is rare (Bajulaiye & Addonizio, 1992), a minority of cases present late, and many elderly patients with long-standing disorders have never been adequately treated (Jenike, 1989). Therefore, it is important that all elderly patients receive thorough evaluation and treatment when they come to the notice of services. The development of obsessional orderliness and preoccupation with routines may presage the onset of dementia. Obsessional symptoms may appear at any age following head injury or cerebral tumour.

Somatoform disorders

Somatisation

The somatisation of psychological distress usually starts in early adult life, and once established, has a chronic, fluctuating course showing little improvement with age (Pribor *et al*, 1994). Somatising patients are skilled at seeking medical treatment and avoiding psychiatrists, and it is not uncommon for these individuals to present to psychiatric services for the first time in old age. They come with a very extensive history of complaints, referrals and investigations; are usually depressed and anxious; and the clinical picture is often complicated by the presence of true physical illness. They are the epitome of the 'heartsink' patient, and a significant challenge to all involved in their care.

Hypochondriasis

In contrast to somatisation, hypochondriacal patients usually restrict physical complaints to one or two body organs or systems. Typically they are preoccupied with the possibility of serious physical illness and their demand is for investigation rather than treatment (World Health Organization, 1992). In the elderly, primary hypochondriasis is usually long-standing; hypochondriacal preoccupations that present for the first time in late life are more likely to be a secondary manifestation of depression or anxiety.

Malingering

Malingering is an abnormal illness behaviour that has yet to be dignified as a disorder by any psychiatric nosology. It is largely unresearched and there are no formal diagnostic criteria; nevertheless, it is well recognised and disapproved of by doctors who tend to ignore or dismiss what lies behind it. Doctors and other carers find malingering particularly irritating because the malingerer is clearly physically ill, or disabled, and yet the complaints and crises, such as breathlessness, falls or episodes of incontinence, are timed to cause distress and inconvenience to those responsible for their care. It is important to understand what is being communicated by such behaviour, such as distress, anger, fear or depression. Failure to address this can result in rejection by carers, and institutionalisation, with subsequent escalation in the patient's distress and disruptive behaviour.

Dissociative disorders

Elderly patients occasionally manifest what appear to be hysterical dysmnesias and conversion reactions to stressful experiences, and it is important to know what these represent. As a rule the appearance of such symptoms in late life is due to organic disease, or the release of hysterical tendencies in vulnerable personalities, by cerebral pathology or functional psychiatric disorder. As Bergmann (1978) said, "It is best to assert dogmatically that primary hysterical illness does not begin in old age".

Management

Psychological

Although the behavioural and cognitive approaches to psychological treatment are theoretically distinct, in practice most interventions involve elements of both. Cognitive–behavioural therapy is of proven effectiveness in the treatment of conditions such as phobias and OCD, in younger adults (Marks, 1978). Case reports and small series indicate that they are just as effective in the elderly (Leng, 1985; Woods & Britton, 1985; Woods, 1995). Anxiety management training, involving instruction, relaxation and other control techniques (McCarthy *et al*, 1991) is an important approach to anxiety symptoms in the elderly, which can be applied in a wide range of settings to both groups and individuals. Further research is needed to establish which strategies are most effective in this age group; while the principles of cognitive–behavioural therapy are the same at all ages, the goals and techniques may need to be modified to make allowance for physical disabilities (see Chapter 17).

Physical

Despite the effectiveness of behavioural, training and cognitive strategies in the management of neurotic disorders, most elderly patients with these conditions are treated with drugs. Sometimes this is appropriate; for example, if depression is a prominent feature then a course of antidepressant treatment should always be considered. However, the pharmacotherapy of neurotic disorders is often merely an easy and convenient means of avoiding a more detailed and painstaking assessment of the patient's symptoms and circumstances.

The greatest problems with inappropriate and excessive drug treatment of neurotic disorders in the elderly have occurred in association with benzodiazepines. In spite of the fact that there have been relatively few formal controlled trials of benzodiazepine treatment in elderly patients, old people are the largest consumers of this class of drugs, particularly as hypnotics. Because of the altered handling of drugs by the body with increasing age, some benzodiazepines and their metabolites accumulate substantially in some elderly patients, with the result that apparently therapeutic doses can eventually cause persistent drowsiness, incontinence, delirium and falls (Evans & Jarvis, 1972; Fancourt & Castleden, 1986). Other problems in the elderly include increased central nervous system sensitivity to the effect of the drug, the presence of physical illness (particularly respiratory disease), interactions with other drugs and alcohol, and non-compliance (Salzman, 1991). At all ages, long-term benzodiazepine use can result in physical dependence, cognitive impairment and paradoxical excitement. In view of all these problems, benzodiazepine prescription in the elderly should be restricted to short courses of short-acting compounds without active metabolites, such as oxazepam. As a rule, long-term benzodiazepine users should be encouraged to withdraw from their medication, particularly if they have continuing neurotic symptoms (see Chapter 11).

There is evidence that some of the new generation of anxiolytics and antidepressants are more effective in providing relief in neurotic disorders without unacceptable side-effects. Buspirone is an azapirone anxiolytic drug whose pharmacokinetics, safety and efficacy in the elderly, are similar to those in younger adults (Robinson *et al*, 1988). It is well tolerated by this age group, and it appears that short-term use is not associated with rebound, dependence or misuse (Lader, 1991). Unlike other anxiolytics it takes two to three weeks to have an effect, so it is not useful in the management of acute anxiety states. Neuroleptic drugs have only a limited role in the management of anxiety because of the risk of disabling extrapyramidal side-effects. Antihistamine drugs such as hydroxyzine have a history of use as anxiolytics in elderly patients, and they may be useful when respiratory depressant drugs are contraindicated.

Conclusion

Neurotic disorders are more common in the elderly than generally realised. Faced with the urgent demands of dementia and depression, it is understandable that some hard-pressed old age psychiatric services might regard the treatment of neurotic disorders as a relatively low priority. While it is true that services should aim to have a limited role in the long-term management of these conditions, they should nevertheless be proficient in their assessment and acute treatment, and be able to advise primary care teams, physicians and others responsible for the continuing care of these patients, in appropriate management strategies.

References

American Psychiatric Association (1994) *Diagnostic and Statistical Manual of Mental Disorders* (4th edn) (DSM–IV). Washington, DC: APA.
Andrews, G., Pollack, C. & Stewart, G. W. (1990) Genetics of six neurotic disorders: a twin study. *Journal of Affective Disorders*, 19, 23–29.

Ballard, C., Boyle, A., Bowler, C., *et al* (1996) Anxiety disorders in dementia sufferers. *International Journal of Geriatric Psychiatry*, 11, 987–990.

Bajulaiye, R. & Addonizio, C. (1992) Obsessive compulsive disorder arising in a 75-year-old woman. *International Journal of Geriatric Psychiatry*, 7, 139–142.

Beitman, B. D., Kushner, M. & Grossberg, G. T. (1991) Late onset panic disorder: evidence from a study of patients with chest pain and normal cardiac evaluations. *International Journal of Psychiatry in Medicine*, 21, 29–35.

Bergmann, K. (1972) The neuroses of old age. In *Recent Developments in Psychogeriatrics* (eds D. W. K. Kay & A. Walk), pp. 39–50. Ashford: Headley Bros.

—— (1978) Neurosis and personality disorder in old age. In *Studies in Geriatric Psychiatry* (eds A. D. Isaacs & F. Post), pp. 41–75. London: Wiley.

Blazer, D., George, L. K. & Hughes, D. (1991) The epidemiology of anxiety disorders: An age comparison. In *Anxiety in the Elderly* (eds C. Salzman & B. D. Lebowitz), pp. 17–30. New York: Springer Publishing.

Boyd, J. H., Burke, J. D., Gruenberg, E., *et al* (1984) Exclusion criteria of DSM–III: a study of the co-occurrence of hierarchy-free syndromes. *Archives of General Psychiatry*, 41, 983–989.

Brown, G. W. (1993) Life events and psychiatric disorder: replications and limitations. *Psychosomatic Medicine*, 55, 248–259.

——, Bifulco, A. & Harris, T. O. (1987) Life events, vulnerability and onset of depression: some refinements. *British Journal of Psychiatry*, 150, 30–42.

Copeland, J. R. M., Dewey, M. E., Wood, N., *et al* (1987*a*) Range of mental illness among the elderly in the community: Prevalence in Liverpool using the GMS/AGECAT package. *British Journal of Psychiatry*, 150, 815–823.

——, Gurland, B. J., Dewey, M. E., *et al* (1987*b*) Is there more dementia, depression and neurosis in New York? A comparative study of the elderly in New York and London using the computer diagnosis AGECAT. *British Journal of Psychiatry*, 151, 466–473.

Evans, J. G. & Jarvis, E. H. (1972) Nitrazepam and the elderly. *British Medical Journal, iv*, 487.

Fancourt, G. & Castleden, M. (1986) The use of benzodiazepines with particular reference to the elderly. *British Journal of Hospital Medicine*, 5, 321–325.

Fattah, E. A. & Sacco, V. F. (1989) *Crime and Victimization in the Elderly*. New York: Springer-Verlag.

Goldberg, D. P., Bridges, K., Duncan-Jones, P., *et al* (1987) Dimensions of neurosis in primary care. *Psychological Medicine*, 17, 461–470.

Goodman, W. K., Price, L. H., Rasmussen, S. A., *et al* (1989) Efficacy of fluvoxamine in obsessive-compulsive disorder. A double-blind comparison with placebo. *Archives of General Psychiatry*, 46, 36–44.

Himmelfarb, S. & Murrell, S. A. (1984) The prevalence and correlates of anxiety symptoms in older adults. *Journal of Psychology*, 116, 159–167.

Insel, T. R. (1992) Neurobiology of obsessive-compulsive disorder: a review. *International Clinical Psychopharmacology*, 7 (suppl. 1), 31–33.

Jenike, M. A. (1989) *Geriatric Psychiatry and Psychopharmacology: A Clinical Approach*, Mosby Year Book. St Louis, MO: Mosby.

Kay, D. W. K. & Bergmann, K. (1966) Physical disability and mental health in old age. *Journal of Psychosomatic Research*, 10, 3–12.

Kendler, K. S., Heath, A. C., Martin, N. G., *et al* (1987) Symptoms of anxiety and symptoms of depression. Same genes, different environments? *Archives of General Psychiatry*, 122, 451–457.

Kennedy, G. J., Kelman, H. R. & Thomas, C. (1989) Hierarchy of characteristics associated with depressive symptoms in an urban elderly sample. *American Journal of Psychiatry*, 146, 220–222.

Knoff, W. F. (1970) A history of the concept of neurosis, with a memoir of William Cullen. *American Journal of Psychiatry*, 127, 80–84.

Lader, M. (1991) Can buspirone induce rebound, dependence or abuse? *British Journal of Psychiatry*, 159 (suppl. 12), 45–51.

Leng, N. (1985) A brief review of cognitive-behavioural treatments in old age. *Age and Ageing*, 14, 257–263.

Lindesay, J. (1990) The Guy's/Age Concern Survey: physical health and psychiatric disorder in an urban elderly community. *International Journal of Geriatric Psychiatry*, 5, 171–178.

—— (1991) Phobic disorders in the elderly. *British Journal of Psychiatry*, 159, 531–541.

—— (ed.) (1995) *Neurotic Disorders in the Elderly*. Oxford: Oxford University Press.

——, Briggs, K. & Murphy, E. (1989) The Guy's / Age Concern Survey: Prevalence rates of cognitive impairment, depression and anxiety in an urban elderly community. *British Journal of Psychiatry*, 155, 317–329.

Manela, M., Katona, C. & Livingston, G. (1996) How common are the anxiety disorders in old age? *International Journal of Geriatric Psychiatry*, 6, 65–70.

McCarthy, P. R., Katz, I. R. & Foa, E. B. (1991) Cognitive-behavioural treatment of anxiety in the elderly: A proposed model. In *Anxiety in the elderly* (eds C. Salzman & B. D. Lebowitz), pp. 197–214. New York: Springer Publishing.

Macdonald, A. (1986) Do general practitioners 'miss' depression in elderly patients? *British Medical Journal*, 292, 1365–1367.

Mackinnon, A., Christiansen, H., Jorm A. F., *et al* (1994) A latent trait analysis of an inventory designed to detect symptoms of anxiety and depression in an elderly community sample. *Psychological Medicine*, 24, 977–986.

Marks, I. (1978) Behavioural therapy of the neuroses. In *Handbook of Psychotherapy and Behaviour Therapy* (eds S. L. Garfield & A. E. Bergin), pp. 493–547. New York: Wiley.

Montgomery, S. (1980) Clomipramine in obsessional neurosis: A placebo-controlled trial. *Pharmacological Medicine*, 1, 189–192.

Philpot, M. (1995) Biological factors. In *Neurotic Disorders in the Elderly* (ed. J. Lindesay), pp. 73–96. Oxford: Oxford University Press.

Pitt, B. (1995) Neurotic disorders and physical illness. In *Neurotic Disorders in the Elderly* (ed. J. Lindesay), pp. 46–55. Oxford: Oxford University Press.

Pribor, E. F., Smith, D. S. & Yutzt, S. H. (1994) Somatization disorder in elderly patients. *American Journal of Geriatric Psychiatry*, 2, 109–117.

Rasmussen, S. A. & Tsuang, M. T. (1986) Clinical characteristics and family history in DSM–III obsessive compulsive disorder. *American Journal of Psychiatry*, 143, 317–322.

Regier, D. A., Boyd, J. H., Burke, J. D., *et al* (1988) One-month prevalence of mental disorders in the United States. *Archives of General Psychiatry*, 45, 977–986.

Robins, L. N. & Regier, D. A. (1991) *Psychiatric Disorders in America*. New York: Free Press.

Robinson, D., Napoliello, M. J. & Shenck, J. (1988) The safety and usefulness of buspirone as an anxiolytic drug in elderly versus young patients. *Clinical Therapeutics*, 10, 740–746.

Salzman, C. (1991) Pharmacologic treatment of the elderly anxious patient. In *Anxiety in the Elderly* (eds C. Salzman & B. D. Lebowitz), pp. 149–174. New York: Springer Publishing.

Shamoian, C. A. (1991) What is anxiety in the elderly? In *Anxiety in the Elderly* (eds C. Salzman and B. D. Lebowitz), pp. 3–16. New York: Springer Publishing.

Sheikh, J. I., King, R. J. & Barr Taylor, C. (1991) Comparative phenomenology of early-onset versus late-onset panic attacks: a pilot survey. *American Journal of Psychiatry*, 148, 1231–1233.

Snaith, P. (1991) *Clinical Neurosis* (2nd edn). London: Oxford University Press.

Thompson, J. W., Burns, B. J., Bartko, J., *et al* (1988) The use of ambulatory services by persons with and without phobia. *Medical Care*, 26, 183–198.

Tyrer, P. (1985) Classification of anxiety. *British Journal of Psychiatry*, 144, 78–83.

Wands, K., Merskey, H., Hachinski, V., *et al* (1990) A questionnaire investigation of anxiety and depression in early dementia. *Journal of the American Geriatrics Society*, 36, 535–538.

Weissman, M. M. & Merikangas, K. R. (1986) The epidemiology of anxiety and panic disorders: an update. *Journal of Clinical Psychiatry*, 47, 11–17.

Woods, R. T. (1995) Psychological treatments I: behavioural and cognitive approaches. In *Neurotic Disorders in the Elderly* (ed. J. Lindesay), pp. 97–113. Oxford: Oxford University Press.

—— & Britton, P. G. (1985) *Clinical Psychology with the Elderly*. London: Croom Helm.

World Health Organization (1992) *The Tenth Revision of the International Classification of Diseases and Related Problems* (ICD–10). Geneva: WHO.

Zahner, G. E. P. & Murphy, J. M. (1989) Loss in childhood: anxiety in adulthood. *Comprehensive Psychiatry*, 30, 553–563.

10 Late paraphrenia

Osvaldo Almeida

Historical context ● *Psychiatric signs and symptoms* ● *Classification*
● *Prevalence and incidence* ● *Risk factors* ● *Divisions* ● *Management*
● *Conclusion*

Historical context

The term 'paranoid' has its origin in the ancient Greek words 'paranoia' and 'paranoeo', which were commonly used to express the idea of madness or being out of one's mind. In the 18th century the term was incorporated into medical terminology to describe a number of mental disorders that included mood disorders and dementia. By the end of the 19th century, paranoia was part of the medical vocabulary, although controversy surrounded its use and definition.

Kraepelin introduced the term 'paraphrenia', and in 1913, described it as a condition which occurred in patients with well-preserved personalities, no disturbance of will and good affective response. He identified four forms:

(a) Systematica: an insidious development of delusions of persecution and exaltation.
(b) Expansiva: exuberant ideas of grandiosity and mild excitement.
(c) Confabulaloria: falsifications of memories.
(d) Phantastica: extraordinary, incoherent and changeable delusional ideas.

The first systematic description of paranoid features with onset in later life was published under the title of *Involutional Paranoia* (Kleist, 1913). Kleist speculated on the possible contribution of organic factors to the development of psychotic symptoms, and concluded that involutional paranoia was unlikely to be caused by a primary degenerative or vascular dementia. He remarked that the clinical features were very similar to those described by Kraepelin as paraphrenia.

In 1952, Roth & Morrisey described a group of elderly patients with a well-organised system of paranoid delusions in whom signs of organic dementia, sustained confusion or affective disorder were absent. The authors emphasised that the disorder developed in the setting of a well-preserved intellect and personality, was often primary in character, and was usually associated with hallucinations, passivity phenomena and other volitional disturbances.

148

A few years later, Fish (1960) challenged the use of the term late paraphrenia. He believed that the condition Roth had described represented nothing more than a senile form of schizophrenia. Fish advocated the use of Leonhard's confusing classification of schizophrenia (Fish, 1958) and, by an inexplicable paradox, chose to allocate his patients into six different subtypes of the very diagnosis he had just rejected: affect-laden, hypochondriacal, fantastic, incoherent, phonemic and confabulatory.

Since the early 1960s, discussions about the nature of late paraphrenia and related disorders have focused on two conflicting views:

(a) Late paraphrenia is nothing more than the expression of schizophrenia in the elderly (Fish, 1960; Gold, 1984; Grahame, 1984).
(b) The paranoid symptoms of late life are genetically different from schizophrenia and arise from the complex interaction of various pathogenic factors associated with old age (Funding, 1961; Post, 1966; Herbert & Jacobson, 1967; Almeida *et al*, 1992).

Psychiatric signs and symptoms

Delusions and hallucinations

Delusions and hallucinations usually dominate the clinical picture. Kay & Roth (1961) offered a vivid description:

> "Neighbours, landlords, or relatives are implicated in plots to be rid of the patients, or to annoy or interfere with them through jealousy or simply for amusement... Patients feel drugged, hypnotised, have their thoughts read, their minds or bodies worked upon by rays, machines or electricity, complain that they are spied upon, can get no privacy in thought or act... (auditory hallucinations) consist of threatening, accusing, commanding or cajoling voices, jeering commentaries, screams, shouts for help, obscene words and songs, music, loud bangs, rappings, shots or explosions... their thoughts are repeated aloud... God, spirits, distant or deceased relatives, or most often, jealous, hostile neighbours are held responsible (for these phenomena)".

A wide range of delusions have been observed in late-onset paranoid states (Box 10.1). Persecutory delusions are possibly the most consistent and frequent; they are found in around 90% of patients (Almeida *et al*, 1995a) (Table 10.1). Auditory hallucinations are detected in about three-quarters of patients. Visual, olfactory, tactile and somatic hallucinations are less common, but not rare. Visual hallucinations, for instance, have been observed in up to 60% of patients. Other frequent symptoms include first rank symptoms of Schneider (Post, 1966; Holden, 1987). A similar type and frequency distribution of psychotic symptoms has been found in schizophrenia of early onset (Andreasen, 1990a), which seems to

---

Box 10.1 Types of delusions found in late paraphrenia

Persecution
Reference
Misidentification
Control
Hypochondriasis
Grandiosity
Gender
Religion

---

indicate that late paraphrenia and schizophrenia are the same condition. However, there is more to schizophrenia than delusions and hallucinations.

Other schizophrenic symptoms

ICD–10 (World Health Organization, 1992) and DSM–IV (American Psychiatric Association, 1994) include thought disorder, catatonic symptoms and negative symptoms as important clinical features of schizophrenia. Thought disorder is present in up to 60% of early-onset people with schizophrenia (Wing *et al*, 1974; Andreasen, 1990*b*; Menezes, 1992), and catatonic symptoms are observed in up to a quarter of patients (Creer & Wing, 1975; Andreasen, 1990*b*). In addition, typical negative symptoms such as lack of speech inflection, reduced speech output, reduced facial expression, reduced gestures and affective blunting are found in up to 85% of early-onset people with schizophrenia (Andreasen *et al*, 1990).

These findings contrast with late paraphrenia. Thought disorder, catatonic symptoms and negative symptoms are extremely uncommon

Table 10.1 Psychiatric symptoms in late paraphrenia

	%
Persecutory delusions	83
Auditory hallucinations	77
First rank symptoms	46
Delusions of reference	33
Delusions about mind reading	17
Visual hallucinations	13
Somatic/tactile hallucinations	12
Somatic delusions	9
Grandiose delusions	6
Thought broadcast	4
Olfactory hallucinations	4
Delusions of sin or guilt	2

in late-onset cases. Even in the few instances when such symptoms are reported, they are not described as severe (Kay & Roth, 1961; Pearlson *et al*, 1989; Almeida *et al*, 1995*a*). By emphasising the similarities between the delusions and hallucinations of late paraphrenia and schizophrenia, sight may be lost of important psychopathological differences. In fact, the two disorders show very different symptomatological profiles.

Other psychiatric symptoms

There are few references to other psychiatric symptoms in the late paraphrenia literature. Almeida *et al* (1995*a*) found irritability, social unease, loss of interest and concentration, self-neglect and obsessive features associated with the typical psychotic symptoms of late paraphrenia.

Classification

The classification of the paranoid states of late life has been the subject of an intense, and sometimes emotive, controversy (Levy *et al*, 1987; Grahame, 1988). ICD–10 (Boxes 10.2 and 10.3) and DSM– III–R (American Psychiatric Association, 1987) introduced further problems by not including a diagnosis of late paraphrenia. In ICD–10 some people with late paraphrenia are diagnosed with schizophrenia, while others are

---

Box 10.2 Summary of ICD–10 diagnostic guidelines for schizophrenia (World Health Organization, 1992)

The presence for one month or more, of at least one very clear symptom (and usually two or more if less clear cut) belonging to (a) to (d) or symptoms from at least two groups of (e) to (h)
(a) thought echo, insertion, withdrawal or broadcasting
(b) delusions of passivity, delusional perception
(c) hallucinatory voices giving a running commentary, discussing the patient or coming from some part of the body
(d) persistent delusions of other kinds such as superhuman abilities
(e) persistent hallucinations in any modality
(f) thought disorder
(g) catatonic behaviour
(h) negative symptoms such as marked apathy, paucity of speech, blunting of emotion, lowering social performance
(i) a significant and consistent change in quality of personal behaviour with loss of interest and social withdrawal

---

Box 10.3 Summary of ICD–10 diagnostic guidelines for delusional disorder (World Health Organization, 1992)

Delusions are the most conspicuous or only clinical characteristic, present for at least three months
Depression may be present but only intermittently
No evidence of brain disease
No or only occasional auditory hallucinations
No history of schizophrenic symptoms

---

classified as delusional disorder, schizoaffective disorder, or other types of psychoses (Rabins *et al*, 1984; Quintal *et al*, 1991).

There is little evidence (Quintal *et al*, 1991; Howard *et al*, 1994; Almeida *et al*, 1995a) to suggest that people with late paraphrenia are better classified under the headings 'persistent delusional disorder' or 'schizophrenia' (Grahame, 1984; Harris & Jeste, 1988; Jeste, 1993). The use of the diagnosis of delusional disorder seems inappropriate because most people with late paraphrenia display symptoms such as prominent hallucinations. Similarly, there are limitations to the use of the diagnosis of schizophrenia:

(a) There is poor agreement on how to define it.
(b) The diagnosis of schizophrenia fails to take into account the associated factors of late paraphrenia.
(c) It is unlikely that the neurodevelopmental basis postulated for schizophrenia (Weinberger, 1987; Bloom, 1993) plays an important pathogenic role in late-onset cases.

Prevalence and incidence

People with late paraphrenia represent approximately 10% of the elderly population of psychiatric hospitals. The reported prevalence of the disorder among the elderly living in the community ranges from 0.1 to 4% and its incidence has been estimated to be between 10–26 per 100 000 per year. On average only 1.5% of those diagnosed with schizophrenia have an onset of illness after the age of 60, in contrast to 23 and 16% of patients with other paranoid states and reactive psychoses (Almeida *et al*, 1992).

Risk factors

It is difficult to think about lung cancer without immediately associating it with smoking. Similarly, a number of risk factors are important in late paraphrenia (Box 10.4).

Box 10.4 Factors associated with late paraphrenia

Female gender
Hearing loss
Visual impairment
Social isolation
Brain disease
Not marrying (may be a weaker factor)
Family history

Gender

Late paraphrenia is more common in women than men. Ratios have been reported between three to one, and 20 to one (Kay *et al*, 1964; Herbert & Jacobson, 1967). Compared to men the onset of schizophrenia in women is delayed by three to four years (Bland, 1977; Keith *et al*, 1991; Häfner *et al*, 1993). The later preponderance of women is unlikely to be due merely to some protective factor delaying the onset of illness in this population. Indeed, Castle & Murray (1991) showed that the incidence of schizophrenic symptoms in women after the age of 55 clearly exceeds the frequency expected if the incidence curve had been simply shifted to the right. In other words, early (with a predominance of men) and very late-onset cases (with a clear predominance of women) may represent distinct diseases.

Theories to explain the later onset of schizophrenia in women include:

(a) There is a separate disorder genetically related to mood disorders, rather than schizophrenia (Castle & Murray, 1991), which explains why these patients show a better prognosis and response to treatment (Hogarty *et al*, 1974).

(b) The condition is associated with a concurrent decline of oestrogen levels, and a relative excess of dopamine D_2 receptors (Pearlson & Rabins, 1988; Seeman & Lang, 1990).

(c) Psychosocial factors, such as better use of coping behaviour strategies and social support schemes, delay the onset of schizophrenic symptoms among women (Riecher *et al*, 1990).

Sensory deficits

Hearing impairment has been experimentally (Zimbardo *et al*, 1981) and clinically (Moore, 1981) associated with the development of paranoid symptoms. Almeida *et al* (1995*b*) estimated that the risk of hearing impairment among people with late paraphrenia was four times greater than that of age- and gender-matched controls. Cooper *et al* (1974) showed that this hearing loss is usually caused by conductive, rather than degenerative, mechanisms. Late paraphrenia was associated with deafness of early onset, long duration and profound auditory loss (Cooper, 1976). Unfortunately, interpreting these associations is far from simple because most elderly individuals with hearing problems do not become psychotic (Corbin & Eastwood, 1986). Moreover, hearing impairment in the elderly has been more frequently associated with depression and decreased self-sufficiency in daily living activities (Carabellese *et al*, 1993) than with paranoid symptoms.

Cooper & Porter (1976) suggested that hearing deficits may have a pathogenic role by reinforcing a pre-existing tendency to social isolation, withdrawal and suspiciousness. However, it is not suspiciousness but auditory hallucinations that have been most frequently connected to hearing impairment (Corbin & Eastwood, 1986). The symptomatological relief reported by some of these patients after the fitting of a hearing aid (Khan *et al*, 1988; Almeida *et al*, 1993) highlights the contribution made by deafness to the production of auditory hallucinations. David & Lucas (1992) propose a cognitive model in which auditory hallucinations result from a failure to recognise internal auditory input at the auditory analysis system level. This model suggests that a defective auditory analysis system might lead to impaired discrimination of spoken material. This has been confirmed by the preliminary work of Stein & Thienhaus (1993).

The diagnosis of late paraphrenia has also been associated with visual impairment (Kay & Roth, 1961; Post, 1966; Herbert & Jacobson, 1967). Major ocular pathology (predominantly cataracts) was found in over half of people with late paraphrenia, significantly more than in elderly depressive controls (Cooper & Porter, 1976). However, the mechanisms by which visual impairment could produce psychotic symptoms are still unclear.

Social isolation

Kay & Roth (1961) pointed out that people with late paraphrenia were socially isolated, and that 40% of them lived alone. A more systematic assessment of social isolation was reported by Almeida *et al* (1995*b*) who evaluated the frequency of contacts with friends during the six months prior to the interview. They found that 79% of people with late paraphrenia were socially isolated, compared with 18% of age- and gender-matched controls. The role of social isolation in late paraphrenia is uncertain, but there have been suggestions that deafness, deviant personality, and few surviving relatives may contribute (Kay & Roth, 1961; Post, 1966; Herbert & Jacobson, 1967).

Brain disease

Evidence for an association between late paraphrenia and brain dysfunction comes from clinical, neurological, psychological, imaging and pathological studies.

Clinical

The concept of late paraphrenia emerged as an attempt to address the contribution of brain disease to the late-onset psychotic states (Roth & Morrisey, 1952). Kay & Roth (1961) found that 21% of their patients showed evidence of organic disease, although organic factors had bearing on the later course of the illness in only 5% of subjects.

Neurological

Almeida *et al* (1995*b*) found two main types of neurological signs in late paraphrenia: (a) abnormal and dyskinetic movements, which were associated with the use of neuroleptics; and (b) neurological soft signs.

Neurological soft signs do not have the same localising power as hard signs (Cadet *et al*, 1986), although their presence can often be related to impaired performance on cognitive tests (Förstl *et al*, 1992*a*; Liddle *et al*, 1993), and may indicate the presence of brain disease or dysfunction (Förstl *et al*, 1992*a*; Manschreck, 1986).

Psychological

Naguib & Levy (1987) found deficits in a group of people with late paraphrenia on the Mental Test Score and a mild deterioration on scores at 3.7 year follow-up, although they remained above the cut-off point for dementia (Hymas *et al*, 1989). Almeida *et al* (1995*c*) found that performance on tests assessing memory was fairly well preserved, although executive functions (frontal tests) and general mental skills (Wechsler, 1981; Roth *et al*, 1988) were worse than matched controls.

Imaging

A number of computerised tomography and magnetic resonance imaging studies have looked at the association between late paraphrenia and brain pathology (Almeida *et al*, 1992) (see Chapter 12). Their results can be summarised by three main findings:

(a) Late life psychosis is often associated with cerebrovascular pathology, either in the form of white matter changes or infarcts.
(b) People with late paraphrenia with first rank symptoms of Schneider, have more cortical atrophy than patients without first rank symptoms.
(c) Patients with late life psychosis show mild ventricular enlargement compared to controls. Ventricular enlargement has been observed in late paraphrenia and late-onset schizophrenia (Naguib & Levy, 1987; Rabins *et al*, 1987; Burns *et al*, 1989; Krull *et al*, 1991; Howard *et al*, 1992).

Pathological

Blessed *et al* (1968) published the only available quantitative neuropathological study of late paraphrenia. They examined the brains of five people with late paraphrenia and found that the mean number of plaque counts was much lower than in people with dementia, and not significantly different from those observed in elderly with depression or controls.

Marriage

Some reports suggested that people with late paraphrenia were more likely to be unmarried than elderly people with depression or normal age matched controls (Post, 1966; Herbert & Jacobson, 1967). Furthermore, married patients with late paraphrenia have a lower fertility rate than control groups (Kay & Roth, 1961; Herbert & Jacobson, 1967). More recent investigations suggest that these associations are not as consistent as female gender, hearing impairment, social isolation and brain damage (Rabins *et al*, 1984; Pearlson *et al*, 1989; Almeida *et al*, 1995*b*).

Family history

A family history of schizophreniform disorder is another factor frequently associated with the diagnosis of late paraphrenia. Kay (1972) reported that the risk of developing schizophrenia among first degree relatives of people with late paraphrenia was 3.4%, a rate intermediate between that described for the general population (less than 1%) and for the families of young people with schizophrenia (5.8%). Naguib *et al* (1987) used the human leucocytic antigen system to look at the association between late paraphrenia and genetic markers. There was no obvious relationship between the disorder and the antigens investigated although the authors proposed the HLA-B37 as a possible marker candidate for late paraphrenia. More recently Howard *et al* (1995) reported no difference in ApoE4 frequency rates between people with late paraphrenia and controls.

Divisions

A number of attempts have been made to subdivide the paranoid states of late life. Kay & Roth (1961) allocated patients to three different groups according to their symptoms and aetiology. Other subdivisions have included those of Post (1966, 1980) and Holden (1987). Howard *et al* (1994) divided a group of 101 people with late paraphrenia using ICD–10 criteria and a cluster analysis of symptoms. They found poor agreement between the two groupings (Table 10.2).

More recently, Almeida *et al* (1995*d*) divided people with late paraphrenia into two groups by a cluster analysis of cognitive test scores.

Table 10.2 Divisions of patients with late paraphrenia

	%
ICD–10 diagnoses	
Paranoid schizophrenia	61
Delusional disorder	31
Schizoaffective disorder	8
Cluster analysis of symptoms	
Schneider's first rank symptoms	35
Prominent auditory hallucinations, few delusional experiences	27
Older age at onset, marked delusions, but few hallucinations	38

These groups need to be tested against clinical outcomes, functional neuroimaging and neuropathology:

(a) A more 'functional' group which showed cognitive deficits restricted to executive functions and a high prevalence of positive psychotic symptoms, including first rank symptoms of Schneider.
(b) A more 'organic' group which exhibited generalised cognitive decline and a relatively high frequency of neurological signs.

Management

Patients with late paraphrenia rarely seek help spontaneously, but may request action from their relatives, police or other authorities against their persecutors. Many are maintained in the community with support from families, friends and social workers, but the effectiveness of this form of management has not been evaluated. Doctors tend to see these patients only when these measures fail and behaviour becomes disruptive.

These patients rarely agree to attend a psychiatric appointment in an out-patient clinic, and a home visit is often necessary. A successful first medical contact may prove crucial in overall treatment. The psychiatrist should try to establish a good rapport with the patient, and be sympathetic to his or her complaints. They must also ensure that late paraphrenia is the correct diagnosis (investigate cognitive decline, neurological signs or symptoms, associated affective symptoms, etc.), and further interviews should be organised to establish the patient's good compliance with the therapeutic strategy. Antipsychotic medication can be rationalised for the patient as a way of lessening distress. Unfortunately, compulsory admission may be necessary with non-compliant subjects. In these cases the medical team should try to regain confidence in order to guarantee an effective future management.

Box 10.5 Management

Home visit
Establish rapport
Exclude other illnesses
Develop a therapeutic alliance
Reduce isolation
Antipsychotics
Compulsory admission sometimes necessary

Antipsychotics

The use of antipsychotics for the treatment of late paraphrenia is widely accepted, although no controlled trials have been reported. The risk of side-effects (mainly extrapyramidal) favours the use of oral medication, although Howard & Levy (1992) have suggested that depot intramuscular medicine may improve compliance and reduce the required antipsychotic dose. Post (1966) looked at patients who had received 10–30 mg of trifluoperazine or 40–500 mg of thioridazine per day. Nine per cent showed no response, 31% showed some signs of improvement and 60% presented a complete response to treatment. Less optimistic results were reported by Rabins *et al* (1984) and Pearlson *et al* (1989), who found that 15 and 24%, respectively, failed to improve after neuroleptic treatment. Howard & Levy (1992) reported that after at least three months of treatment, 42% of patients showed no response, 31% improved partially and 27% presented symptomatological remission. Several factors may be involved with failure to respond to the medication side-effects, and the presence of concomitant organic factors.

Outcome

Post (1966) suggested a number of good prognostic features: immediate response to treatment; development of insight; younger age; and being married. Psychological, social and occupational support are also important for a good outcome. Early interactions are important. Untreated patients may pursue an unremitting chronic course and once the symptoms have fully developed they are unlikely to change substantially until the patient's death.

Conclusion

The aetiology of late paraphrenia is complex, and includes the interaction of ageing, female gender, social isolation, hearing impairment, subtle brain lesions and cognitive decline. There is evidence that the division of late paraphrenia into delusional disorder and schizophrenia is unsatisfactory. The term 'late paraphrenia' may still be the best option available. However, increasing evidence from neuroimaging and neuropsychological studies may help subdivide late paraphrenia into a functional group and an organic group. Few studies have looked at treatment for this condition but there is evidence that neuroleptics benefit a majority of patients. Attempts should always be made to form a therapeutic alliance with the patient. A multi-disciplinary approach offers the best hope for successful treatment and outcome.

References

Almeida, O. P., Howard, R., Förstl, H., *et al* (1992) Late paraphrenia: a review. *International Journal of Geriatric Psychiatry*, 7, 543–548.

——, Förstl, H., Howard, R., *et al* (1993) Unilateral auditory hallucinations. *British Journal of Psychiatry*, 162, 262–264.

——, Howard, R., Levy, R., *et al* (1995*a*) Psychotic states arising in late life – psychopathology and nosology. *British Journal of Psychiatry*, 166, 205–214.

——, ——, ——, *et al* (1995*b*) Psychotic states arising in late life – the role of risk factors. *British Journal of Psychiatry*, 166, 215–228.

——, ——, ——, *et al* (1995*c*) Cognitive features of psychotic states arising in late life (late paraphrenia). *Psychological Medicine*, 25, 685–698.

——, ——, ——, *et al* (1995*d*) Clinical and cognitive diversity of psychotic states arising in late life (late paraphrenia). *Psychological Medicine*, 25, 699–714.

American Psychiatric Association (1987) *Diagnostic and Statistical Manual of Mental Disorders* (3rd edn, revised) (DSM–III–R). Washington, DC: APA.

—— (1994) *Diagnostic and Statistical Manual of Mental Disorders* (4th edn) (DSM–IV). Washington, DC: APA.

Andreasen, N. C. (1990*a*) Methods for assessing positive and negative symptoms. In *Schizophrenia: Positive and Negative Symptoms and Syndromes. Modern Problems in Pharmacopsychiatry*, Vol. 24 (ed. N. C. Andreasen), pp. 73–88. Basel: Karger.

—— (1990*b*) Positive and negative symptoms: historical and conceptual aspects. In *Schizophrenia: Positive and Negative Symptoms and Syndromes. Modern Problems in Pharmacopsychiatry*, Vol. 24 (ed. N. C. Andreasen), pp. 1–42. Basel: Karger.

——, Flaum, M., Swayze, V. W., *et al* (1990) Positive and negative symptoms in schizophrenia: a critical appraisal. *Archives of General Psychiatry*, 47, 615–621.

Bland, R. C. (1997) Demographic aspects of functional psychoses in Canada. *Acta Psychiatrica Scandinavica*, 55, 369–380.

Blessed, G., Tomlinson, B. E. & Roth, M. (1968) The association between quantitative measures of dementia and of senile change in the cerebral grey matter of elderly subjects. *British Journal of Psychiatry*, 114, 797–811.

Bloom, F. E. (1993) Advancing a neurodevelopmental origin for schizophrenia. *Archives of General Psychiatry*, 50, 224–227.

Burns, A., Carrick, J., Ames, D., *et al* (1989) The cerebral cortical appearance in late paraphrenia. *International Journal of Geriatric Psychiatry*, 4, 31–34.

Cadet, J. L., Rickler, K. C. & Weinberger, D. R. (1986) The clinical examination in schizophrenia. In *Handbook of Schizophrenia, Vol. 1: The Neurology of Schizophrenia* (eds H. A. Nasrallah & D. R. Weinberger), pp. 1–47. Amsterdam: Elsevier.

Carabellese, C., Appollonio, I., Rozzini, R., *et al* (1993) Sensory impairment and quality of life in a community elderly population. *Journal of the American Geriatric Society*, 41, 401–407.

Castle, D. J. & Murray, R. M. (1991) The neurodevelopmental basis of sex differences in schizophrenia. *Psychological Medicine*, 21, 565–575.

Cooper, A. F. (1976) Deafness and psychiatric illness. *British Journal of Psychiatry*, 129, 216–226.

——, Cuny, A. R., Kay, D. W. K., *et al* (1974) Hearing loss in paranoid and affective psychoses of the elderly. *Lancet*, *ii*, 851–854.

—— & Porter, R. (1976) Visual acuity and ocular pathology in the paranoid and affective psychoses of later life. *Journal of Psychosomatic Research*, 20, 107–114.

Corbin, S. L. & Eastwood, M. R. (1986) Sensory deficits and mental disorders of old age: causal or coincidental associations? *Psychological Medicine*, 16, 251–256.

Creer, C. & Wing, J. K. (1975) Living with a schizophrenic patient. *British Journal of Hospital Medicine*, 14, 73–82.

David, A. S. & Lucas, P. A. (1992) Neurological models of auditory hallucinations. In *Delusions and Hallucinations in Old Age* (eds C. Katona & R. Levy), pp. 57–83. London: Gaskell.

Fish, F. (1958) Leonhard's classification of schizophrenia. *Journal of Mental Science*, 104, 943–971.

—— (1960) Senile schizophrenia. *Journal of Mental Science*, 106, 938–946.

Förstl, H., Burns, A., Levy, R., *et al* (1992) Neurologic signs in Alzheimer's disease: results of a prospective clinical and neuropathologic study. *Archives of Neurology*, 49, 1038–1042.

Funding, T. (1961) Genetics of paranoid psychoses in later life. *Acta Psychiatrica Scandinavica*, 37, 267–282.

Gold, Jr, D. D. (1984) Late age of onset schizophrenia: present but unaccounted for. *Comprehensive Psychiatry*, 25, 225–237.

Grahame, P. S. (1984) Schizophrenia in old age (late paraphrenia). *British Journal of Psychiatry*, 145, 493–495.

—— (1988) Late paraphrenia. *British Journal of Psychiatry*, 152, 289.

Harris, A. E. & Jeste, D. V. (1988) Late onset schizophrenia: an overview. *Schizophrenia Bulletin*, 14, 39–55.

Herbert, M. E. & Jacobson, S. (1967) Late paraphrenia. *British Journal of Psychiatry*, 113, 461–469.

Häfner, H., Maurer, K., Löffler, W., *et al* (1993) The influence of age and sex on the onset and early course of schizophrenia. *British Journal of Psychiatry*, 162, 80–86.

Hogarty, G. E., Goldberg, S. C. & Schooler, N. R. (1974) Drugs and sociotherapy in the after care of schizophrenic patients: adjustment of nonrelapsed patients. *Archives of General Psychiatry*, 31, 609–618.

Holden, N. L. (1987) Late paraphrenia or the paraphrenias? A descriptive study with a 10-year follow-up. *British Journal of Psychiatry*, 150, 635–639.

Howard, R. & Levy, R. (1992). Which factors affect treatment response in late paraphrenia? *International Journal of Geriatric Psychiatry*, 7, 667–672.

Howard, R., Castle, D., O'Brien, J., *et al* (1992) Permeable walls, floors, ceilings and doors: partition delusions in late paraphrenia. *International Journal of Geriatric Psychiatry*, 7, 719–724.

——, Almeida, O. P. & Levy, R. (1994) Phenomenology, demography and diagnosis in late paraphrenia. *Psychological Medicine*, 24, 397–410.

——, Dennehey, J., Lovestone, S., *et al* (1995) Apolipoprotein E genotype and late paraphrenia. *International Journal of Geriatric Psychiatry*, 10, 147–150.

Hymas, N., Naguib, M. & Levy, R. (1989) Late paraphrenia: a follow-up study. *International Journal of Geriatric Psychiatry*, 4, 23–29.

Jeste, D. V. (1993) Late-onset schizophrenia. *International Journal of Geriatric Psychiatry*, 8, 283–285.

Kay, D. W. K. (1972) Schizophrenia and schizophrenia-like states in the elderly. *British Journal of Hospital Medicine*, 8, 369–376.

—— & Roth, M. (1961) Environmental and hereditary factors in schizophrenias of old age ("late paraphrena") and their bearing on the general problem of causation in schizophrenia. *Journal of Mental Science*, 107, 649–686.

——, Beamish, P. & Roth, M. (1964) Old age disorders in Newcastle upon Tyne. Part 1: a study of prevalence. *British Journal of Psychiatry*, 110, 146–158.

Keith, S. J., Regier, D. A. & Rae, D. S. (1991) Schizophrenic disorders. In *Psychiatric Disorders in North America. The Epidemiological Catchment Area Study* (eds L. N. Robins & D. A. Regier), pp. 33–52. New York: Free Press.

Khan, A. M., Clark, T. & Oyebode, F. (1988) Unilateral auditory hallucinations. *British Journal of Psychiatry*, 152, 297–298.

Kleist, K. (1913) Is involutional paranoia due to an organic-destructive brain process? (partially translated by: Förstl, H., Howard, R., Almeida, O. P., *et al* in 1992 from the German paper: 'Die involutionsparanoia. Allgenteine Zeitschriff für Psychiatrie., 70, 1-64'). In *Delusion and Hallucination in Old Age* (eds C. Katona & R. Levy), pp. 165–166. London: Gaskell.

Kraepelin, E. (1913) *Dementia Praecox and Paraphrenia* (trans. by R. M. Barclay in 1919 from the German 8th edition of the "Psychiatrie, eine Lebrbuch für Studierende und Arzte", vol. 111, part 2). Edinburgh: Livingstone.

Krull, A. J., Press, G., Dupont, R., *et al* (1991) Brain imaging in late-onset schizophrenia and related disorders. *International Journal of Geriatric Psychiatry*, 6, 651–658.

Levy, R., Naguib, M. & Hymas, N. (1987) Late paraphrenia. *British Journal of Psychiatry*, 151, 702.

Liddle, P. F., Haque, S., Moffis, D. L., *et al* (1993) Dyspraxia and agnosia in schizophrenia. *Behavioural Neurology*, 6, 49–54.

Manschreck, T. C. (1986) Motor abnormalities in schizophrenia. In *Handbook of Schizophrenia, Vol. 1. The Neurology of Schizophrenia* (eds H. A. Nasrallali & D. R. Weinberger), pp. 65–96. Amsterdam: Elsevier.

Menezes, P. R. (1992) *The Outcome of Schizophrenia in São Paulo, Brazil: Preliminary Results of a 2-Year Follow-Up Study.* MSc thesis, London School of Hygiene and Tropical Medicine, Department of Epidemiology and Population Sciences, University of London.

Moore, N. C. (1981) Is paranoid illness associated with sensory defects in the elderly? *Journal of Psychosomatic Research*, 25, 69–74.

Naguib, M. & Levy, R. (1987) Late paraphrenia: neuropsychological impairment and structural brain abnormalities on computed tomography. *International Journal of Geriatric Psychiatry*, 2, 83–90.

Naguib, M., McGuffin, P., Levy, R., *et al* (1987) Genetic markers in late paraphrenia: a study of HLA antigens. *British Journal of Psychiatry*, 150, 124–127.

Pearlson, G. & Rabins, P. (1988) The late-onset psychoses: possible risk factors. In *Psychosis and Depression in the Elderly, The Psychiatric Clinics of North America*, Vol. 11 (eds D. V. Jeste & S. Zisook), pp. 15–32. Philadelphia, PA: W. B. Saunders.

Pearlson, G. D., Kreger, L., Rabins, P. V., *et al* (1989) A chart review study of late-onset and early-onset schizophrenia. *American Journal of Psychiatry*, 146, 1568–1574.

Post, F. (1966) *Persistent Persecutory States of the Elderly.* Oxford: Pergamon Press.

—— (1980) Paranoid, schizophrenia-like, and schizophrenic states in the aged. In *Handbook of Mental Health and Aging* (eds J. E. Birren & R. B. Sloane), pp. 591–615. Englewood Cliffs: Prentice Hall.

Quintal, M., Day-Cody, D. & Levy, R. (1991) Late paraphrenia and ICD–10. *International Journal of Geriatric Psychiatry*, 6, 111–116.

Rabins, P., Pauker, S. & Thomas, J. (1984) Can schizophrenia begin after age 44? *Comprehensive Psychiatry*, 25, 290–295.

——, Pearlson, G., Jayaram, G., *et al* (1987) Increased ventricle-to-brain ratio in late-onset schizophrenia. *American Journal of Psychiatry*, 142, 557–559.

Riecher, A., Maurer, K., Löffler, W., *et al* (1990) Gender differences in age at onset and course of schizophrenic disorders: a contribution to the understanding of the disease? In *Search for the Causes of Schizophrenia*, Vol.II (eds H. Häfner & W. F. Gattaz), pp 14–33. Berlin: Springer-Verlag.

Roth, M. & Morrisey, J. (1952) Problems in the diagnosis and classification of mental disorders in old age. *Journal of Mental Science*, 98, 66–80.

——, Huppert, F. A., Tyin, E., *et al* (1988) CAMDEX – The Cambridge Examination for Mental Disorders of the Elderly. Cambridge: Cambridge University Press.

Seeman, M. V. & Lang, M. (1990) The role of estrogens in schizophrenia gender differences. *Schizophrenia Bulletin*, 16, 185–195.

Stein, L. M. & Thienhaus, O. J. (1993) Hearing impairment and psychosis. *International Psychogeriatrics*, 5, 49–56.

Wechsler, D. (1981) *Wechsler Adult Intelligence Scale-Revised.* New York: The Psychological Corporation.

Weinberger, D. R. (1987) Implications of normal brain development for the pathogenesis of schizophrenia. *Archives of General Psychiatry*, 44, 660–669.

Wing, J. K., Cooper, J. E. & Sartorius, N. (1974) *Measurement and Classification of Psychiatric Symptoms. An Instruction Manual for the PSE and CATEGO Program.* Cambridge: Cambridge University Press.

World Health Organization (1992) *The ICD–10 Classification of Mental and Behavioural Disorders: Clinical Descriptions and Diagnostic Guidelines.* Geneva: WHO.

Zimbardo, P. G., Anderson, S. M. & Kabat, L. G. (1981) Induced hearing deficit generates experimental paranoia. *Science*, 212, 1529–1531.

11 Personality disorders and alcohol dependence

John Wattis

Personality disorder • *Ageing and behaviour* • *Prevalence* • *Association with other diagnoses* • *Management of personality disorder* • *Outcome* • *Sexuality* • *Alcohol dependence* • *Epidemiology* • *Aetiology* • *Medical complications* • *Presentation* • *Management of alcohol dependence* • *Other drug dependence* • *Conclusion*

Personality traits describe habitual clusters of behaviour. If one cluster of behaviour is dominant (e.g. depressive or obsessional behaviours) then that may justify the description of a personality type. Many different personality traits and types have been described by various authors. There is a debate over how constant styles of behaviour are, and how far they are influenced by situations.

Personality is likely to be determined by a mixture of genetics and life experience, particularly from childhood. In younger people the concept of personality is linked to development through stages of maturation. Beyond early adulthood theories about the maturation of personality are sparse. The core maturational task of later life has been defined by Erikson (1965) as establishing ego-integrity to avoid facing despair.

Personality disorder

Personality disorder is difficult to define. The most useful short definition, from a clinical point of view, may be a long-standing pattern of maladaptive, interpersonal behaviour (Kroessler, 1990). It is unclear whether it is best to regard personality disorder as a range of abnormality, which merges gradually from personality difficulties into mild and severe personality disorders, or to make a simple separation between those with and without personality disorder. A personality disorder is sometimes said to occur when behaviour resulting from personality causes damage to the person or others. Behaviour is an important marker of personality because it can be observed and does not have to be inferred, leading to more reliable diagnoses. In DSM–IV (American Psychiatric Association, 1994) a separate axis (axis II) is reserved for disorders of personality or development, while mental state disorders are classified as axis I disorders.

ICD–10 classification

ICD–10 (World Health Organization, 1992) defines personality disorders as deeply ingrained and enduring behaviour patterns, manifesting themselves as inflexible responses to a broad range of personal and social situations. The following points are made: (a) personality disorders start in childhood or adolescence; (b) they are not secondary to other disorders; (c) there are overlaps between different types; and (d) a diagnosis should be based on as many sources of information as possible. ICD–10 specific personality disorders are listed in Box 1.1.

Ageing and behaviour

As people age, changes in physical health reduce the likelihood of some behaviours associated with personality disorder in younger people. Impulsive behaviour, law-breaking, initiating fights, promiscuity and aggression to children are all less likely for a variety of reasons. While some behaviour which acts as a marker of disorder in younger people is less likely to be found in older people, other 'marker' behaviour, such as social withdrawal, may become more likely because of physical or sensory disabilities or undiagnosed illness, including depressive illness. Valliant & Valliant (1990) found that antisocial behaviour at college was not associated, 45 years later, with any important psychosocial adjustment at the age of 65.

Social expectations of behaviour also change. An old man who strikes another person is less likely to be charged with assault than a young man who does the same. An old woman who behaves histrionically is less likely to be labelled 'hysterical' than a young woman. There are socially conditioned expectations about what is 'normal' for people in different age groups, which influence where the line is drawn between 'normal' and 'abnormal'. These changing standards make the concept of personality disorder particularly difficult to define in old age.

Box 11.1 Specific personality disorders in ICD–10 (World Health Organization, 1992)

Paranoid
Schizoid
Dissocial
Emotionally unstable (impulsive type and borderline type)
Histrionic
Anankastic
Anxious (avoidant)
Dependent

Personality disorders in older people

There are a number of practical problems in diagnosing personality disorders in older people:

(a) It is often difficult to trace behaviour back to childhood or adolescence.
(b) Older patients may live alone so it is difficult to find an informant.
(c) Informants, when available, may be biased in their reporting (such as long suffering partners).

Prevalence

Early studies found a community prevalence, in old age, of 4% for 'character disorders' including paranoid states (Kay *et al*, 1964). The prevalence of personality disorder is probably lower in old age than middle age, but it is associated with a higher psychiatric referral rate. Hospital prevalence has been found to be between 6 and 50%, depending upon the methodology used (Fogel & Westlake, 1990; Kunik *et al*, 1994). Abrams (1996) looked at 23 studies published between 1980 and 1994, and concluded that the overall prevalence rate for personality disorders in the over 50 age group is around 10%.

Association with other diagnoses

Depression

In younger patients, the presence of a personality disorder significantly affects the treatment outcome of axis I (mental state) symptoms (Peselow *et al*, 1994). It is likely the same is true in the elderly. About a third of elderly depressed patients have a personality disorder, and this is associated with a chronic outcome for depression and poor social support. Personality disorder is more common in older people with early-onset depression than late-onset depression. It may therefore reflect post-depressive personality change, predisposition to depression or a low-grade depressive subtype. Avoidant, dependent and compulsive traits are particularly likely to occur in patients with a depressive illness, irrespective of age. There may be an increase in compulsive traits in old age (Fogel & Westlake, 1990; Kunik *et al*, 1994).

Schizophrenia

The relationship between personality and schizophrenia, in old age, has not been examined recently, although there is a link between paranoid personality types and the development of late paraphrenia. There is a strong association between schizophrenia and personality disorders in younger patients. Many patients with late paraphrenia have never married and have lived alone for some time, suggesting that there may have been personality problems predating the paraphrenia.

Somatisation disorder

Hypochondriacal personality disorder is associated with psychotic depression. One early study found 'hypochondria' in two-thirds of depressed elderly in-patients (De Alarcon, 1964). The main source of preoccupation was with bowels. In 30% of patients, hypochondriacal ideas preceded depressive symptoms by two to three months, demonstrating the importance of considering depressive illness in older people presenting with health anxiety, somatic preoccupation or hypochondria. Somatoform disorders are also common in older adults and are complicated by the frequency of concurrent physical illness. In some cases, antidepressants and psychological management, including a clear explanation and a planned physical examination, are important (Wattis & Martin, 1993).

Diogenes' syndrome

Diogenes was a Greek philosopher, living in the fourth century B.C., who became famous for living in a barrel. When Alexander, the warlord, asked him if there was anything he could do to help, Diogenes asked Alexander to 'step out of the light'. Diogenes believed happiness could only be achieved through contemplation of oneself, and consequently, there was no need to involve others. The 'Diogenes syndrome' refers to a syndrome of self-neglect in older people, unaccompanied by a medical or psychiatric condition sufficient to account for the situation. It can be seen as the response of someone with a particular personality type to the hardships of old age and loneliness (Howard & Bergmann, 1993). Management is notoriously difficult as it is often impossible to form a therapeutic alliance with the patient.

Dementia

Personality changes occur in organic disorders (Petry *et al*, 1989; Dian *et al*, 1990; Burns, 1992), although these changes are not classified as personality disorders. Negative personality changes are reported by relatives in two-thirds of people with dementia. Four patterns of personality change have been reported: alteration at onset of dementia, with little subsequent change; ongoing change with disease progression; regression to previously disturbed behaviours; and no change.

Negative personality traits such as being more out of touch, reliant on others, childish, listless, changeable, unreasonable, lifeless, unhappy, cold, cruel, irritable and mean, tend to be attributed to people with dementia. Some of these perceived changes may be due to other person's reaction to the illness; some might be directly determined by organic change; and others may mark a reaction of the person, with dementia, to their experience.

Management of personality disorder

When a personality disorder is associated with a functional mental illness, the first concern must be to treat the latter. Many personality 'traits' will resolve with treatment of the underlying functional disorder (Peselow *et al*, 1994). However, when a patient has persistent or residual symptoms of a personality disorder, a consistent approach from an experienced therapist will bring most benefit. As with younger patients, forming a therapeutic alliance with a patient whose early life experience may have taught him or her to distrust authority figures is difficult (Norton, 1996). Supportive, dynamic and cognitive approaches can all play a role, depending on present symptoms. It is particularly important to ensure a consistency of approach between involved professionals, and this requires good communication. Efforts may also be helpful at modifying the reaction of significant other people to unwanted behaviour.

When changes of personality are secondary to dementia, the increased dependence of the person with dementia on the environment, including care-givers, means management is often through changing that environment. This could involve an analysis of unwanted behaviour and contingency management. More general advice can be given to care-givers to help them become more aware of changes in personality and the best ways of dealing with them (see Chapter 6). Management is summarised in Box 11.2.

Outcome

Abnormal personality traits, by definition, are relatively stable. However, since they represent maturational defects they might be expected to resolve with age. Longitudinal studies show that while personality tends

---

Box 11.2 Management of personality disorders

Treat any mental state disorder
Consistent, long-term approach
Form a therapeutic alliance
Supportive, dynamic or cognitive psychotherapy
Good communication between professionals
Involve significant others

to be stable throughout life, introversion increases with age (Howard & Bergmann, 1993). Changes in the health of the individual, or changes of environment (e.g. moving to residential care), may sometimes precipitate maladaptive behaviour that is taken to signify personality disorder. Personality may also continue to develop abnormally with increasing age, perhaps undergoing a transformation into frank illness, as in the development of paraphrenia in someone with a previous tendency to be isolated and suspicious of others. Borderline personality disorder, in later life, may involve an inability to formulate future plans or pursue goal directed activity, and elderly patients with severe personality disorders may disrupt nursing homes and other service delivery systems.

Sexuality

Research into the important topic of sexual behaviour in old age is still limited. A steep decline in marital sexual activity occurs in extreme old age (Marsiglio & Donnelly, 1991). Attitudes and health are likely to contribute to this as much as simple ageing. There is a place for sexual therapy with older couples which include such practical remedies as hormone replacement therapy, intracavernosal prostaglandins and vaginal lubricants. The place of the new drug sildenafil has yet to be established. Other considerations include the treatment of remedial disorders (like depression) and an exploration of the relationship and inhibitions.

Problems may occur with inappropriate sexual activity in older people in residential and nursing home care (Barker & Wattis, 1991). Of course, whereas public masturbation is unlikely to be acceptable, a sexual relationship between unattached older people may only be a problem because of staff and family disapproval. Sympathetic understanding is the basis of all management, whether behavioural or pharmacological (Seymour, 1990).

Alcohol dependence

Definition

Alcohol is a unique drug in terms of its ready availability 'over the counter' and its social acceptability. Many terms have been used to describe those who come to harm through the use of alcohol but 'alcohol dependence' (Edwards & Gross, 1976) and 'harmful drinking' are perhaps the most useful. Alcohol dependence is defined as a serious medical and psychiatric disorder, characterised by certain features (Box 11.3). Harmful drinking is defined as a pattern of alcohol use that causes damage to physical or mental health. There is considerable overlap between the two terms.

ICD–10 includes the following clinical conditions within the classification of mental and behavioural disorders due to psychoactive

---

Box 11.3 Summary of the ICD–10 criteria for dependence (World Health Organization, 1992)

Three or more of the following in the last year:
(a) A strong desire or sense of compulsion to take the substance
(b) Difficulties in controlling substance taking behaviour
(c) A physiological withdrawal state, on reducing or stopping the substance
(d) Evidence of tolerance
(e) Progressive neglect of other pleasures
(f) Persisting despite harm

---

substance use, acute intoxication, harmful use, dependence syndrome and withdrawal state.

Effect of ageing on alcohol metabolism

The College guidelines for 'safe' drinking are 14 units of alcohol a week for women and 21 units a week for men (Chick & Cantwell, 1994). These upper limits take no account of age, and such drinking may harm an older person. With age, body water content declines and body fat content increases, so that lean body mass decreases by about 10% between the ages of 20 and 70. This results in altered distribution and increased blood alcohol levels for a given dose of alcohol (Vestal *et al*, 1977). Ageing organs, including the brain, are less able to withstand the toxic effects of alcohol. Drug interactions with benzodiazepines (Cook *et al*, 1984), neuroleptics or opiates are more common.

Epidemiology

Surveys, in the elderly, are limited by several factors:

(a) under-reporting of current consumption occurs because of cultural factors;
(b) 'retrospective bias' is stronger in older people;
(c) screening tools may not be appropriate for old age;
(d) the heaviest drinkers may be missed; and
(e) broad categories, such as 'heavy drinking', are of limited relevance in older people.

Some research has attempted to identify problem drinkers and follow patterns of alcohol consumption longitudinally (Mishara & Kastembaum, 1992). It appears that alcohol intake remains relatively high in the 65–75 age range but falls markedly in the 75–85 age range. There are large differences in age-related intake and dependence in different cultural settings, even within the same country. Men are more likely to be regular drinkers, although if women do drink regularly, they are as likely as men to exceed 'sensible' limits. In some cultures, older women have higher rates of misuse than younger women (Seymour & Wattis, 1992). Community surveys such as the Epidemiological Catchment Area study (Holzer *et al*, 1984), probably underestimate the proportion of older alcoholism, at just under two per cent for men, and less than one per cent in women. About half the over 65-year-old population drink alcohol (Jones & Joseph, 1997).

Trends in consumption

The per capita consumption varies over time and between countries. Generally, there is a higher consumption of alcohol in countries that are richer. National trends conceal a multitude of cultural and ethnic effects. People born at different times may have different patterns of alcohol intake. For example, prohibition in the US may have influenced subsequent drinking habits in those people who were children or adolescents during that era, by placing a taboo on drinking during formative years (Knupfer & Room, 1970). There is a relationship between per capita alcohol consumption and the numbers of people developing alcohol-related problems (Leifman & Romelsjö, 1997).

Aetiology

Elderly people with alcoholism who were dependent in younger life (early onset) have different characteristics from those who started drinking heavily in later life (late onset) (Atkinson *et al*, 1990). Early-onset dependent drinkers are more likely to have a family history of alcohol misuse, a history of smoking and a greater alcohol intake. Late-onset drinkers are more likely to have an obvious precipitant for drinking; a milder, more circumscribed drink problem; and greater premorbid psychological stability. Drinking may start or escalate after a bereavement. Sometimes elderly people resort to alcohol to help them sleep or mask pain.

Medical complications

All systems of the body may be affected by alcohol (Box 11.4). A direct causal link between alcohol dependence and pathology is clear in some conditions (e.g. pancreatitis (Singh & Simsek, 1990) and liver cirrhosis (Groover, 1990)), but less clear when the aetiology is complex and multifactorial. For example, high alcohol intake is linked with hypertension

(Marmot *et al*, 1994), but other risk factors may be involved such as smoking, obesity, family history, diet or exercise. Smoking is a particular confounding factor. Many people who drink heavily also smoke, and many of the pathological processes caused or exacerbated by alcohol are also caused or exacerbated by smoking (e.g. peptic ulcers or ischaemic heart disease).

Nutrition

Alcohol dependence is associated with poor nutrition in older people. Factors include a neglected diet; poor appetite due to medical complications; malabsorption; the increased dietary demands of metabolising large quantities of alcohol; and the toxic effects of alcohol on cell metabolism. Alcohol dependence can lead to severe deficiencies of vitamins, most notably vitamins C and B group (Barburiak & Rooney, 1985).

Immune system

Heavy drinking impairs the immune system, resulting in increased susceptibility to infection, including tuberculosis. The mechanisms are complex, and at present poorly understood, although alcohol probably affects T cells and cell-mediated immunity. Alcoholic liver disease further impairs immunity (Dunne, 1989).

Cancer

Excess alcohol is a known risk factor for cancer in most regions of the gastrointestinal tract. Alcohol is also implicated in the aetiology of breast cancer (Bowlin *et al*, 1997), perhaps mediated by reduced immune surveillance.

Liver disease

Alcohol dependence results in a spectrum of liver disorders, ranging from fatty liver to cirrhosis. Liver cirrhosis is a disease of the late middle aged, or slightly older, and prognosis is worse in old age (Potter & James, 1987).

Heart disease

Dependence is associated with higher mortality from hypertension, haemorrhagic stroke and cardiomyopathy (Peacock, 1990). High alcohol intake (above safety guidelines) is probably associated with increased ischaemic heart disease. It remains unclear whether a small intake of alcohol has a cardioprotective effect.

Box 11.4 Medical complications of alcohol dependence

Vitamin deficiencies, especially B and C
Infections
Cancer, especially of the gastrointestinal tract
Liver disease
Heart disease
Drug interactions

Drug interactions

Alcohol has an additive, sedative effect to benzodiazepines, barbiturates, chloral hydrate and tricyclic antidepressants. Alcohol reduces their metabolism and raises their serum concentrations. There may also be pharmacodynamic interactions. Conversely, the metabolism of barbiturates, tolbutamide, phenytoin and warfarin may be increased as the result of enzyme induction in the liver, or reduced by liver damage. Alcohol influences compliance with medication. Elderly people may omit medication as they fear an interaction with alcohol, or elect not to take medication at all if they want to carry on drinking.

Neuropsychiatric complications

Acute intoxication

Older people rarely present in an alcoholic coma. An elderly patient presenting to casualty in a coma and smelling of alcohol may have concurrent pathology, for example, a drug overdose or a subdural haematoma. Pathological drunkenness is rare, but may occur in older people, especially men with brain damage who can behave completely out of character after a small amount of alcohol.

Withdrawal syndrome

A withdrawal syndrome, ranging from anxiety to fully developed delirium tremens with epileptic fits and coma, can largely be prevented by good management. Delirium tremens is a medical emergency demanding immediate sedation and the possible use of anti-epileptic drugs (CRAG/SCOTMEG, 1994).

Wernicke–Korsakoff syndrome

Wernicke's encephalopathy is characterised by the clinical triad of: opthalmoplegia, ataxia and delirium. It is caused by an acute deficiency of thiamine (vitamin B1) (Perkin & Hondler, 1983). Wernicke's encephalopathy is a medical emergency which requires intravenous administration of thiamine. Treatment delay increases the risk of permanent damage with Korsakoff's psychosis (Anonymous, 1990). Even with treatment only a fifth of patients with Wernicke's encephalopathy fully recover, and over half are left with Korsakoff's psychosis.

Korsakoff's psychosis is characterised by apathy, the inability to learn or form new memories, loss of insight and confabulation. Patients are otherwise mentally intact and may survive many years into old age. On CT scan, frontal brain shrinkage is particularly pronounced, suggesting a dual aetiology: thiamine deficiency and a direct neurotoxic effect of ethanol on the brain, particularly the frontal lobes. With time, up to a quarter of Korsakoff's patients make a complete recovery and half show some improvement.

Alcoholic cerebellar degeneration

This condition tends to arise in binge drinkers and so called 'skid row' populations of deteriorated long-term misusers of alcohol, and is not commonly diagnosed in the elderly (Victor *et al*, 1959). The clinical picture is identical to subacute cerebellar degeneration secondary to carcinoma of the bronchus, so a chest X-ray should always be performed in the elderly. There is a progressive ataxia of gait (without incoordination of the limbs), dysarthria and gaze-evoked nystagmus. Cerebellar damage probably arises from the direct toxic effect of very high levels of alcohol rather than a nutritional effect, as alcohol produces (lesser degrees of) cerebellar ataxia in normal subjects and there is a poor response to treatment with thiamine.

Alcoholic hallucinosis

These are persistent auditory hallucinations, usually derogatory or hostile in nature, in the context of prolonged heavy drinking. Alcoholic hallucinosis is rare in old people.

Morbid jealousy

This usually occurs in men and is characterised by paranoid delusions concerning infidelity. The delusions may be refractory to neuroleptics and stopping alcohol. Patients are often a danger to their partner or ex-partner. It is rare for this condition to arise *de novo* in old age, but it may persist into old age.

Alcoholic dementia and cortical atrophy

Increasing age is a major risk factor for alcoholic dementia. Alcohol in large quantities causes a decrease in brain size, widening of sulci and

---

Box 11.5 Neuropsychiatric complications of alcohol dependence

Acute intoxication
Withdrawal syndrome and delirium tremens
Wernicke–Korsakoff syndrome
Cerebellar degeneration
Alcoholic hallucinosis
Morbid jealousy
Dementia

---

enlargement of ventricles. There is neuronal loss affecting principally neocortex, basal ganglia, hippocampus and reticular activating system: the same areas affected principally in normal ageing. This macroscopic and microscopic brain damage is reflected in impaired performance on tests of cognition and motor skills (Lishman, 1990).

So-called 'social drinking' within the safety guidelines may affect cognitive function (Robertson, 1984). Problem-solving, abstraction abilities and memory and psychomotor abilities have been shown to be affected. There may be a continuum of cognitive deficit directly related to alcohol intake, ranging from barely detectable or no deficit (social drinking) through to Korsakoff's psychosis (very high alcohol intake). Brain damage may also result indirectly from alcohol misuse. For example, hypertension and other cardiovascular changes resulting from alcohol misuse, may cause a vascular dementia. Whenever alcohol misuse and a dementing illness coexist they pose particular problems, since the patient's impaired memory and judgement make it impossible to control his own alcohol intake. Neuropsychiatric complications are summarised in Box 11.5.

Presentation

Alcohol dependence, in older age, often presents indirectly with confusion, falls, self-neglect or associated medical problems (Wattis, 1981, 1983). Alcohol problems are often undetected as appropriate questions are not asked of older people. Information on alcohol intake must be sought, it is rarely volunteered. Patients may underestimate their weekly intake, be unaware of harmful effects or deny the link between alcohol and harmful effects. A history from an informant is vital, although the informant may have a vested interest in minimising consumption, especially if he or she is also a heavy drinker. The CAGE questionnaire (Ewing, 1984) is a useful short screening instrument (see Chapter 1).

Physical examination may reveal the medical complications of alcohol misuse. Laboratory results including a raised mean corpuscular volume or liver function tests should alert the physician to the possibility of alcohol misuse. Hyperuricaemia, hypertriglyceridaemia and hypoglycaemia may be caused or exacerbated by alcohol misuse.

Management of alcohol dependence

The principles of management are the same in the elderly as they are for younger age groups. They include the recognition of a problem (by patient, carers, doctor); the acceptance of treatment; detoxification; treatment of concurrent psychiatric and medical disorders; rehabilitation; and continuing support. Management is summarised in Box 11.6.

Therapeutic nihilism should be avoided. 'It's too late for her to change her drinking habits now' or 'beer is one of his few pleasures left in life' are ageist statements. Older alcohol misusers may find it particularly difficult to change their drinking habits if there are younger alcohol misusers colluding with them. Hospital admission is often necessary. It breaks the pattern of consumption; enables full medical assessment; treatment of any complications; assessment of mood and cognitive functioning; and the supervised initiation of treatment for concurrent psychiatric disorders.

Withdrawal regime

Admission to hospital for detoxification is often necessary as out-patient detoxification can be hazardous. Sometimes the person refuses hospital admission. Compulsory admission under the mental health legislation is often not appropriate (the Mental Health Act specifically excludes alcohol misuse as a reason for compulsory admission). In that case attempts should be made to build a relationship with the person until the need for change is accepted or the home situation deteriorates to the point that hospital admission becomes inevitable.

The alcohol withdrawal regime pays particular attention to fluid and electrolyte balance, and concurrent medical conditions. Shorter acting sedatives, such as chlormethiazole, are recommended for old people, often in reduced doses, rather than longer acting benzodiazepines such as chlordiazepoxide, although opinion is divided (CRAG/SCOTMEG, 1994). Phenytoin should be used prophylactically if there is a history of epilepsy or withdrawal fits, in which case the duration of the withdrawal regime may need to be slightly extended. Vitamin supplements are important, especially thiamine which should be given orally or parenterally with suitable precautions for anaphylaxis where Wernicke's encephalopathy is suspected.

> **Box 11.6 Summary of management**
>
> Recognition of a problem
> Acceptance of treatment
> Detoxification
> Treatment of concurrent psychiatric and medical disorders
> Rehabilitation
> Continuing support

Rehabilitation

After detoxification, rehabilitation is essential and increased social contacts may prevent recurrence. Education about the alcohol content of different drinks is necessary and a switch to low or no alcohol beers may help. Local facilities (e.g. day centres, and visits from members of the multi-disciplinary team) may provide alternatives to drinking. Alcoholics Anonymous can offer considerable support and there are related support groups for partners and children. At this stage, the emphasis is on social intervention rather than on medical treatments, such as disulfiram (antabuse), which may be dangerous in older people. For a fuller review of alcohol dependence in old age see *A Handbook of Nutrition in the Elderly* (Wattis & Seymour, 1993).

Other drug dependence

The therapeutic use of narcotics increases with age, but non-therapeutic misuse declines (Dunne, 1994). It may be that the non-therapeutic use of drugs in old people will increase as the 'hippies' and 'flower people' of the 1960s grow older (cohort effect). For now, a more urgent problem is the number of older people who are dependent on benzodiazepine, usually prescribed as sleeping tablets, but sometimes as anxiolytics (Dunne, 1994; McInnes & Powell, 1994). The longer-acting hypnotics have 'hang-over' effects on cognitive function and some of the benzodiazepines appear to interfere

> **Box 11.7 Withdrawal of benzodiazepines**
>
> Educate and inform the patient, and other involved individuals
> Change to a long-acting benzodiazepine
> Gradually reduce over several weeks
> Closely monitor the patient
> Offer therapeutic help including relaxation therapy

with memory. Evidence is emerging that benzodiazepine dependence is associated with increased hospital admissions and length of stay. Withdrawal regimes are available, the principles of which are in Box 11.7.

Conclusion

Personality disorder, sexual problems and alcohol dependence present differently in older people. This is partly due to social and cultural differences and partly due to age-related changes in the body, including the central nervous system. In particular, physical illness and drug interactions are more common in older people and these are often important. Although it is obvious that older people have these problems, they have traditionally been neglected. Now that a growing body of research has demonstrated their significance to old age psychiatry, they may be taken more seriously.

References

Abrams, R. C. (1996) Personality disorders in the elderly. *International Journal of Geriatric Psychiatry*, 11, 759–763.

American Psychiatric Association (1994) *Diagnostic and Statistical Manual of Mental Disorders* (4th edn) (DSM–IV). Washington, DC: APA.

Anonymous (1990) Korsakoff's syndrome. *Lancet*, 336, 873.

Atkinson, R. M., Tolson, R. L. & Turner, J. A. (1990) Late versus early onset problem drinking in older men. *Alcoholism, Clinical and Experimental Research*, 14, 574–579.

Barburiak, J. J. & Rooney, C. B. (1985) Alcohol and its effects on nutrition in the elderly. In *Handbook of Nutrition in the Aged* (ed. R. R. Watson), pp. 215–248. Boca Raton, FL: CRC Press.

Barker, G. & Wattis, J. P. (1991) Dangerous liaisons? *Nursing the Elderly*, April, 23–24.

Bowlin, S. J., Leske, M. C., Varma, A., *et al* (1997) Breast cancer risk and alcohol consumption: results from a large case control study. *International Journal of Epidemiology*, 26, 915–923.

Burns, A. (1992) Psychiatric phenomena in dementia of the Alzheimer type. *International Psychogeriatrics*, 4 (suppl. 1), 43–54.

Chick, J. & Cantwell, R. (eds) (1994) *Seminars in Alcohol and Drug Misuse*. London: Gaskell.

Cook, P. J., Flanagan, R. & James, I. M. (1984) Diazepam tolerance: effect of age, regular sedation and alcohol. *British Medical Journal*, 289, 351–353.

CRAG/SCOTMEG Working Group on Mental Illness (1994) *The Management of Alcohol Withdrawal and Delirium Tremens*. Edinburgh: Scottish Office.

De Alarcon, R. (1964) Hypochondriasis and depression in the aged. *Gerontologia Clinica*, 6, 266–277.

Dian, L., Cummings, J. L., Petry, S., *et al* (1990) Personality alterations in multi-infarct dementia. *Psychosomatics*, 31, 415–419.

Dunne, F. J. (1989) Alcohol and the immune system. *British Medical Journal*, 298, 543–544.

—— (1994) Misuse of alcohol or drugs by elderly people. *British Medical Journal*, 308, 608–609.

Edwards, G. & Gross, M. M. (1976) Alcohol dependence: provisional description of a clinical syndrome. *British Medical Journal, i*, 1058–1061.

Erikson, E. H. (1965) *Childhood and Society*. Harmondsworth: Penguin Books.

Ewing, J. (1984) Detecting alcoholism: the CAGE questionnaire. *Journal of the American Medical Association*, 252, 1905–1907.

Fogel, B. S. & Westlake, R. (1990) Personality disorder diagnoses and age in inpatients with major depression. *Journal of Clinical Psychiatry*, 51, 232–235.

Groover, J. R. (1990) Alcoholic liver disease. *Emergency Medicine Clinics of North America*, 8, 887–902.

Holzer, H., Robins, L. N., Myers, J. K., *et al* (1984) Antecedents and correlates of alcohol misuse and dependence in the elderly. In *Nature and Extent of Alcohol Problems Among the Elderly* (eds G. Maddox, L. N. Robins & N. Rosenberg), National Institute on Drug Abuse Research Monograph No 14. Rockville, MD: DHHS, US Government Printing Office.

Howard, R. & Bergmann, K. (1993) Personality disorders in old age. *International Review of Psychiatry*, 5, 455–460.

Jones, T. V. & Joseph, C. (1997) *Alcohol Use Disorders in Older Adults: Clinical Guidelines*. New York: American Geriatrics Society.

Kay, D. W., Beamish, P. & Roth, M. (1964) Old age mental disorders in Newcastle-upon-Tyne. Part I: A study of prevalence. *British Journal of Psychiatry*, 110, 146–158.

Knupfer, G. & Room, R. (1970) Abstainers in a metropolitan community. *Quarterly Journal of Studies in Alcohol*, 31, 108–131.

Kroessler, D. (1990) Personality disorder in the elderly. *Hospital and Community Psychiatry*, 41, 1325–1329.

Kunik, M. E., Mulsant, B. H., Rifai, A. H., *et al* (1994) Diagnostic rate of comorbid personality disorder in elderly psychiatric inpatients. *American Journal of Psychiatry*, 151, 603–605.

Leifman, H. & Romelsjö, A. (1997) The effect of changes in alcohol consumption on mortality and admisssions with alcohol-related diagnoses in Stockholm county – a time series analysis. *Addiction*, 92, 1523–1536.

Lishman, W. A. (1990) Alcohol and the brain. *British Journal of Psychiatry*, 56, 635–644.

Marsiglio, W. & Donnelly, D. (1991) Sexual relations in later life: a national study of married persons. *Journal of Gerontology*, 46, S338–S344.

Marmot, M. G., Elliott, P., Shipley, M. J., *et al* (1994) Alcohol and blood pressure: the INTERSALT study. *British Medical Journal*, 308, 1263–1267.

McInnes, E. & Powell, J. (1994) Drug and alcohol referrals: are elderly substance abuse diagnoses and referrals being missed? *British Medical Journal*, 308, 444–446.

Mishara, B. L. & Kastenbaum, R. (1992) *Alcohol and Old Age*. New York: Grune and Stratton.

Norton, K. (1996) Management of difficult personality disorder patients. *Advances in Psychiatric Treatment*, 2, 202–210.

Peacock, W. F. (1990) Cardiac disease in the alcoholic patient. *Emergency Medicine Clinics in North America*, 8, 775–791.

Perkin, G. D. & Hondler, C. E. (1983) Wernicke–Korsakoff syndrome. *British Journal of Hospital Medicine*, 30, 331–334.

Peselow, E. D., Sanfilipo, M. P., Fieve, R. R, *et al* (1994) Personality traits during depression and after clinical recovery. *British Journal of Psychiatry*, 164, 349–354.

Petry, S., Cummings, J. L., Hill, M. A., *et al* (1989) Personality alterations in dementia of the Alzheimer type: a three year follow-up study. *Journal of Geriatric Psychiatry and Neurology*, 2, 203–207.

Potter, J. F. & James, O. W. F. (1987) Clinical features and prognosis of alcoholic liver disease in respect of advancing age. *Gerontology*, 33, 380–387.

Robertson, I. (1984) Does moderate drinking cause mental impairment? *British Medical Journal*, 289, 711–712.

Seymour, J. (1990) Sexuality in the elderly. *Care of the Elderly*, 2, 315–316.

—— & Wattis, J. P. (1992) Alcohol abuse in old age. *Reviews in Clinical Gerontology*, 2, 141–150.

Singh, M. & Simsek, H. (1990) Ethanol and the pancreas: current status. *Gastroenterology*, 98, 1051–1062.

Valliant, G. E. & Valliant, C. O. (1990) Natural history of male psychosocial health. XII. A 45 year study of predictors of successful aging at age 65. *American Journal of Psychiatry*, 147, 31–37.

Vestal, R. E., McGuire, E. A., Tobin, J. D., *et al* (1977) Ageing and ethanol metabolism. *Clinical Pharmacology and Therapeutics*, 21, 343–354.

Victor, M., Adams, R. D. & Mancall, E. L. (1959) A restricted form of cerebellar cortical degeneration occurring in alcoholic patients. *Archives of Neurology*, 1, 579–585.

Wattis, J. P. (1981) Alcohol problems in the elderly. *Journal of the American Geriatrics Society*, 3, 131–134.

—— (1983) Alcohol and old people. *British Journal of Psychiatry*, 143, 306–307.

—— & Martin, C. (1993) *Practical Psychiatry of Old Age*. London: Chapman and Hall.

—— & Seymour, J. (1993) Alcohol abuse in elderly people: medical and psychiatric consequences. In *A Handbook of Nutrition in the Elderly* (2nd edn). Boca Raton, FL: CRC Press.

World Health Organization (1992) *The Tenth Revision of the International Classification of Diseases and Related Health Problems* (ICD–10). Geneva: WHO.

12 Imaging

John Besson

Structural imaging

Computerised tomography (CT), developed in the 1970s, allows a black and white image to be computed from multiple beams of X-rays. Magnetic resonance imaging (MRI) uses powerful magnets to alter the spin of hydrogen atoms. This allows mapping of their distribution. CT and MRI can be used to identify intracranial lesions such as tumours, abscesses, haematomas, haemorrhages, infarcts and normal pressure hydrocephalus. Quantification of changes in brain atrophy can be carried out using linear or area measurements of brain compartments. Computerised three dimensional displays of the brain allow the volumes of brain structures, like the hippocampus or temporal lobes, to be measured. Changes within the parenchyma of the brain, including white matter lesions, can be identified with MRI.

Box 12.1 Advantages and disadvantages of magnetic resonance imaging

Advantages
Distinguishes between temporal lobe and posterior fossa structures
Gives a three dimensional display of the brain
Sensitive to white matter lesions, distinguishes between grey and white matter
Does not expose subjects to ionising radiation, particularly useful for repeated imaging

Disadvantages
Some patients are unable to tolerate the claustrophobic scanners
Magnets may displace pacemakers or metal in the body
Calcified lesions are poorly visualised on MRI but clearly seen on CT
MRI costs more than CT

Functional imaging

Single photon emission computed tomography (SPECT) is a technique which involves intravenously injecting a radio-labelled tracer, and mapping its distribution in the brain. The radio-labelled compounds, depending on blood flow, are taken up and trapped by brain cells allowing a scanner to map their distribution. The scans can either be looked at, or quantities can be measured by comparing the radioactivity in different areas of the brain. Often the regions under study are compared with standards, such as 'total brain activity' or the activity of a 'neutral region', such as the occipital lobe in Alzheimer's disease. This gives a measure of regional cerebral blood flow (rCBF). Receptor populations can be mapped by injecting radio-labelled isotopes (radioligands) which bind to specific neurochemical receptors.

Positron emission tomography (PET) uses injected, radio-labelled material to measure blood flow, regional metabolism and receptor populations. The half-lives of the radio-labels used in PET are much shorter than in SPECT (^{15}O has a half-life of two minutes while ^{18}F has a half-life of 110 minutes), and therefore need to be made on site, using a cyclotron. This makes PET extremely expensive and only available to a few centres. Using ^{15}O labelled water, subjects can be imaged repeatedly in the same session, under different states. This allows brain activity to be measured in response to external sensory stimuli, voluntary movement, cognitive tasks and drugs.

Magnetic resonance spectroscopy (MRS) is a technique used to measure metabolites in the brain, giving the concentrations in the regions studied. It has the advantage of being a functional scanner which does not expose the subjects to radiation, so it is useful for repeated imaging. It has the disadvantage of being claustrophobic for some patients. At present it is exclusively a research tool.

Box 12.2 Advantages and disadvantages of positron emission tomography

Advantages
Higher resolution and greater sensitivity than SPECT
Shorter half-life radio-labels allow more activation studies to be carried out in a session
More precisely quantified, whereas SPECT is used qualitatively or semi-quantitatively

Disadvantages
Very much more expensive than SPECT
Only available in a few specialist centres
Less patient friendly

Table 12.1 Brain-imaging techniques and main uses

	Techniques	Main use
Computed tomography	Structural	Diagnosis
Magnetic resonance imaging	Structural	Diagnosis
Single photon emission computed tomography	Functional	Diagnosis and research
Positron emission tomography	Functional	Research
Magnetic resonance spectroscopy	Functional	Research

Dementia

Computerised tomography

The main value of CT in dementia is to exclude intracranial pathology. Space occupying lesions such as tumours, abscesses or haematomatas, and lesions giving rise to altered ventricular size such as normal pressure hydrocephalus, can be identified. About 5% of patients with dementia have these lesions (Philpot & Burns, 1989).

The presence of infarcts has been used to differentiate vascular dementia from Alzheimer's disease. There are more white matter lesions in patients with Alzheimer's disease than in normal subjects, although this differentiation is not absolute and normal subjects often have vascular lesions.

In ageing and dementia, the brain atrophies (shrinks). Atrophy is identified by measuring the size of the ventricles and sulci in one of four ways: visually; linear changes on a standard section; area changes; and volume changes of the relevant spaces.

CT studies usually use linear or area measures, the latter being more sensitive. With ageing there is cortical atrophy and lateral ventricular enlargement. These tend to be greater after the age of 60, and correlate with age and cognitive impairment. In dementia, the third ventricle also enlarges and this correlates with cognitive impairment. Although measures of atrophy are greater in patients with dementia than controls, there is an overlap, and a diagnosis cannot be made on CT alone. However, follow-up CT scans, after a year, show that ventricular size increases much more rapidly in dementia than in normal ageing. A sensitivity and specificity of diagnosis approaching 100% can be made on serial scans (Luxenberg *et al*, 1987).

Specific syndromes in Alzheimer's disease may be associated with regional atrophy, such as delusional misidentification and accentuated right frontal degeneration. In Creutzfeldt–Jakob disease, atrophy is found in around 80% of cases.

Magnetic resonance imaging

MRI is more sensitive than CT at detecting white matter lesions. In Alzheimer's disease grey matter volumes are reduced, while white matter volumes are unchanged. This is particularly marked in the temporal lobe, which is consistent with the cortical cell loss found in pathological studies.

Hippocampal volumes

MRI is used to measure the volumes of the hippocampus, amygdala and temporal lobe. These volumetric measurements, corrected for brain size, are smaller in disease, and have been shown to accurately distinguish Alzheimer's disease from normal ageing, without overlap (Kesslak *et al*, 1991). Furthermore, hippocampal volumes are smaller in patients with age associated memory impairment than in normal ageing, and are similar to patients with Alzheimer's disease.

Hippocampal atrophy also occurs in vascular dementia, Parkinson's disease with dementia, and to a lesser degree, in Parkinson's disease without dementia. Hippocampal volume correlates with memory scores in Alzheimer's disease and Parkinson's disease with dementia, but not in vascular dementia or Parkinson's disease without dementia. This may reflect the presence of Alzheimer's disease pathology, in dementia associated with Parkinson's disease (Laasko *et al*, 1996).

Apolipoprotein E4 alleles appear to predispose people to Alzheimer's disease. They are also associated with more severe neuropathological changes, particularly amyloid deposition. MRI studies have shown that Apo E4 alleles are associated with greater volume loss in the hippocampus and amygdala, but not the frontal lobes (Lehtovirta *et al*, 1996).

White matter lesions

The image in MRI is compiled from measurements of proton behaviour following excitation by magnetic pulses. The behaviour of greatest interest is the 'relaxation time', which is the time taken for excited protons to return to their pre-stimulus positions. Relaxation time reflects the water content of tissue, and is altered in a number of diseases. In Alzheimer's disease it is prolonged in the hippocampus, although there is significant overlap with controls.

White matter lesions, associated with long relaxation times, are found more often in vascular dementia than Alzheimer's disease (Erkinjuntti *et al*, 1987). The lesions are more severe. White matter lesions in Alzheimer's disease tend to be associated with vascular risk factors, particularly hypertension, and are also found in normal ageing. Hypertension is itself associated with brain atrophy and white matter abnormalities. Furthermore, hypertensive patients, without severe white matter changes, have reduced cerebral metabolism, but normal neuropsychological performance. The reduction in metabolism is small, and greatest in the vascular water-shed regions of the brain, a distribution different from the metabolic pattern seen in Alzheimer's disease. This evidence suggests that white matter lesions can be helpful in the diagnosis of dementia.

In Creutzfeldt–Jakob disease MRI shows diffuse cerebral atrophy and deep white matter lesions. There are bilateral, symmetrical, paired areas of increased signal in the lentiform nucleus. Regions of bilateral, increased relaxation times occur in hypoxic and ischaemic damage, such as carbon monoxide poisoning.

Single photon emission computed tomography

Alzheimer's disease

Regional cerebral blood flow reflects the severity of dementia. In Alzheimer's disease there is a characteristic picture of reduced rCBF in the temporal and posterior parietal lobes. This is consistent with neuropathological changes and neuropsychological testing (Burns *et al*, 1989). In early Alzheimer's disease these changes may be undetectable, or confined to the temporal lobes. As the disease progresses reduced rCBF is seen in the temporal and posterior parietal cortex, then more globally. In more severe Alzheimer's disease reduced rCBF is found in the frontal cortex.

Reduced rCBF correlates with deficits on neuropsychological testing. In the early stages, the most profound correlations involve temporal and posterior parietal rCBF, and global scores of dementia, praxis and language (Burns *et al*, 1989). As the disease progresses, reduced frontal rCBF correlates with neuropsychology (Brown *et al*, 1996). Using clinical criteria the rate of accurate diagnosis of Alzheimer's disease is around 75%. With SPECT this increases to over 90% (Read *et al*, 1995).

Physostigmine (a short acting acetylcholinesterase inhibitor) increases performance in some memory tasks in Alzheimer's disease. SPECT studies have shown that it is associated with increased left cortical and frontal rCBF. Tacrine (another acetylcholinesterase inhibitor) increases right temporal rCBF in Alzheimer patients whose performance improves on memory tasks (O'Brien, 1996). These studies suggest SPECT can play an important role in providing objective evidence of improvement with the new acetylcholinesterase inhibitors, such as donepezil.

Patients with Alzheimer's disease and delusions, have reduced temporal rCBF compared to non-delusional patients with the same severity of disease. Patients with hallucinations have relatively increased parietal rCBF (Kotrla *et al*, 1995).

Age associated memory impairment

In age associated memory impairment there are perfusion deficits between those of Alzheimer's disease and controls. The reduced rCBF correlates with global cognitive impairment. This finding, together with the finding that hippocampal volumes are similar to Alzheimer's disease, suggests that the two conditions are on a continuum rather than being distinct entities (Parnetti *et al*, 1996).

Vascular dementia

Multi-infarct dementia is associated with focal deficits of rCBF, corresponding to ischaemic lesions. The contrast between the temporal and parietal reduced rCBF found in Alzheimer's disease, and the irregular perfusion deficits found in vascular dementia, mean that SPECT can play a role in the differentiation between these two conditions.

Lewy body dementia

Lewy body dementia is a relatively new type of dementia characterised by a fluctuating cognitive impairment, visual hallucinations and marked sensitivity to the extrapyramidal side-effects of neuroleptics. Preliminary data suggest that patients with Lewy body dementia show reduced temporal and parietal rCBF, in a similar picture to Alzheimer's disease (Read *et al*, 1995).

Frontotemporal dementia

Frontotemporal dementia accounts for around 15% of primary degenerative dementia. It is characterised by behavioural changes and frontal lobe neuropsychological deficits. Patients with this condition have reduced frontal or frontotemporal rCBF. Post-mortem pathology demonstrates an absence of plaques and tangles, but marked frontal gliosis and neuronal loss. Pick bodies are found in a quarter to a half of cases. In Creutzfeldt–Jakob disease, irregular dispersed mottled deficits are found.

Positron emission tomography

Coupling

PET allows CBF and cerebral metabolic rates for oxygen and glucose to be measured. Generally speaking, CBF and cerebral metabolism change together (i.e. they are coupled). However, in ageing (which is associated with declining blood flow and metabolism), the blood flow declines faster. This is because neurones relatively increase their oxygen extraction from the blood. Uncoupling can also occur in certain pathological processes, the principal one being vascular disease.

CBF and oxygen metabolism decline in Alzheimer's disease and vascular dementia, and this decline is more severe as the dementia advances. In vascular dementia, oxygen extraction increases in order to meet the oxygen requirements of active tissue, in the presence of a declining blood supply. In Alzheimer's disease reduction in the metabolic requirements of the ailing neurones means that lower blood flow adequately meets the oxygen demand.

In other words, the decline is coupled in Alzheimer's disease, but uncoupled in vascular dementia. This is useful in differentiating the two conditions. It also demonstrates the complex relationship between blood flow, metabolism and disease.

Alzheimer's disease

In Alzheimer's disease the cerebral metabolic rate for glucose is reduced by 20 to 30%. The reduction correlates with cognitive impairment. The pattern of impairment in glucose and oxygen metabolism mirrors that of cerebral blood flow (i.e. reductions occur in the temporal and posterior parietal lobes). Deficits in early dementia may be asymmetrical. Longitudinal studies, one to two years apart, show that in mild to moderate dementia, metabolism in the parietal cortex decreases faster than in the frontal cortex. In the severely demented, metabolism in the frontal cortex falls faster (Jagust, 1988).

Patients with familial Alzheimer's disease show no difference in regional glucose metabolism from sporadic cases. However, patients with early-onset Alzheimer's disease show different patterns of regional glucose metabolism to late-onset Alzheimer's disease. Metabolic impairment is found mainly in the frontal and parietotemporal cortices in the early-onset group, whereas there are more global reductions in the late-onset group (Guze *et al*, 1992).

Extrapyramidal signs, particularly rigidity and tremor, are found in some patients with Alzheimer's dementia. Dopamine receptor imaging, using 18-fluorodopa, shows no difference in basal ganglia uptake between normal controls and rigid, and non-rigid, patients with Alzheimer's disease. In contrast, patients with Parkinson's disease show a marked reduction in 18-fluorodopa uptake in the basal ganglia, demonstrating that the extrapyramidal syndrome in Alzheimer's disease may have a different pathogenesis to Parkinson's disease (Tyrrel *et al*, 1990). In Creutzfeldt–Jakob disease, areas of diffuse hypometabolism occur, corresponding to spongiform changes.

Magnetic resonance spectroscopy

MRS allows a number of brain metabolites to be measured. Proton spectroscopy and phosphorus spectroscopy are the two most commonly used techniques.

Proton spectroscopy

Proton spectroscopy is used to measure N-acetylaspartate, which is a marker of neuronal damage and the most commonly studied metabolite.

Box 12.3 Imaging in Alzheimer's disease

CT: trophy, including third ventricle, correlates with cognitive impairment, increases rapidly

MRI: reduced grey matter, hippocampus, amygdala and temporal lobes volumes

SPECT: characteristic reduction in blood flow in temporal and parietal regions

PET: reduced blood flow and metabolism in temporal and parietal regions

MRS: abnormal synthesis of membrane phospholipids early in the disease

---

N-acetylaspartate is reduced in patients with Alzheimer's disease and this correlates with the number of senile plaques and neurofibrillary tangles. N-acetylaspartate is also reduced in Creutzfeldt–Jakob disease.

Phosphorus spectroscopy

Phosphorus spectroscopy allows the direct measurement, *in vivo*, of brain membrane phospholipid metabolism. Phosphomonoesters reflect the rate of synthesis of membrane phospholipids, and phosphodiesters reflect the rate of degeneration of membrane phospholipids. In ageing, phosphomonoesters decrease while phosphodiesters increase. In Alzheimer's disease, phosphomonoesters increase early in the course of the disease. Later, phosphomonoester levels correlate negatively, and phosphodiester levels correlate positively, with the number of senile plaques (Pettegrew *et al*, 1988). This suggests that abnormalities in the synthesis of membrane phospholipids occur early in Alzheimer's disease. This technique may help to differentiate Alzheimer's disease and vascular dementia.

Box 12.4 Imaging in vascular dementia

CT: increased number of infarcts

MRI: white matter lesions are more numerous and severe than in Alzheimer's disease

SPECT: irregular perfusion deficits

PET: cerebral blood flow and metabolism reduced and uncoupled

MRS: absence of phospholipid changes allow differentiation from Alzheimer's disease

---

Affective disorders

Computerised tomography

Late-onset depression is associated with cortical atrophy and ventricular enlargement. The CT scan appearances are closer to subjects with dementia than controls. Cortical CT density is reduced, while caudate density is increased. Patients with greater cortical atrophy have a reduced life expectancy. Patients with depressive pseudo-dementia have increased lateral ventricular size and decreased tissue density counts.

Magnetic resonance imaging

MRI shows elderly depressed patients to have more atrophy than controls. Changes include: sulcal atrophy; larger Sylvian fissures; larger ventricles; more basal ganglia lesions; smaller caudate nuclei, putamen and hippocampal volumes; and more subcortical hyperintensities.

Hippocampal atrophy increases with age in Alzheimer's disease and depression (O'Brien *et al*, 1994). Using visual semi-quantitative measures of hippocampal atrophy it is possible to differentiate up to 90% of patients with Alzheimer's disease from major depression. Depressed patients with delusions do not differ from those without delusions on any MRI measure (Rabins *et al*, 1991).

White matter lesions

There are two types of white matter lesions: those adjacent to the ventricular system, periventricular white matter lesions, and those separate from the ventricles, in deep white matter.

Periventricular white matter lesions and deep white matter lesions are both more common in depression. However, periventricular white matter lesions occur more frequently in Alzheimer's disease than depression, and deep white matter lesions are found in a number of conditions including multi-infarct dementia, multiple sclerosis, hydrocephalus and Binswanger's disease

In depression, deep white matter lesions tend to occur in the left basal ganglia and, to a lesser extent, the right frontal area. They are associated with sporadic, late-onset depression, psychomotor retardation and poor prognosis (O'Brien *et al* , 1996). Deep white matter lesions may represent a biological factor predisposing the elderly to depression.

Some studies have linked deep white matter lesions with cognitive impairment, but this is not a universal finding. Deep white matter lesions are significantly increased in late-onset mania. Lesions occur in equal frequency in both hemispheres. Otherwise, there is no difference from controls in terms of ventricular size or the presence of periventricular white matter lesions.

Box 12.5 Imaging in depression

CT: cortical atrophy and ventricular enlargement
MRI: atrophy, ventricular enlargement, basal ganglia and white
    matter lesions
SPECT: reduced rCBF, sparing the posterior parietal cortex

Single photon emission computed tomography

SPECT studies in elderly patients with depression have found reduced global blood flow and reduced rCBF in the anterior cingulate, frontal and temporal areas, but no reduction in the posterior parietal cortex. This may be helpful in distinguishing patients with depression from Alzheimer's disease (Curran *et al*, 1993). Depressed patients who have larger areas of white matter intensity on MRI have lower rCBF.

Paraphrenia

Computerised tomography

CT studies have found that in paraphrenia there is dilation of the lateral ventricles, but the degree of cortical atrophy is normal for the patient's age. People with paraphrenia with Schneiderian first rank symptoms have more cerebral atrophy, particularly in the left frontal lobe (Howard *et al*, 1992).

Magnetic resonance imaging

Patients with paraphrenia have greater lateral and third ventricular volumes than controls. When patients are subdivided into schizophrenia or delusional disorder, enlargement is slightly more marked in the delusional disorder group. Temporal lobe volumes were smaller in patients with delusional disorder than with schizophrenia, or controls (Howard *et al*, 1994).

White matter lesions are not found more frequently in paraphrenia. Periventricular white matter and subcortical grey matter hyperintensities are associated with raised blood pressure. Furthermore, these lesions and deep white matter lesions are associated with increasing age (Howard *et al*, 1995).

Conclusion

The role of imaging is shifting from predominantly research, to clinical investigation and diagnosis. Structural imaging remains of greatest clinical value in identifying brain lesions in the elderly such as tumours, infarcts, vascular malformations and hydrocephalus. CT and MRI are also useful at measuring focal and global atrophy and the volumes of specific brain regions. This is particularly informative when done serially. Functional imaging offers the promise of a greater understanding of the physiological processes in mental illnesses in the elderly. SPECT is the most widely available technique and can offer information to aid diagnosis and treatment plans. Imaging is increasingly becoming part of a full, clinical assessment in old age psychiatry.

References

Brown, D. R. P., Hunter, R., Wyper, D. J., *et al* (1996) Longitudinal changes in cognitive function and regional cerebral function in Alzheimer's Disease: A SPECT blood flow study. *Journal of Psychiatric Research*, 30, 109–126.

Burns, A., Philpot, M. P., Costa, D. C., *et al* (1989) The investigation of Alzheimer's disease with single photon emission tomograph. *Journal of Neurology, Neurosurgery and Psychiatry*, 52, 248–253.

Curran, S. M., Murray, C. M., Van-Beck, M., *et al* (1993) A single photon emission computed tomograph study of regional brain function in elderly patients with major depression and with Alzheimer type dementia. *British Journal of Psychiatry*, 163, 155–165.

Erkinjuntti, T., Ketonen, L., Sulkava, R., *et al* (1987) Do white matter changes on MRI and CT differentiate vascular dementia from Alzheimer's disease? *Journal of Neurology, Neurosurgery and Psychiatry*, 50, 37–42.

Guze, B. H., Hoffinann, J. M. & Mazziotta, J. C. (1992) Positron emission tomograph and familial Alzheimer's Disease: a pilot study. *Journal of the American Geriatrics Society*, 40, 120–123.

Howard, R. J., Forstl, H., Naguib, M., *et al* (1992) First rank symptoms of Schneider in late paraphrenia. Cortical structural correlates. *British Journal of Psychiatry*, 160, 108–109.

——, Almeida, O., Levy, R., *et al* (1994) Quantitative magnetic resonance imaging volumetry distinguishes delusional disorder from late onset schizophrenia. *British Journal of Psychiatry*, 165, 474–480.

——, Cox, T., Almeida, O., *et al* (1995) White matter signal hyperintensities in the brains of patients with late paraphrenia and the normal community living elderly. *Biological Psychiatry*, 38, 86–91.

Jagust, W. J., Freidland, R. P. & Budinger, T. F. (1988) Longitudinal studies of regional cerebral metabolism in Alzheimer's disease. *Neurology*, 38, 909–1012.

Kesslak, J. P , Nalcioglu, O. & Cotman, C. W. (1991) Quantification of magnetic resonance scans for hippocampal and parahippocampal atrophy in Alzheimer's disease. *Neurology*, 44, 51–54.

Kotrla, K., Chacko, R. C., Harper, R. G., *et al* (1995) SPECT findings in psychosis in Alzheimer's disease. *American Journal of Psychiatry*, 152, 1470–1475.

Laasko, M. P., Partanen, K., Riekkinen, P., *et al* (1996) Hippocampal volumes in Alzheimer's disease, Parkinson's disease with and without dementia, and in vascular dementia: an MRI Study. *Neurology*, 46, 678–681.

Lehtovirta, M., Soininen, H., Laakso, M. P., *et al* (1996) SPECT and MRI analysis in Alzheimer's disease: Relation to apolipoprotein E e4 allele. *Journal of Neurology, Neurosurgery and Psychiatry*, 60, 644–649.

Luxenberg, J., Haxby, J., Creasey, H. *et al* (1987) Rate of ventricular enlargement in dementia of Alzheimer type correlates with the rate of psychological deterioration. *Neurology*, 37, 1135–1140.

O'Brien, J. T. (1996) SPET Scaning in Alzheimer's disease and the effects of tacrine on regional cerebral blood flow. *International Journal of Geriatrics Psychiatry*, 11, 343–348.

——, Desmond, P., Ames, D., *et al* (1994) The differentiation of depression from dementia by temporal lobe magnetic resonance imaging. *Psychological Medicine*, 24, 633–640.

——, ——, ——, *et al* (1996) A magnetic resonance imaging study of white matter lesions in depression and Alzheimer's disease. *British Journal of Psychiatry*, 168, 477–485.

Pametti, L., Lowenthal, D. T., Presciutti, O., *et al* (1996) MRI-based hippcampal volumetry and 99m Tc HMPAO-SPECT in normal aging: Age associated memory impairment and probable Alzheimer's disease. *Journal of the American Geriatric Society*, 44, 133–138.

Pettegrew, J. N. V., Moossy, J., Withers, G., *et al* (1988) Nuclear magnetic resonance study of the brain in Alzheimer's disease. *Journal of Neuropathology and Experimental Neurology*, 47, 235–248.

Philpot, M. & Burns, A. (1989) Reversible dementias. In *Dementia Disorders: Advances and Prospects* (ed. C. Katona), pp. 142–149. London: Chapman and Hall.

Rabins, P. V., Pearlson, G. D., Alyward, E., *et al* (1991) Cortical magnetic resonance imaging changes in elderly inpatients with major depression. *American Journal of Psychiatry*, 148, 617–620.

Read, S. L., Miller, B. C., Mena, I., *et al* (1995) SPECT in dementia: clinical and pathological correlation. *Journal of the American Geriatrics Society*, 43, 1243–1247.

Tyrrel, P. J., Swale, G. V., Ibanez, V., *et al* (1990) Clinical and positron emission tomographic studies in the 'extra pyramidal syndrome of dementia of the Alzheimer Type'. *Archives of Neurology*, 47, 1318–1323.

Further reading

Abou-Saleh, M. T. & Geaney, D. P. (1993) Single photon emission computed tomography. In *Principles and Practice of Geriatric Psychiatry* (ed. J. R. M. Copeland, M. T. Abou-Saleh & D. Blazer), pp. 495–502. London: John Wiley and Sons.

Besson, J. A. O. (1993) Magnetic resonance imaging. In *Principles and Practice of Geriatric Psychiatry* (eds J. R. M. Copeland, M. T. Abou-Saleh & D. Blazer), pp. 473–482. London: John Wiley and Sons.

Burns, A. (1993) Computed tomography. In *Principles and Practice of Geriatric Psychiatry* (eds J. R. M. Copeland, M. T. Abou-Saleh & D. Blazer), pp. 467–472. London: John Wiley and Sons.

Liddle, P. F. (1993) Positron emission tomography. In *Principles and Practice of Geriatric Psychiatry* (eds J. R. M. Copeland, M. T. Abou-Saleh & D. Blazer), pp. 489–494. London: John Wiley and Sons.

Locke, T., Abou-Saleh, M. T. & Edwards, R. H. T. (1993) Magnetic resonance spectroscopy. In *Principles and Practice of Geriatric Psychiatry* (eds J. R. M. Copeland, M. T. Abou-Saleh & D. Blazer), pp. 483–488. London: John Wiley and Sons.

Maier, M. (1995) *In vivo* magnetic resonance spectroscopy. Applications in Psychiatry. *British Journal of Psychiatry*, 167, 299–306.

13 Services

Colin Godber and Henry Rosenvinge

Development of services ● *Range of services available* ● *Links with other services* ● *Conclusion*

Development of services

Psychiatry was slow to respond to the challenge of an ageing population. The growth of specialised services for the elderly was essentially a grass roots response to local problems. From this emerged a generally accepted model of service. The way this operates has been strongly affected by increasing private institutional care during the 1980s, and has changed again with the renewed Government emphasis on community care in the 1990s.

The pre-specialist era – the 1960s

In the 1960s, a handful of major figures in psychiatry put the elderly on the map (Roth, 1955; Macmillan, 1960; Robinson, 1962; Post, 1965). However, the speciality as a whole found old people an encumbrance, particularly if they suffered from dementia (see Box 13.1). Functional illness was undertreated, and the standard response to a presentation of dementia was avoidance, or consideration solely of the option of institutional care. In some districts, geriatric services elected or found themselves obliged to help out from their already overstretched resources. Sometimes they were offered beds and staff by the psychiatrists to run the dementia service for them (Portsmouth, 1973). Generally, the scenario was one of great strain on families, with little support from the psychiatric service.

General practitioners (GPs) saw little point in early referral, often waiting until things were so bad that the psychiatric service was forced to respond, or intercurrent illness justified an acute medical admission. In the latter case the extra leaning power of the physicians often brought the patient rapidly to the top of the psychiatric or geriatric waiting list (whichever was the shorter or least stoutly defended). In the year or two before the establishment of the psychogeriatric unit in which we work, the general psychiatrists had embargoed admission of confused elderly people to their acute beds, leaving an already overstretched and under-resourced geriatric unit to pick up the pieces.

This sort of situation resulted in extra pressure on residential homes, which frequently found themselves admitting people with whom they could not cope, and without recourse to help or admission from the

---

Box 13.1 Psychogeriatrics in the 1960s

Dementia avoided and sometimes banned from psychiatric
    wards
Functional illness in the elderly undertreated
GPs saw little point in referring patients; instead patients
    admitted to medical wards with intercurrent illness
Residential homes admitting patients for whom they could not
    cope
Well patients 'banned' from homes, and living on long-stay wards
A few key figures such as Roth, MacMillan, Robinson and Post

---

psychiatric service if they became acutely disturbed. Not surprisingly this undermined trust, and when such patients eventually gained admission, the home would refuse to have them back even if they had considerably improved. As a result, the hospital long-stay beds often housed many patients who required little nursing care, while the homes carried many patients with dependency and behaviour more suited to long-stay hospital care (Clarke *et al*, 1979; Wilkin *et al*, 1985).

Emergence of a 'comprehensive' psychogeriatric service – the 1970s

Joint psychogeriatric assessment units

By the early 1970s, psychiatry was coming under increasing pressure to put its house in order with regard to the elderly. With many geriatric units tackling the needs of the physically disabled elderly in a much more effective manner, the Department of Health began to encourage psychiatrists to learn from them, and establish a partnership in the management of patients with dementia. In two important circulars (Department of Health and Social Security, 1970, 1972) it proposed that at least one psychiatrist in each district should take responsibility for liaising with the geriatric and social services, and that the focus of their collaboration should be a joint psychogeriatric assessment unit (see Box 13.2). Patients admitted to such a unit would have their psychiatric, medical and social needs assessed and treated, after which they would return home, or be placed in long-stay psychiatric, geriatric or residential care, according to guidelines laid down in the circular. The idea was a good one, but the guidelines were too simplistic and too susceptible to different interpretation by the respective agencies, as they attempted to protect their overstretched resources. Joint units would often clog up because one or more party failed to transfer patients when their assessment was complete. Where there was firm adherence to the operational policy, and the geriatric and psychiatric services worked well, they could prove a valuable asset (Donovan *et al*, 1971; Arie & Dunn, 1973; Godber, 1978).

Pioneers

Although the joint unit was not a panacea, the early 1970s did see an increasing number of psychiatrists electing to focus on the elderly, though widening their brief to include functional illness in a 'comprehensive' psychogeriatric service (as opposed to the 'dementia' service envisaged by the department). A cluster of pioneers (e.g. Arie, 1970; Whitehead, 1972; Pitt, 1974) described the establishment of such services, and demonstrated how much could be achieved therapeutically in the support of caring families, by an enthusiastic community-oriented approach, coupled with more effective use of beds. Many psychiatric trainees were stimulated by these accounts, or by direct exposure to such services, to move into the field themselves. An active peer support and pressure group began to meet at the Royal College of Psychiatrists and was later to metamorphose into the present Old Age Faculty. This group agreed on a number of guidelines and policies, on a range of important service issues, many of which are referenced in Arie & Jolley's article (1983).

Home assessments

In contrast to the Department of Health's model, most psychogeriatricians based their assessment in the patient's home, or secondarily in the clinic or day hospital. This enabled many patients to be treated without recourse to hospital admission. Those needing residential, geriatric or other specialist care could be referred directly to the appropriate service, without interposing what might be an unnecessary or lengthy period in the assessment unit. Those requiring psychogeriatric admission would come in with a specific plan for treatment, and with preparations for discharge already set in train. This reduced pressure on beds, making it easier to admit urgent cases without delay, and to achieve the trust and cooperation of carers with a high rate of acceptance by them for discharge. This capacity for quick response and rescue in a crisis came to be seen as the crucial hallmark of an effective psychogeriatric service, and an essential back-up to its support work in the community.

Against the background of previously severely unmet needs, the novelty of a responsive service inevitably increased referral rates and the demand for short-term care. Likewise, the more optimistic approach to functional illness in the elderly shown by most psychogeriatricians, and the demonstration to GPs that many patients they had previously seen as 'demented' or intractably or 'understandably' depressed could be treated successfully, increased demand on that front too. This change in work pattern usually resulted in a steady shift in bed use from long to short stay, with shorter spells

---

Box 13.2 Psychogeriatrics in the 1970s

Department of Health and Social Security recommended joint
    psychogeriatric assessment units
Group meeting regularly at the Royal College of Psychiatrists
Domiciliary-based assessments
Proving to GPs that treating depression was necessary and
    effective
Pioneers such as Arie, Whitehead and Pitt

---

in the latter. Eventually there was enough turnover to meet all acute needs, which in turn reduced the demand for long stay further. In our district, the existence of a case register enabled us to monitor this shift in work pattern. This showed much higher admission rates, and lower long-stay occupancy, than in districts without specialised psychogeriatric services (Jennings, 1984).

Fruition of the district psychogeriatric service – the 1980s

The impact of the early services led many districts to follow suit by setting up their own psychogeriatric posts (see Box 13.3). By 1981 the number of consultants working in the field had risen to 106 (Wattis *et al*, 1981) and by 1985 the figure was just under 250 (Wattis, 1988). The spread was most marked in the regions in which the earlier services had been set up. The resources offered with these posts were variable and often quite inadequate. The Old Age Section of the College produced guidelines for the resourcing of new posts, and identified a psychogeriatrician in each region to brief regional advisers and health authorities on new posts as they arose. It also established links with the British Geriatric Society, and jointly agreed a code for collaboration between old age psychiatrists and geriatricians, an interface all too prone to conflict (Royal College of Psychiatrists, 1979; Royal College of Psychiatrists & British Geriatric Society, 1992).

For some years the Department of Health dragged its feet in acknowledging these developments, though the Health Advisory Service publication *The Rising Tide* (1983) laid down some important guidelines for district provision for the elderly, and stimulated the Government to invest money to promote "demonstration services" and examples of good practice. However, it was not until a joint working party of the Royal College of Physicians and Psychiatrists (1989) published its report that the extent and patchiness of the development of old age psychiatry was recognised by the department and the colleges. This report endorsed the comprehensive model of psychogeriatric service, and listed the resources and working relationships necessary to achieve a good district service. It

---

Box 13.3 Psychogeriatrics in the 1980s

Expansion in consultant numbers

Old Age Section of the Royal College of Psychiatrists links with British Geriatric Society

Health Authority Service, in their report *The Rising Tide* (1983), suggest "demonstration services"

Joint report from the Royal Colleges of Physicians and Psychiatrists recommend a "comprehensive model"

---

recommended the establishment of old age psychiatry as a speciality with specific higher training requirements. This was accepted by the department. It was estimated that a further 250 consultant posts would be needed by the end of the century to bring every district up to what was currently regarded as an adequate level.

Community care – the 1990s

It was hoped that the purchaser–provider split, introduced by the NHS reforms, would enable health authorities to reduce the extent to which they were constantly having to bale out over expenditure on acute services. This would enable the promised investments in the 'Cinderella services', such as the elderly and mental health. Unfortunately the political imperative to cut waiting lists, and a succession of resultant crises in emergency services, resulted in the black hole of acute care continuing to suck in the greater part of any new investment (see Box 13.4).

Psychogeriatricians have had to fight harder than ever to hang onto the resources for their patients. They have had to second guess their health authorities purchasing plans (because they are seldom nowadays asked to participate in local planning and strategic development) in order to be ready to shape their services accordingly. They have also had to work to contract activity targets that have virtually no relevance to the quality of service being provided. With health authorities generally anxious to reduce their expenditure on such important areas as respite and continuing care, psychogeriatricians have had to make a careful judgement as to how much of these they can afford to stockade. If they aim too high, they invite competitive tendering with a private sector that will invariably undercut them. Those who have kept their continuing care units intact have usually done so on the basis of a much smaller number of beds, focusing on patients requiring very skilled care and multi-disciplinary review of a type seldom achievable by the private sector. Although the old norms of three longer-stay beds per thousand elderly still apply in Scotland, something around one bed per thousand is seen as more realistic in England.

Following National Health Service Executive guidance (Department of Health,1995), health authorities have had to be much more specific about who qualifies for different aspects of continuing health care. Fortunately, they usually involved local clinicians in drawing up their criteria. This has been effective in stemming the tide of NHS disinvestment in these areas, and has given clinicians a better chance of justifying continuing specialist care for their clients. Nevertheless, it leaves a health–social care divide which is entirely artificial, but very firmly maintained because of the different financial rules that operate on either side. The House of Commons Select Committee on Health (1996) urged the Government to require health authorities to pay for the nursing element of care in nursing homes. An authoritative Joseph Rowntree Foundation working party (1996) went further and supported a European model of social insurance, whereby an earnings-related levy would fund social care in the event of chronic disability or old age. If politicians find the courage to promote such a system, we might get closer to the integrated care management that was implied in the rhetoric with which the Government launched the Community Care Act.

The implementation of the Act was anticipated with trepidation. It was feared that the inadequate funding of social services, the unpreparedness of social workers for the purchasing role and the lack of providers of domiciliary care, would lead to a rapid silting up of hospital beds, such as occurred in the late 1970s. The picture has turned out better, initially at least, than feared. Certainly, social services have not had enough money, a problem exacerbated by the political difficulty of charging more than a nominal rate for domiciliary and day care services (which means that they are subsidising these in a way that they are not with residential and nursing home care). Generally, however, they have managed their budgets well, and care managers have shown increasing skill in putting together imaginative and effective packages of care for their clients, and linking these in with those provided by the NHS. The Government's hopes that the vacuum in domiciliary care would be filled by the entrepreneurial independent sector, have been substantially justified, though the quality of care is certainly variable.

People with dementia living on their own are still prone to require residential care at a rather earlier stage than their physically disabled counterparts. Nevertheless, the use of domiciliary carers to make sure that they are getting meals, medication and attending day centres, has certainly kept many people going much longer in their homes, and within acceptable limits of risk than was feasible in the past. The delay in hospital discharge that was anticipated has taken some years to become apparent; and it has often been related to disputes by reluctant purchasers over who pays for what, at the health–social care boundary. It is certainly pleasing to see many more patients now supported at home who, in the 1980s, were consigned to residential care.

Box 13.4 Old age psychiatry in the 1990s

Acute care continues to take resources
Old age services have to compete for resources
Local guidelines for continuing care
Social services budgets remain restricted
Private sector offering domiciliary care
More patients staying in the community

Range of services available

Psychogeriatric services only deal with a small proportion of mental illness in old people. Our quite busy service is in contact with just over 3.5% of those over 65 in the catchment area. Comparing this with actual prevalence rates for the psychiatric illnesses of old age means that we see under half of those with moderate or severe dementia, and a much smaller proportion of those with major functional illness (although the latter constitute over half of referrals). Clearly it is important to educate those in primary care to identify patients most in need of specialist referral, and to manage the rest.

The introduction of annual screening of the over 75s as part of the GPs contract, has provided an opportunity for dialogue. In our district, many GPs have adopted a screening instrument whose design was shared with geriatricians and psychogeriatricians, who also contributed a set of algorithms for the management of identified 'cases'. Such a partnership may be improved through the Care Programme Approach (CPA), and the participation by community mental health nurses (CMHNs) and primary care nurses in care management. Building links with social services and primary care teams improves their care of mental illness in older people and their selection of which patients to refer on.

Old age psychiatrists

Most psychogeriatricians prefer to assess patients at home, feeling that this gives a clearer picture of the patient's environment and support, better access to the ambivalent patient, and the opportunity to establish a plan of management before the patient, or the service, is otherwise committed (see Chapter 1). It has been suggested that another motivation is the domiciliary visit fee. Clearly, if the policy of the psychogeriatric service is that all patients will be assessed at home, it behoves the consultant only to claim such a fee if the GP specifically requests a home visit. The great variability in the extent to which such fees are claimed, and the increasing insistence by employers that they should only reflect out of hours work, makes it likely that they will be replaced by a more appropriate

---

Box 13.5 Advantages of home assessments

Offers a clearer picture of environment and support
Better access to the patient
Avoids difficult travel for the patient
Results in a fee (likely to be phased out)
Teaching experience for junior doctors and medical students

---

way of recognising the extra effort of taking the service to the community. There is certainly a need for proper evaluation of medical home assessment, and of the sharing of this work between members of a multi-disciplinary community team, and closer joint working with GPs through regular visits or clinics in surgeries.

Our service assesses all new cases at the point of referral, and carry out most follow-ups at home. Junior staff are involved in this work, which offers them an insight into the natural history and community impact of their patients' illnesses, an experience which has drawn many into subsequent careers in psychogeriatrics. Extending this to medical students during their psychiatry attachment has greatly enhanced their experience and enjoyment of the placement. Generally, the aim is to follow patients only as frequently and as long as specialist input is required. In the case of patients with dementia where surveillance, carer support, help in managing behaviour problems and liaison with primary care, social and voluntary services are the main requirements, the ongoing involvement of the CMHN is more effective.

Community mental health nurses

The CMHN is the lynch pin of the community psychogeriatric team, with a particular remit in the support of patients with dementia and their carers. Carers rarely take in all that is told to them at the time of the initial assessment, and they usually rely on the CMHN for information and counselling about dementia, and the task that faces them. The CMHN also acts as an advocate, a guide to services and benefits, and as a bridge between the specialist and primary care services. They will monitor the health of the patient and carers, encouraging involvement with support groups (which the CMHNs often help to run), and local organisations such as the Alzheimer's Disease Society. As the illness progresses, CMHNs can offer extra respite and domiciliary services, and alert the GP or psychogeriatrician if reassessment and treatment are needed.

CMHNs can play a similar monitoring and advisory role with residential homes and develop training courses for staff. CMHNs may be aligned to

---

Box 13.6 Roles of community mental health nurses

Key members of multi-disciplinary teams
Offer information and support to patients and carers
Monitor the health of patient and carer
Offer training to residential and other staff
Offer advice to primary health care teams

---

particular general practices, acting as a specialist resource within the primary care team, whose members may consult them, without the need for a formal referral to the service. Our community service operates in two teams, one of two consultants, and one of three consultants (also GP linked); each consultant's patch comprises the practices of three to five CMHNs. This offers familiarity with local conditions and resources, and close links with services, such as day centres or social services teams. Another advantage of sectorisation is that it allows the CMHNs and consultants to relate their use of beds and day places to the size of the population they serve.

Other members of the team

There has been a trend for occupational therapists and psychologists to extend their work outside the hospital or day hospital, both to facilitate discharge, and to widen the range of assessment and treatment available to patients referred to the service. In many services, multi-disciplinary teams have been set up to operate solely in the community, sometimes incorporating staff from social services (social workers, home care manager, home carers and occupational therapists) and the primary care team (health visitor, district nurses). While recognising individual specialist skills teams often encourage a generic approach to assessment with keyworkers. Team meetings are used to allocate and review clients, and to make referrals between members of the team when specialised skills are needed (Coles *et al*, 1991; Lindesay *et al*, 1991). This model is felt to work well by most who have adopted it, and it has been favourably evaluated by MacDonald and colleagues (1994). Exponents of the different models tend to support their particular approach with great conviction. Dening (1992) attempted a more dispassionate review in his commentary on a number of services he had visited prior to taking up his own consultant post.

A variety of other methods have been adopted to extend support to psychogeriatric patients and their carers. Some CMHNs have auxiliaries giving direct care in the home. Under the auspices of MIND, in Southampton we have established a sitting service to widen the range of respite offered to carers, especially when admission or day care was unacceptable (Rosenvinge *et al*, 1986). This service now offers 20 000 hours of care a year, and apart from enhancing the quality of care, it has paid its way financially in terms of reduced demand for long-stay beds. More recently this project has been extended to people with dementia living alone, in a way which dovetails with the home care service, often succeeding where the latter has been refused entry. This has led to an extension of the service to support patients with chronic functional illness.

Day care

Day care is an area in which psychogeriatricians have made the best use of the opportunities and resources they have available, rather than designing to a set plan. Although some have used day hospital as a major part of the assessment process (Bergmann *et al*, 1978) and a few for the treatment of acute illness (Whitehead, 1972), the most usual functions have been longer term support for the most vulnerable and respite for carers.

Our day hospital operates four types of service:

(a) Providing psychotherapy and behavioural intervention to tackle specific problems.
(b) Longer term support to those with relapsing illness or poor response in the first setting.
(c) Assessment, rehabilitation and respite for patients with dementia.
(d) A travelling day hospital taking a mixed clientele from rotating venues in the more distant parts of the catchment area.

Doubts have been expressed as to the specific function and cost-effectiveness of day hospitals in the care of older people (Royal College of Physicians, 1994). A debate in the *International Journal of Geriatric Psychiatry* (Fasey, 1994; Howard, 1994) concluded that there was need for further evaluation. It is important to see the role of the day hospital as potentially very different from a day centre. It can be the focus for assessment and treatment, as well as providing respite for the most dependent patients (Rosenvinge, 1994). The influence of day hospital treatment on the long-term use of the psychogeriatric service needs to be evaluated. One difficult to measure group are chronic functionally ill patients who comply poorly with treatment, and have a high risk of relapse. This group are only manageable with the high level of nursing and medical supervision that the day hospital provides.

Our own unpublished audit of day hospital care showed benefit to patients, as perceived by their carers, referrers and GPs, as well as by themselves. GPs, if they are fundholders, are now in a position to purchase day hospital care for their patients. It is important that they appreciate what an active day hospital can offer. By having special links with the community, the day hospital is well placed as a flexible resource centre, a liaison facility

---

Box 13.7 Roles of day hospitals

Long-term support for patients and carers including respite
Assessment
Treatment of acute illness
Psychotherapy and behavioural interventions
Rehabilitation
Opportunity for teaching professionals and volunteers

---

with primary care and social service departments. It therefore makes an excellent venue for teaching professionals and volunteers (see Box 13.7).

In-patient care

The more positive approach to functional illness and the relatively high rate of use of electroconvulsive therapy in the elderly has created the need for more acute beds than recognised in the old Department of Health and Social Security norms (Department of Health and Social Security, 1975). In our service, functional illness beds comprise about a third of the 90 short-stay beds operating for the catchment area population of 60 000 people over 65. Although seasonal peaks of affective illness sometimes result in an overflow to the organic wards, it is much better to separate the two, whose nursing and therapeutic needs are very different.

The acute organic ward is undoubtedly the most demanding on staff, and requires close integration of nursing, remedial therapy and medical skills. Department of Health and Social Security norms for so called 'assessment' beds generally underestimated the need for such acute care in an active psychogeriatric service. Beds are needed for respite care in an environment that is gently rehabilitative and avoids disruption to the patient as much as possible. Despite undue alarm raised by Rai *et al* (1986) on the basis of so called 'social admissions' to their geriatric unit, others have found no increase in mortality from planned respite care (Selley & Campbell, 1989), and clear benefit to carers (Pearson, 1988; Levin, 1991) (see Chapter 18). It is important to be able to admit patients without delay, and to honour planned respite admissions. Equally important is careful preparation for discharge, with involvement of the CMHNs, carers and those responsible for the social care at home.This includes follow-up at home within a day or two by a designated member of the team. Preparatory home visits are used with increasing frequency.

One way of responding to the demand for more extensive and flexible day care (with the capacity for longer hours and availability seven days a week), is to make the day hospital the main focus of non-domiciliary care (Baldwin, personal communication). Taken to its logical conclusion this would enable patients to be cared for through crises or episodes of illness as day patients, with overnight stay as an optional extra (e.g. at the height of the episode or perhaps the night before electroconvulsive therapy). This would undoubtedly reduce the number of nights spent in hospital and help to avoid the disruption and dependency that tends to occur with spells of in-patient care. It would require closer day-to-day review of the progress of in-patients and day patients than is customary. It would also need to be backed up by a more flexible transport system, enhanced CMHN input and the availability of 'getting up' and 'tucking in' services.

There is still a definite role for the psychogeriatric service in the continuing in-patient care of a hard core of disturbed patients. At the same time there is a need to replace the old warehousing model with a more homely environment in which the patients' choice and dignity is respected. Placing responsibility for the longer stay patients in a unit with a highly respected nursing officer committed to this approach can achieve a remarkably changed 'nursing home unit' (Norman, 1987; Hargreaves, 1989; Murphy, 1989; Lindesay *et al*, 1991). A major task in the future will be to impress on health authorities, the need to maintain such provision within the NHS, but ensure that its cost is not seen as too prohibitive.

Links with other services

Geriatric services

Efforts have been made with geriatric medicine to achieve joint working and planning at national and local levels (Royal College of Psychiatrists & British Geriatrics Society, 1992). Joint clinics are frequent, and in many districts one specialist will visit the other's unit on a regular basis, or joint assessment units have been established. Collaboration can be enhanced if consultant catchment areas are the same, or both units have beds on the same site. Overlapping needs of many patients receiving day, respite and long-term care justifies the extension of joint care to these areas, especially for poorly mobile patients with functional or organic illness. In some centres the logical step has been taken of merging the two services, such as the joint department of Health Care of the Elderly in Nottingham (Arie, 1983). In many districts the merging of units, following the NHS reforms, has brought the two services closer managerially.

Social services

Another important interface is with the providers of social care (see Box 13.8). The importance of support to residential homes and day centres has already been mentioned, and probably reaches its closest level in the context of specialised homes for the elderly mentally ill where psychogeriatricians have often been involved in both selection and ongoing review of residents. A close working relationship with social services is essential and is facilitated if they have their own 'elderly' teams.

The principles of the CPA were well established in old age psychiatry before it became a formalised process. For patients at risk, or requiring mixed health and social care input, the CPA assessments and reviews can be helpful in coordinating support, and clarifying responsibilities, as well as making contingency plans to cope with crises or the breakdown of care at home. The meetings are time-consuming, but are helpful to families and other grass roots carers and serve to forge links between the CMHNs and their other community colleagues. It is important for consultants to participate when needed, and can be a useful exposure for trainees; the infrequency of attendance by GPs is regrettable. Use of supervision orders and supervised discharge tends to be much less in old age than general psychiatry. We, at the time of writing, have used these procedures only seven times and once respectively (see Chapter 19).

Domiciliary care agencies

The proliferation of the independent provision of domiciliary care since the implementation of community care has increased the complexity of monitoring patients and their carers in the community. Responsibility for care management usually lies with a social worker, but it is often the CMHNs who have the skills to guide carers confronted with, sometimes difficult, patients with dementia. CMHNs often act as care managers, in all but name. An increasing proportion of domiciliary care is now provided by private agencies (some diversifying from residential care) whose staff selection and training may be far from rigorous. This is obviously an area of risk for vulnerable people with dementia, particularly if they live alone and have little family contact. This underlines the need for vigilance by CMHNs.

Voluntary services

The Alzheimer's Disease Society plays an invaluable role as a self-help organisation, and a source of information to patients and their carers, when first confronted by a dementing illness. At both local and national levels it has been very effective as a pressure group, and as a fundraiser for research or local service projects. Like Age Concern, it also provides some domiciliary and day care services (see Appendix for a list of useful addresses).

Conclusion

Services for the elderly mentally ill have evolved rapidly since the 1960s. They have often been developed at a local level by committed individuals. They have had to reflect changes in Government policy, and have been

---

Box 13.8 Links with other services

Geriatric medicine, nationally (British Geriatrics Society) and
   locally
Social services, including care programme approach meetings
General practitioners
Community psychiatric nurses
Private sector, including residential home staff
Voluntary agencies, including the Alzheimer Disease Society

---

consistently underfunded. Present services are based around the multi-
disciplinary team, where community psychiatric nurses play a central
role. Day care and in-patient care can complement each other. Better
links with other agencies are important for future development.

References

Arie, T. (1970) The first year of the Goodmayes psychiatric service for old people.
   Lancet, *ii*, 1179–1182.
Arie, T. (1983) Organisation of services for the elderly: implications for education
   and patient care – experience in Nottingham. In *Geropsychiatric Diagnosis
   and Treatment* (ed. M. Bergener), pp. 189–195. New York: Springer.
—— & Dunn, T. (1973) A 'do-it-yourself' psychiatric-geriatric joint patient unit.
   Lancet, *ii*, 1313–1316.
——— & Jolley, D. (1983) Making services work: organisation and style of
   psychogeriatric services. In *Psychiatry of Late Life* (eds R. Levy & F. Post), pp.
   222–251. Oxford: Blackwell.
Bergmann, K., Foster, E. M., Justin, A. W., *et al* (1978) Management of the demented
   elderly patient in the community. *British Journal of Psychiatry*, 132, 441–447.
Clarke, M. G., Hughes, A. & Dodd, K. (1979) The elderly in residential care: patterns
   of disability. *Health Trends*, 2, 17–20.
Coles, R. G., von Abendorff, R. & Herzberg, J. L. (1991) The impact of a new
   community mental health team on an inner city psychogeriatric service.
   International Journal of Geriatric Psychiatry, 6, 31–39.
Dening, T. (1992) The community psychiatry of old age: a UK perspective.
   International Journal of Geriatric Psychiatry, 7, 757–766.
Department of Health (1995) *NHS Responsibilities for Meeting Continuing Health
   Care Needs*, HSG(95)8 LAC(95)5. London: Department of Health.
Department of Health and Social Security (1970) *Psychogeriatric Assessment
   Units*, circular HM 70 (II). London: HMSO.
—— (1972) *Service for Mental Disorder Related to Old Age*, Circular HM 72 (71).
   London: HMSO.
—— (1975) *Better Services for the Mentally Ill*. London: HMSO.
Donovan, J. F., Williams, I. E. L. & Wilson, T. S. (1971) A fully integrated
   psychogeriatric service. In *Recent Developments in Psychogeriatrics* (eds D.
   W. K. Kay & A. Walk), pp. 113–123. Ashford: RMPA.

Fasey, C. (1994) The day hospital in old age psychiatry: the case against. *International Journal of Geriatric Psychiatry*, 9, 519–523.

Godber, C. (1978) Conflict and collaboration between geriatric medicine and psychiatry. In *Recent Advances in Geriatric Medicine* (ed. B. Isaacs), pp. 131–142. London: Churchill Livingstone.

Hargreaves, S. (1989) A model for long term care – assessment at 2 years. *Geriatric Medicine*, 19 (5), 55.

Health Advisory Service (1982) *The Rising Tide: Developing Services for Mental Illness in Old Age*. London: HMSO.

House of Commons Select Committee on Health (1996) *Long Term Care: Future Provision and Funding, Third Report*, HCP 59/95/96. London: HMSO.

Howard, R. (1994) Day hospitals: the case in favour. *International Journal of Geriatric Psychiatry*, 9, 525–529.

Jennings, C. (1984) *Psychiatric Care in Eight Register Areas: Statistics from Eight Psychiatric Case Registers in Great Britain 1976–1981*. Southampton: University of Southampton.

Joseph Rowntree Foundation (1996) *Meeting the Costs of Continuing Care: Recommendations*. York: Joseph Rowntree Foundation.

Levin, E. (1991) Carers – problems, strains and services. In *Psychiatry in the Elderly* (eds R. Jacoby and C. Oppenheimer), pp. 301–312. Oxford: Oxford University Press.

Lindesay, J. (ed.) (1991) *Working Out: Setting Up and Running Community Psychogeriatric Teams*. London: Research and Development for Psychiatry.

——, Briggs, K., Lawes, M., *et al* (1991) The Domus philosophy: a comparative evaluation of a new approach to residential care for the elderly. *International Journal of Geriatric Psychiatry*, 6, 727–736.

Macdonald, A., Goddard, C. & Poynton, A. (1994) The impact of 'Open Access' to specialist services – the case of community psychogeriatrics. *International Journal of Geriatric Psychiatry*, 9, 709–714.

Macmillan, D. (1960) Preventive geriatrics. *Lancet, ii*, 1439–1440.

Murphy, E. (1989) *Home or Away?* London: National Unit for Psychiatric Research.

Norman, A. (1987) *Severe Dementia: The Provision of Long-Stay Care*. London: Centre for Policy on Ageing.

Pearson, N. D. (1988) An assessment of relief hospital admission for elderly people with dementia. *Health Trends*, 20, 120–121.

Pitt, B. (1974) *Psychogeriatrics* (1st edn). Edinburgh: Churchill Livingstone.

—— (1992) Damning evidence. *British Medical Journal*, 304, 323.

Portsmouth, O. H. D. (1973) The organisation of psychogeriatric care. *Modern Geriatrics*, 3, 553–556.

Post, F. (1965) *Clinical Psychiatry of Late Life*. Oxford: Pergamon.

Rai, G. S., Bielawska, C., Murphy, P. J., *et al* (1986) Hazards for elderly people admitted for respite ('holiday admissions') and social care ('social admissions'). *British Medical Journal*, 292, 240.

Robinson, R. A. (1962) The practice of a psychiatric geriatric unit. *Gerontologia Clinica*, 1, 1–19.

Rosenvinge, H. P. (1994) The role of the psychogeriatric day hospital. *Psychiatric Bulletin*, 18, 733–736.

——, Dawson, J. & Guion, J. (1986) Sitting service for the elderly confused. *Health Trends*, 18, 47.

Roth, M. (1955) The natural history of mental disorder in old age. *Journal of Mental Science*, 101, 281–301.

Royal College of Physicians (1994) *Geriatric Day Hospital: Their Role and Guidelines for Good Practice. Report of the Research Unit of the Royal College of Physicians and the British Geriatrics Society.* London: Royal College of Physicians.

—— & Royal College of Psychiatrists (1989) *Care of Elderly People with Mental Illness: Specialist Service and Medical Training.* London: Royal College of Physicians.

Royal College of Psychiatrists (1979) Guidelines for collaboration between geriatric physicians and psychiatrists in the care of the elderly. *Bulletin of the Royal College of Psychiatrists*, 3, 168.

Royal College of Psychiatrists & British Geriatrics Society (1992) Revised guidelines for collaboration between physicians in geriatric medicine and psychiatrists of old age. *Psychiatric Bulletin*, 16, 583–584.

Selley, C. & Campbell, M. (1989) Relief care and risk of death in psychogeriatric patients. *British Medical Journal*, 298, 1223.

Wattis, J. P. (1988) Geographical variations in the provision of psychogeriatric services for old people. *Age and Ageing*, 17, 171–180.

—— (1989) A comparison of 'specialised' and 'non-specialised' psychiatric services for old people in the United Kingdom. *International Journal of Geriatric Psychiatry*, 4, 59–62.

——, Wattis, L. & Arie, T. (1981) Psychogeriatrics: a national survey of a new branch of psychiatry. *British Medical Journal*, 282, 1529–1533.

Whitehead, J. A. (1972) Services for older people with mental symptoms. *Community Health*, 4, 83–86.

Wilkin, D., Hughes, B. & Jolley, D. J. (1985) Quality of care in institutions. In *Recent Advances in Psychogeriatrics* (ed. T. Arie), pp. 103–118. Edinburgh: Churchill Livingstone.

Additional reading

Age Concern (1991) *Issues in Financing Residential and Nursing Home Care.* London: Age Concern.

Department of Health and Social Security (1989) *Caring for People: Community Care into the Next Decade and Beyond.* London: HMSO.

Levin, D. (1991) Psychiatric services for the elderly carers – problems, strains and services. In *Psychiatry in the Elderly* (eds R. Jacoby & C. Oppenheimer), pp. 301–312. Oxford: Oxford University Press.

Murphy, E. (1997) Dementia care in the UK: loking towards the millenium. In *Advances in Old Age Psychiatry* (eds C. Holmes & R. Howard), pp. 128–134. Bristol, PA: Wrightson Biomedical Publishing.

Norman, A. (1982) *Mental Illness in Old Age: Meeting the Challenge.* Policy Studies in Ageing No. 1. London: CPA.

14 Liaison

Brice Pitt

Epidemiology ● Psychiatric disorders ● Screening ● Attitudes ●
Liaison practice ● Relationship between geriatric physicians and old
age psychiatrists ● Conclusion

Much of the psychiatry of old age takes place in the general hospital. This is because a large proportion of patients on these wards are elderly, and their morbidity for psychiatric disorder is high. There is also a high morbidity for physical illness and disability in those who present with psychiatric disorder in late life; so these patients might be seen as having the first claim to accommodation on a general hospital site.

Epidemiology

The consensus from several studies is that dementia prevails in up to 30% of those over 65 in general hospital wards (Feldman *et al*, 1987; Johnston *et al*, 1987; Pitt 1991*a*); that is six times the rate in the community.

Between 10 and 20% of elderly patients on medical wards have delirium (Bergmann & Eastham, 1974; Seymour *et al*, 1980; Cameron *et al*, 1987; Rockwood, 1989). The nature of the ward and the procedures to which the patient is subjected affects the frequency. Gustafson *et al* (1988) found delirium in 61% of patients operated on for fractured neck of femur. Delirium may be present on admission or arise later, a quarter of patients judged to be cognitively intact on admission may be expected to develop delirium in the ensuing month (Hodkinson, 1973).

It might be expected that the prevalence of depression in general hospital wards would be a good deal higher than in the community but not all surveys agree that this is markedly so. Studies show a range from 5% to more than 40% (Pitt, 1991*c*). The variation may be due to different screening instruments, different cut-off points on the same instruments or different diagnostic criteria; to whether or not cognitively impaired patients were excluded; to the nature of the area served by the hospital and its alternative resources; and to whether the hospital is acute or long-stay, and takes its patients from a defined catchment area or selectively from further afield.

Psychiatric disorders

Dementia

People with dementia fail to look after themselves adequately, to take prescribed medications, and are at risk of accidents and hypothermia. Therefore, while admission to hospital is usually for a sufficient medical reason, it may also reflect the limitations of care; hence the (often pejorative) label 'social admission'. Once the medical problem has been solved, there is the need to establish that adequate care will be available. The momentum of previous support may have been lost and former carers may be reluctant to take up the burden again, which may mean discharge to a home or transfer to a longer-term ward. The time this takes increases the prevalence of patients with dementia on general hospital wards.

Delirium

Delirium is far more common in hospital than in the community, being associated with the serious physical illnesses, pneumonia, metabolic upsets, major surgery, for which admission is required (see Chapter 3). A major risk factor for delirium, as well as severity of physical illness, is pre-existing dementia. Koponen *et al* (1989) looked at the computerised tomography scans of the brains of delirious elderly patients and found significantly more cortical atrophy, focal changes and ventricular dilatation than in controls. It is generally expected that patients will either recover from their delirium or die (Bedford, 1959), though there is rather more information about mortality than recovery (Pitt, 1991*b*). Rockwood & Fox (1992) point out that some features of delirium are less transitory than others (e.g. memory impairment lasted a mean 28 days in their study).

Depression

Depressive illness may cause or arise from physical illness, or may lead to deliberate self-harm (Pitt & Nowers, 1986); all of which may result in admission to general hospital wards. Severe depression may result in malnutrition and dehydration from food and fluid refusal, gross self-neglect and failure to take medication for concomitant physical disorders such as heart failure and diabetes. Deliberate self-harm (unlike suicide) is much less common in the elderly than in young adults, but is still not rare as a cause of admission to medical or surgical wards.

Physical illness has long been identified as a major factor in late-life depression (Post, 1962; Murphy, 1982). Stroke (Robinson *et al*, 1983; Dam *et al*, 1989), malignant disease (Evans *et al*, 1991), myocardial infarction (Koenig *et al*, 1988) and chronic obstructive airways disease (Kukull *et al*, 1986; Borson & McDonald, 1989) seem to be especially depressing.

Box 14.1 Physical illnesses associated with depression

Stroke
Cancer
Myocardial infarct
Chronic obstructive airways disease
Cushing's syndrome
Hypothyroidism
Hypoparathyroidism

Usually the depression is an adjustment disorder (American Psychiatric Association, 1980) or a major depressive illness precipitated by the stress of physical illness, but occasionally it is intrinsic to the physical disorder: endocrine disease such as Cushing's syndrome (Cohen, 1980; Haskett, 1985), hypothyroidism (Tappy *et al*, 1987) and hyperparathyroidism (McAllion & Paterson, 1989); occult carcinoma (Whitlock & Siskind, 1979); and stroke where the cerebral lesion is in the anterior left hemisphere (Robinson *et al*, 1984).

Iatrogenic factors related to the treatment of depression or physical illness are considered below. Other ways in which depression could contribute to admission to general hospital wards are by the prominence of such somatic symptoms as atypical pain, anorexia and weight loss, which may suggest physical illness; and by lowering the threshold for physical illness, possibly by effects on the immune system (Anonymous, 1987).

Anxiety

Anxiety is rife in a hospital, at all ages (and not only among the patients). Apart from the reason for being in hospital, there are unfamiliar procedures, possibly uncomfortable investigations, strange staff and fellow patients and considerable scope for distorted communication. Bigger fears are of pain, disability, dependence and death. Anxiety contributes to insomnia, and the panacea of a hypnotic has often in the past led to habituation. On the other hand, the unwitting withdrawal of a sedative (including alcohol) after admission to hospital may precipitate acute anxiety, if not a fit. Anxiety is a common legacy of myocardial infarction and probably contributes much to the 'fear of falling' syndrome (Isaacs, 1992) where, after an attack of giddiness, dizziness or a transient ischaemic attack the patient is afraid of walking without having something or someone to hold on to. Anxiety may arise from thyrotoxicosis, hypoxia in those with cardiorespiratory disease (Schiffer *et al*, 1988) and cardiac arrhythmias, and the manifold somatic manifestations of anxiety may suggest a host of physical disorders, through hyperventilation, tachycardia, tachypnoea, diuresis, diarrhoea, pallor, faintness and palpitations.

Alcohol dependence

Alcohol dependence is often overlooked in the elderly (Schiffer *et al*, 1988). Atkinson (1991) points out that clinicians trained with the view that people with lifelong alcohol dependence either die prematurely or recover spontaneously, and that late addiction is rare, do not expect to encounter the disorder in old age. Also the symptoms may mimic the findings of other medical and behavioural disorders, leading to misdiagnosis. Faulty recall and shame limit disclosure by patients and families. Alcohol use contributes to falls, burns, cognitive impairment of various degrees, peripheral neuritis and hepatic cirrhosis, with oesophageal varices and liver failure. The CAGE screening questions (Ewing, 1984) are useful in diagnosis (see Chapter 1).

Iatrogenic comorbidity

Comorbidity may be iatrogenic. Drugs given for psychiatric disorder may cause physical morbidity and vice versa. Tricyclic antidepressants, for example, may cause hypotension and drowsiness (both resulting in falls and other accidents (Blake *et al*, 1988), cardiac arrhythmias, dental problems, glaucoma and retention of urine because of anticholinergic effects and fits. Selective serotonin reuptake inhibitors (SSRIs) may induce hyponatraemia. Steroids, propranolol, some anticonvulsants and anti-cancer drugs may cause depression. Anti-parkinsonian and some hypotensive agents may occasion a variety of psychiatric syndromes, including confusion, visual hallucinations, depression, mania and paranoia.

Box 14.2 Psychiatric disorders found in older patients on general hospital wards

Dementia
Delirium
Depression
Anxiety
Alcohol dependence
Iatrogenic comorbidity
Personality disorders
Paranoid disorders
Graduate schizophrenia

Other disorders

'Difficult' old people, those with personality disorders, paranoid disorders or 'graduate' schizophrenia, though rarely mentioned in morbidity surveys, probably because of the difficulty in devising suitable screening instruments and agreeing diagnostic criteria, are likely to be over-represented in general hospital wards because they neglect themselves or they have alienated or estranged themselves from those who might give care at home. In a prevalence study of patients, over 65, in the general wards of hospitals serving the London Borough of Hackney (Pitt, 1991*a*), 30% of the subjects were single, which might reflect such over-representation.

Screening

Goldberg (1985) explains that the recognition of psychiatric illness in general wards by physicians and surgeons may only come about either because a cue suggests such a disorder, or the patient's complaints cannot be accounted for by a known organic disorder. However, in over half such patients, with illnesses diagnosable according to research criteria, the diagnosis is not made. Goldberg suggests five reasons:

(a) The patients provide no cue (although they will readily describe their symptoms if asked).
(b) The cues are not picked up.
(c) Patients lack privacy.
(d) Having found an organic psychiatric disorder, the doctors look no further.
(e) Even when they suspect psychiatric disorder, the doctors may lack the confidence to pursue the assessment.

Consequently, Goldberg advocates screening tests, with which general hospital doctors may become familiar and comfortable, thus increasing their alertness. Some of the more widely used ones are listed in Box 14.3.

Attitudes

In the general ward, the old person with psychiatric disorder is at risk of getting too little attention or too much of the wrong kind.

Too little results from failure to diagnose the disorder, or labelling and dismissing the patient because of it. Labels such as social admission, bed-blocker, or the adjectives 'geriatric' or 'psychogeriatric' used as nouns, carry the risk that the one so stigmatised will not be seen as a proper patient, let alone a person, and will be abandoned in a corner while there is a long, exasperated and sometimes inept search for 'disposal'. Evidence

---

Box 14.3 Screening instruments

Abbreviated Mental Test Score (AMTS) (Hodkinson, 1972):
cognitive impairment
Mini-Mental State Examination (MMSE) (Folstein *et al*, 1975):
cognitive impairment
Geriatric Depression Scale (GDS) (Yesavage *et al*, 1983):
depression
Brief Assessment Schedule Depression Cards (BASDEC)
(Adshead *et al*, 1992): depression
CAGE (Ewing, 1984): alcohol dependence

---

of consultation with such patients about their future is often lacking and, unwittingly, institutionalisation and dependence are insidiously induced. The momentum of care in the community seems rapidly to be lost once the patient is admitted to hospital, and neither patient nor carers may be very ready to start it up again if at long last there are moves to effect a discharge.

Too much attention takes the form of oversedation, isolation in a side-room and even physical restraint. Binding the elderly, especially those who are confused, even if they are near to death, is not unknown in the USA (Frengley & Mion, 1986; Robbins *et al*, 1987), while in the UK the favoured form of restraint has been the geriatric Buxton chair, which can not only be tilted backwards to thwart attempts to leave it but also has a table which can be locked across the patient's lap. In one of the worst scenarios there is precipitate referral to the psychiatrist who arrives to find the patient unrousable after an intramuscular injection of chlorpromazine, while the notes only record the absence of significant physical signs and the mental state as 'confused', 'restless', 'wandering' or 'aggressive'.

Occasionally psychotropic drugs are peremptorily withdrawn when the patient is admitted, without a proper enquiry into their rationale, the assumption being that they are unnecessary or actually harmful. The attitudes which give rise to these abuses include:

(a) Ignorance: the lessons learnt during a psychiatric attachment or clerkship seem easily forgotten (partly from lack of reinforcement) in the hurly-burly of life on a busy general ward or, in the case of old psychiatry, they may never have been learned in the first place.
(b) Prejudice: 'mental disorder means madness, trouble, unpredictable, erratic behaviour, attention-seeking or even malingering. If the ward is upstairs, then suicidal patients may hurl themselves from the windows. If it is on the ground, restless old people may wander away and get run over or be lost'.

(c) Paranoia: 'we're being used as a dump for problems which belong to the general practitioner, social services, rejecting families, administrators, the geriatricians or the psychiatrists, who do not pull their weight and pass the buck'. The beleaguered house officer (intern) or registrar (resident) subjects the referring doctor to a hostile interrogation if the patient is old, which may leave all parties bruised and aggrieved.

(d) Anxiety: 'we have not the staff, the training or the facilities to deal with these sorts of problems. The other patients, who are really ill, will be upset by noisiness and interference. There will be a disaster, a drip will be pulled down, or someone recovering from a myocardial infarction will have a cardiac arrest, and we will be blamed'.

White's (1990) analysis of why medical patients with psychiatric disorder may not be referred to psychiatrists is worth citing (Box 14.4).

Such attitudes may to some extent be prevented by proper training, and the realisation that in any general hospital two-fifths of the in-patients are likely to be old, and half of these to be confused, depressed or to have

---

Box 14.4 Reasons why medical patients are not referred to psychiatrists (adapted from White, 1990)

The psychiatric service dissatisfies the physician

Psychiatric language is useless to the physician

The physician is unaware of the need for psychiatric intervention

The physician is unaware of the possibility of psychiatric intervention

The physician believes the psychiatric disorder to be incurable.

The physician fears the patient's emotions

The physician feels he or she does not know the patient well enough

The significance of psychological issues is denied

There is a poor working relationship between the physician and the psychiatrist

The physician believes that the patient is disadvantaged by being labelled as a psychiatric case

The patient refuses psychiatric referral

The physician considers the patient too physically ill

The physician believes that every doctor should be able to treat psychiatric illness

The physician cannot or will not spare the time for psychological issues

some other form of psychiatric disorder (Pitt, 1991*a*). A potential corrective is good liaison with the psychiatric services.

Liaison practice

The late Richard Asher, consulting physician at the Central Middlesex Hospital, London, remarked of psychiatrists: "We don't know them – they don't lunch with us!" He was referring to the days when psychiatrists, coming some distance from a mental hospital, would make a 'hit-and-run' ward consultation and be seen by hardly anyone except the patient, leaving just a case note behind them. Now that many psychiatrists are based in general hospitals, there is scope for rather better liaison, though doctors' dining rooms belong to the past, and communications in the hospital canteen tend to be rather rushed and economical.

Ward consultation

At the most basic level there is the ward consultation when the psychiatrist receives a note explaining the problem more or less adequately and goes to see the patient. The psychiatrist may have given notice of the visit, in which case he will hope that the patient will be in the ward, and not at X-ray. He might also meet the house officer or registrar, but almost certainly not the consultant. If in luck, there will be a detailed referral in the case notes explaining how the patient came to be in hospital. Otherwise he may well find the nursing notes more informative than the medical. If very lucky, he will meet a relative who happens to be visiting at the time of the consultation, or has been asked to attend for the occasion. At the end of the consultation he will make a note, indicating the probable diagnosis, how it was reached and what further information and investigations are needed, and make some recommendations, indicating that these are provisional and may be modified after further discussion in the light of better knowledge. The more consultations given, the better the psychiatrist will be known and the more open the ward staff are likely to be.

Box 14.5 Problems which may occur with ward consultations

Inadequate referral
Patient absent, at X-ray etc.
Lack of private, quiet area for interview
Patient frail, fatigued or deaf
Carer not present
Nursing staff unaware of the situation
No direct communication with the referring consultant

Regular meetings

This basic model is enhanced when the psychiatrist has a regular meeting with the medical firms. He or she is unlikely to have the time for this with every consultant whose patients are seen, but should at least aim to meeting the geriatrician. Such meetings may be at set times, or in the context of ward or day hospital rounds or out-patient clinics involving some joint working. It is important that, if possible, the status of those meetings is comparable. For example, if it is always the medical registrar who meets the consultant psychiatrist, then the commitment of the consultant may be in doubt, and while day-to-day problems can be tackled, matters of policy may be hard to resolve. It is good, too, if the respective teams can meet, rather than just representative individuals.

However, less comprehensive liaison can still have measurable effects. Scott *et al* (1988) describe how a senior registrar in old age psychiatry started attending the weekly multi-disciplinary ward round and case conferences and reviews of a geriatric unit. After two years referrals doubled, from the whole hospital, not just the geriatric unit. The recognition and referral of depression, in particular, increased more than five-fold.

Joint wards

Further up the hierarchy of desiderata is the joint geriatric/ psychogeriatric ward. This was commended by the Department of Health and Social Security (1970) Circular HM (70) 11, which was issued in the wake of Kidd's (1962) study suggesting that there was considerable misplacement of old people with psychiatric disorder in geriatric wards, and of those with physical illness in psychiatric wards, and that this was to the patients' disadvantage. These observations were not confirmed by Hodkinson *et al* (1972), but nevertheless the idea of joint units seemed attractive. It was hoped that avoiding misplacement would reduce the need for long-stay beds and that dual expertise would meet the complex needs of older people with their multiple pathology and comorbidity for physical and psychiatric disorder.

Box 14.6 Improved practice

Direct liaison with the medical team.
Full referral with background information.
Arrange appointment with the ward staff.
An unhurried interview in a quiet room.
Speak to carer, general practitioner, social worker and other
    involved individuals.
Liaison clinics can speed up consultations.

An account of the operation of such a unit is given by Pitt & Silver (1980). A joint admission ward in the satellite of a London teaching hospital took all acute geriatric admissions and selected patients with psychiatric disorders. These were:

(a) delirium;
(b) probable dementia;
(c) those with significant comorbidity (e.g. Parkinson's disease and paranoia, severe dehydration and depression); and
(d) patients with non-specific disorders such as not eating, falling, failure to thrive.

These were patients for whom the availability of geriatric expertise was especially relevant. Patients with uncomplicated functional psychiatric disorder and dementia were admitted to a small psychiatric hospital close by.

The consultant geriatrician and psychiatrist each did their own ward round, and they held a joint multi-disciplinary meeting every week. Advantages and disadvantages are listed in Box 14.7. The role of the old age psychiatrist in such a unit is shown in Box 14.8.

Box 14.7 Advantages and disadvantages of a joint medical and psychiatric unit

Advantages

Medicine and psychiatry are simultaneously available to patients who often need both.

The threshold for referral from one service to the other is eliminated.

Psychiatric patients are made more acceptable on the medical wards.

Mutual teaching and training are enhanced.

Liaison and reciprocity are intrinsic to the modus operandi

Patients do not fall between stools – 'too ill for a home, too disturbed for a geriatric ward, too feeble for a psychiatric ward'.

Disadvantages

Considerable senior involvement is required, including time, some spent as a spectator.

Uncertainty about who is in charge.

Mentally normal patients may be upset by those who clearly are not (though this is so on almost any general ward) The unit complements other resources, but does not necessarily replace them.

Box 14.8 The roles of the old age psychiatrist in a liaison service

Identifying psychiatric disorder.
Assessing its relevance to any physical disorder.
Estimating its effect on prognosis.
Implementing its treatment.
Helping staff to understand the possible psychodynamics of dependence, attention-seeking, manipulation, undue disability, aggression and failure to cooperate.
Helping with the management of common losses – dying, bereavement, amputation, being rejected.
Arranging transfer to a psychiatric ward when appropriate.
Arranging follow-up.
Teaching nurses and junior doctors about psychiatric illness in old age.

Joint departments

The ultimate in joint working is the integrated department of health care of the elderly (Arie, 1983), where psychiatrists and physicians work together not only on the same ward but in the same department to provide a seamless service. This adds to the advantages of other forms of joint working: a coherent, comprehensive service for the consumer and the trainee; constant cross-fertilisation, to the advantage of research; and a powerful voice within the health district to assert the needs of the elderly, for whom resources of staffing, expertise and 'real estate' rarely suffice.

Relationship between geriatric physicians and old age psychiatrists

In 1979 a joint committee of the British Geriatrics Society and the Royal College of Psychiatrists approved and published the *Guidelines for Collaboration between Geriatric Physicians and Psychiatrists in the Care of the Elderly*, which had been prepared by Professor Tom Arie (1979). Examples of the clarity and directness of this guidance are:

(a) Services for the elderly should be a unity for 'consumers'... Patients should not be bounced back from one part of the service merely because they seem more appropriate for another part: such distribution of referrals should be the internal responsibility of the service.

(b) Responsibility should be determined by the assessed needs of the patients and not by the quirks of the referral. If a patient with a severe stroke is referred to a psychiatrist, he is no less the responsibility of the medical service through having first made contact with a psychiatrist.

(c) Lack of resources does not alter the definition of responsibility. Once a patient's needs are recognised as falling within the province of one service, that service should support that patient within the limits of the feasible, even if this is less than ideal: a 'psychiatric' patient does not become 'geriatric' simply because there are no psychiatric beds or vice versa.

(d) Experience suggests that the best criterion for the placement of people with dementia needing longer term care is whether they are ambulant or not, always provided that there is flexibility necessary for the odd case that does not fit in.

(e) Patients with a psychiatric history who develop physical illness or gross physical deterioration at home should be assessed again. None should be labelled as a 'psychiatric patient' by virtue merely of some previous psychiatric episode.

Kaufman & Bates (1990) looked at working relations between consultants in the two specialities 10 years later. Opinions were obtained from 30 of 33 consultants in geriatric medicine in two health regions, 25 (83%) of whom were aware of the guidelines. Seventeen (57%) felt that relations were unsatisfactory; this was mainly attributed to lack of resources. Twenty-one (70%) reported particular problems with dementia

---

Box 14.9 Key points for clinical practice

The high comorbidity for physical and psychiatric disorder in late life should always be in the minds of clinicians who work with old people

Screening for psychiatric disorder, mainly depression and dementia, improves its recognition by those who are not psychiatrists

The higher training of specialist psychiatrists for the elderly should include secondments in geriatric medicine

Liaison, especially with general practitioners and physicians in the medicine of the elderly, is an essential component for a psychogeriatric service

An old age psychiatric presence is desirable in any substantial general hospital, not only to ensure proper treatment for elderly psychiatric patients with physical disorder, but also for the larger number of old people with psychiatric problems on the general wards.

beds. The presence or absence of a psychogeriatrician did not necessarily improve relations; if the psychogeriatrician had been given too few beds, problems remained. However, there was a marked association between the presence of collaborative activity (joint meetings or rounds, regular visits to each other's units, research, education, stall rotations) and an absence of substantial problems with demented patients.

Conclusion

Old people with psychiatric disorder form a substantial proportion of the patients in a general hospital. In such a hospital with 500 beds (excluding obstetric, paediatric, psychiatric and geriatric) they could well number 100. Psychiatric disorder is associated with a higher mortality, a longer stay in hospital and less likelihood of being at home after discharge (Pitt, 1991*a*). So, those who deal with older patients in the general hospital need to be trained, and their attitudes and practices adapted, to accept and accommodate these realities. At the same time, psychogeriatric expertise needs to be available for speedy consultation, including diagnosis, treatment, management and placement. There should be an old age psychiatric team in every substantial general hospital, which should be closely affiliated with the department of geriatric medicine.

Acknowledgement

Much of this chapter has been published previously as 'The liaison psychiatry of old age' (1993), in *Recent Advances in Clinical Psychiatry*, No. 8 (ed. K. Granville-Grossman), pp. 91–106. Edinburgh: Churchill Livingstone.

References

Adshead, F., Day Code, D. & Pitt, B. (1992) BASDEC: a novel screening instrument for depression in elderly medical inpatients. *British Medical Journal*, 305, 397.
American Psychiatric Association (1980) *Diagnostic and Statistical Manual of Mental Disorders* (3rd edn) (DSM–III). Washington, DC: APA.
Anonymous (1987) Depression, stress and immunity. *Lancet*, i, 1467–1468.
Arie, T. (1979) Guidelines for collaboration between geriatric physicians and psychiatrists in the care of the elderly. *Bulletin of the Royal College of Psychiatrists*, 3, 168–169.
—— (1983) Organisation of services for the elderly: implications for education and patient care – experience in Nottingham. In *Gerontopsychiatric Diagnostics and Treatment. Multidimensional Approaches* (ed. M. Bergener). New York: Springer.

Atkinson, R. M. (1991) Alcohol and drug abuse in the elderly. In *Psychiatry in the Elderly* (eds R. Jacoby & C. Oppenheimer), pp. 819–851. Oxford: Oxford Medical Publications.

Bedford, P. D. (1959) General medical aspects of confusional states in elderly people. *British Medical Journal, ii*, 185–188.

Bergmann, K. & Eastham, E. J. (1974) Psychogeriatric ascertainment and assessment for treatment in an acute medical ward setting. *Age and Ageing*, 3, 174–188.

Blake, A. J., Morgan, K., Bendall, M. J., *et al* (1988) Falls by elderly people at home – prevalence and associated factors. *Age and Ageing*, 17, 365–372.

Borson, S. & McDonald, G. (1989) Depression and chronic pulmonary disease. In *Depression and Coexisting Disease* (eds R. Robinson & P. Rabins). New York: Igaku-Shoin.

Cameron, D. J., Thomas, R. I., Mulvihill, M., *et al* (1987) Delirium: a test of the diagnostic and statistical manual III on medical in-patients. *Journal of the American Geriatrics Society*, 35, 1007–1110.

Cohen, S. I. (1980) Cushing's syndrome: a psychiatric study of 29 patients. *British Journal of Psychiatry*, 136, 120–124.

Dam, H., Pedersen, H. E. & Ahlgren, P. (1989) Depression among patients with stroke. *Acta Psychiatrica Scandinavica*, 80, 118–124.

Department of Health and Social Security (1970) *Psycho-Geriatric Assessment Units*, Circular RM (70) 11. London: HMSO.

Evans, M. E., Copeland, J. R. M. & Dewey, M. E. (1991) Depression in the elderly in the community: effect of physical illness and selected social factors. *International Journal of Geriatric Psychiatry*, 6, 787–795.

Ewing, J. A. (1984) Detecting alcoholism: the CAGE questionnaire. *Journal of the American Medical Association*, 252, 1905–1907.

Feldman, E., Mayou, R., Hawton, K., *et al* (1987) Psychiatric disorder in medical in-patients. *Quarterly Journal of Medicine*, 240, 301–308.

Folstein, M. F., Folstein, S. E. & McHugh, P. R. (1975) 'Mini-Mental State'. A practical method for grading the cognitive state of patients for the clinician. *Journal of Psychiatric Research*, 12, 189–198.

Frengley, J. D. & Mion, L. C. (1986) Incidence of physical restraints on acute general medical wards. *Journal of the American Geriatrics Society*, 34, 565–568.

Goldberg, D. (1985) Identifying psychiatric illness among general medical patients. *British Medical Journal*, 291, 161–162.

Gustafson, Y., Berggren, D., Brannstrom, B., *et al* (1988) Acute confusional states in elderly patients treated for femoral neck fracture. *Journal of the American Geriatrics Society*, 36, 525–530.

Haskett, R. F. (1985) Diagnostic categorization of psychiatric disturbance in Cushing's syndrome. *American Journal of Psychiatry*, 142, 911–916.

Hodkinson, H. M. (1972) Evaluation of a mental test score for assessment of mental impairment in the elderly. *Age and Ageing*, 1, 233–238.

—— (1973) Mental impairment in the elderly. *Journal of the Royal College of Physicians*, 7, 305–317.

——, Evans, G. J. & Mezey, A. G. (1972) Factors associated with misplacement of elderly patients in geriatric and psychogeriatric wards. *Gerontology Clinics*, 14, 267–273.

Isaacs, B. (1992) *The Challenge of Geriatric Medicine*. Oxford: Oxford Medical Publications.

Johnston, M., Wakeling, A., Graham, N., *et al* (1987) Cognitive impairment, emotional disorder and length of stay of elderly patients in a district general hospital. *British Journal of Medical Psychology*, 60, 133–139.

Kaufman, B. M. & Bates, A. B. (1990) Factors affecting provision of psychogeriatric care: a survey of geriatricians' views. *Care of the Elderly*, 2, 25–27.

Kidd, C. B. (1962) Misplacement of the elderly in hospital. *British Medical Journal*, 2, 1491–1495.

Koenig, H., Meador, K., Cohen, H., *et al* (1988) Self-rated depression scales and screening for major depression in the older hospitalized patient with medical illness. *Journal of the American Geriatrics Society*, 36, 699–706.

Koponen, H., Stenback, U., Mattila, E., *et al* (1989) Delirium among elderly persons admitted to a psychiatric hospital: clinical course during the acute stage and a one year follow-up. *Acta Psychiatrica Scandinavica*, 79, 579–585.

Kukull, W., Koepsell, T., Inui, T. S., *et al* (1986) Depression and physical illness among elderly general medical clinic patients. *Journal of Affective Disorders*, 10, 153–162.

McAllion, S. J. & Paterson, C. R. (1989) Psychiatric morbidity in primary parathyroidism. *Postgraduate Medical Journal*, 65, 628–631.

Murphy, E. (1982) The social origins of depression in old age. *British Journal of Psychiatry*, 141, 135–142.

Pitt, B. (1991*a*) The mentally disordered old person in the general hospital ward. In *Studies on General Hospital Psychiatry* (eds F. K. Judd, G. D. Burrows & D. R. Lipsitt). Amsterdam: Elsevier.

—— (1991*b*) Delirium. *Reviews in Clinical Gerontology*, 1, 147–157.

—— (1991*c*) Depression in the general hospital setting. *International Journal of Geriatric Psychiatry*, 6, 363–370.

—— & Silver, C. P. (1980) The combined approach to geriatrics and psychiatry: evaluation of a joint unit in a teaching hospital district. *Age and Ageing*, 9, 33–37.

—— & Nowers, M. (1986) Elderly would-be suicides are more determined, still treatable. *Geriatric Medicine*, 16, 7–8.

Post, F. (1962) *The Significance of Affective Disorders in Old Age*, Maudsley Monographs 10. London: Oxford University Press.

Robbins, L. J., Boyko, E., Lane, J., *et al* (1987) Binding the elderly: a prospective study of the use of mechanical restraints in an acute care hospital. *Journal of the American Geriatrics Society*, 35, 290–296.

Robinson, R. G., Starr, L. B., Kubos, K. L., *et al* (1983) A two-year longitudinal study of post-stroke mood disorders: findings during the initial evaluation. *Stroke*, 14, 736–741.

——, Kubos, K. L., Starr, L. B., *et al* (1984) Mood disorders in stroke patients: importance of lesion location. *Brain*, 107, 81–93.

Rockwood, K. (1989) Acute confusion in elderly medical patients. *Journal of the American Geriatrics Society*, 37, 150–154.

—— & Fox, R. A. (1992) The duration of delirium. *Age and Ageing*, 21 (suppl. 1), 39.

Schiffer, R. B., Klein, R. F. & Rider, R. C. (1988) *The Medical Evaluation of Psychiatric Patients*. New York: Plenum Medical.

Scott, J., Fairbairn, A. & Woodhouse, K. (1988) Referrals to a psychogeriatric consultation-liaison service. *International Journal of Geriatric Psychiatry*, 3, 131–135.

Seymour, D. G., Henschke, P. J. & Cape, R. D. T. (1980) Acute confusional states and dementia in the elderly: the role of dehydration/volume depletion, physical illness and age. *Age and Ageing*, 9, 137–146.

Tappy, L., Randin, J. P., Schwed, P., *et al* (1987) Prevalence of thyroid disorders in psychogeriatric patients. *Journal of the American Geriatrics Society*, 35, 526–531.

White, A. (1990) Styles of liaison psychiatry: discussion paper. *Journal of the Royal Society of Medicine*, 83, 506–508.

Whitlock, F. A. & Siskind, M. (1979) Depression and cancer: a follow-up study. *Psychological Medicine*, 9, 747–752.

Yesavage, J. A., Brink, T. L., Rose, T. L., *et al* (1983) Development and validation of a geriatric depression screening scale. *Journal of Psychiatric Research*, 17, 37–49.

15 Residential and nursing homes

David Jolley, Simon Dixey and Kate Read

Demographics ● *Historical context* ● *Characteristics of residents* ● *Characteristics of homes* ● *Conclusion*

Residential and nursing homes represent a significant proportion of the resources spent on the care of older people. There have been major changes to these services in recent years, including a large increase in the size of the private sector. To some extent, people living in 'homes' are still set apart. They are the present day successors to the "frail shadows", described in the *The Last Refuge* (Townsend, 1962), who were forced to seek shelter in the workhouses of the 1950s.

Demographics

The developed world is experiencing a rise in the proportion of the older population. This is particularly evident in those aged over 85, and has implications for residential and nursing homes. In 1994 almost half a million older people in England were living in residential homes, nursing homes or long-stay hospital beds (House of Commons Health Committee, 1995) (see Table 15.1). This represents 6% of the older population: a similar proportion of the older population lived in workhouses at the turn of the century (Pelling & Smith, 1991). The major change over the past 20 years has been a substantial rise in the number of private sector places. Over the same period there has been a smaller contraction of hospital and local authority care (Joseph Rowntree Foundation, 1996).

Table 15.1 Long-term care places for elderly people, England (1000s) (adapted from House of Commons Health Committee, 1995)

	General hospital	Psychiatric hospital	Local authority	Voluntary	Private	Total
1977	56	–	113	33	28	229
1980	55	–	114	35	36	240
1985	56	–	116	37	80	316
1990	49	24	105	35	145	448
1994	38	18	69	46	164	483

Historical context

The concept of 'old age' has changed in recent history. Victorian surveys refer to people aged 40 as 'old'. In the 1930s fewer than half of men aged over 65 were retired, compared to around 90% today (Victor, 1994). Old age has been refined so that 'young' old people (50s to mid-70s) are differentiated from the 'old' old (75+) (Laslett, 1989).

Seventeenth century

In the 17th century, children were born at a later stage of the reproductive period, reflecting a tendency for marriages to be somewhat delayed. Additionally, women would continue to have children into their late 30s or early 40s (Stone, 1982). Consequently, there was a strong possibility of having at least one child at home when the parents or parent entered old age (Laslett, 1977). There is evidence that elaborate retirement contracts were made whereby retirees exchanged land and buildings for specific services and support. Living with children or grandchildren was not necessarily considered preferable to an independent household (intimacy at a distance) (Rosenmayr & Kockeis, 1963).

Eighteenth and nineteenth centuries

The main focus of charitable spending on older people during the 18th and 19th centuries was building accommodation. Access to better quality accommodation, such as alms houses, was conditional on good behaviour, sponsorship and good health, shadows of which remain today. The Victorian workhouse was required to accept almost all comers, and has come to represent much of the negative side of institutional care in old age. The proportion of males aged 65 to 74 in poor law institutions rose from 3% in 1851 to 6% in 1901 (the peak of Victorian asylum provision). For females, the comparable figures are 2 and 3% (Pelling & Smith, 1991). Figures from a study in Bedford showed that one in six men and one in 13 women would spend at least one night in a workhouse (Thomson, 1983). One in 10 women would expect to end their lives there (Fennell *et al*, 1988). The stigma associated with the workhouse was powerful, and elements of this remain attached to present day residential care.

1940s

The establishment of the National Health Service led to the demarcation of 'hospitals' from local authority 'residential care' provision. Some former workhouses became hospitals for the long-term sick, and later become part of the geriatric medical services. The remainder fell to the responsibility of local authorities.

1950s

In the 1950s public assistance institutions were spartan, offering dormitories and day rooms which separated the genders, even splitting married couples (Townsend, 1962). Few residents could identify personal possessions, and most spent their days bereft of comforts and satisfactory activities. As a consequence of Townsend's observations and recommendations, authorities spent generously to create a network of smaller homes, either by building new houses, or by refurbishing houses previously occupied by wealthy families. Many public assistance institutions were closed and demolished.

The expectation of the time was that the population, previously subjected to the rigours of workhouse life, would enjoy the advantages of better appointed residential homes. Townsend's hope was that this would improve the general health and well-being of those in residential care, and there would be a shift in their behavioural and dependency problems toward better integrated behaviour and independence in self-care. Unfortunately, this did not happen. Instead, much of the pathological behaviour seen in the workhouse was (almost certainly) derived from underlying mental and physical morbidity compounded by, rather than caused by, the institutions' environment. This morbidity was simply transferred and redistributed within the residential home network (Wilkin *et al*, 1983).

In addition, pressures mounted for the admission of more older people to this form of care. Pressure came from the community, where more people were surviving and being cared for into later life, and from the hospital services which were keen to use their beds for the active assessment, treatment and rehabilitation of patients. Furthermore, hospitals were embarrassed by the poor quality of life they were able to provide for long-term residents in their institutionalised and inappropriately sited wards.

1960s

In the 1960s, older people in care, in most parts of England and Wales, were housed in 'Part III' homes run by local authorities (Audit Commission, 1986; House of Commons Social Security Committee, 1991). There was only a modest contribution from privately run residential or nursing homes, usually accepting people who could pay for their own care, and from charities interested in this work. The pattern of care in Scotland and Northern Ireland was, and has remained, different. The balance of provision in Scotland between Part III homes and the hospital service depends upon a greater level of hospital care than was available in England and Wales. In Northern Ireland, the health and social services are integrated, and this has facilitated the best use of resources with a minimum of friction.

Local authorities wanted to improve the quality of care in their homes, but were keen to offer a 'capacity that was appropriate to demand or need', because they were responsible for a rationed service. It was accepted that a level of 25 beds per thousand people aged over 65 years was desirable. A few determined authorities were able to achieve this. Many could afford only half of this level, and pressures within their communities became intense. Interestingly, the disability profile in well and poorly provided local authorities was similar (McLauchlan & Wilkin, 1982). This suggests that even at this level of provision, there was little room for less disabled residents.

Specialisation

Within the network of homes, the advantages of specialisation was canvassed and explored (Meacher, 1972; Wilkin *et al*, 1983, 1985). Powerful arguments were rehearsed for specialised homes for the elderly mentally ill. These were not universally well received, but in some authorities where close links were forged with psychiatric services for the elderly (notably Newcastle upon Tyne where Gary Blessed and Klaus Bergmann were influential) the system worked very well. Despite claims, and some evidence, for the advantages of mixed 'all comers' homes, the move toward specialised provision gained ground. It is now confirmed, in separate registration arrangements for nursing homes and residential care homes (both of which are for the elderly or the elderly, mentally infirm). This is a pattern seen in the USA, Australia and Europe (Jolley & Arie, 1992).

Alternatives

Townsend's vision of alternative arrangements to cater for older people who require help, supervision and a guarantee of safety from intruders, is being explored in a range of 'sheltered' schemes in this country and in other parts of the world. Whole townships for retired people have been established in the USA, while complexes offering facilities including independent living in bungalows or flats, residential 'hotel' accommodation, and full nursing care have been developed in Europe and parts of the UK. Such initiatives have received the encouragement of governments in some countries (e.g. Denmark) but have usually depended upon voluntary or private sector enthusiasm and sponsorship in the UK. Some local authorities are convinced of their advantages (Wright *et al*, 1981; Bond *et al*, 1989; Copeland *et al*, 1990; Oldman, 1990; Pattie & Moxon, 1991).

1980s

The stranglehold of rationing in the residential care sector, which had restricted Part III development, was released in the 1980s. New legislation allowed the Department of Social Security to make special payments to applicants who required more care and attention than could be provided for them at home because of their age-related frailty or disability (House of Commons Social Security Committee, 1991). These payments (unlike NHS provisions and social service activities) were not subject to rationing by fixed budgets, but were a claimant's right if they fulfilled the necessary criteria. In practice, the criterion was simply that the individual felt they could not cope in their own home.

By moving into care, older people gave up their independence and the pleasures of a home life they had created over a lifetime, and took on a life shared with other older people, under the supervision of staff. However, they and their families were released from the worry of making ends meet financially, and from the vagaries of coping in a world which is sometimes hostile and dangerous to older people, and makes many other demands upon their families. Payments were 'means tested' so that people who had capital resources above £6000, or a substantial pension, would have to pay for their care. For a large section of less well off pensioners these new arrangements opened a door from a world of poverty and hazard into one of security and comfort.

There was a massive increase in the independent sector residential and nursing home availability throughout the country, on a scale not imaginable within the planned budgetary expenditure of the NHS or social services. The capacity of this component of the overall care system expanded dramatically. Flexibility of access and the range of style and quality of care also increased. Indeed, new requirements setting standards for the quality of accommodation and staffing led to an improvement in the facilities. At the same time, the direct provision of services by local authorities came under close scrutiny and intense budgetary pressure, as did the provision for long-stay patients within the NHS.

Many local authorities reduced their own provision of residential care to a minimum, or even ceased provision (Age Concern, 1991; Association of Directors of Social Services, 1994). Health authorities were encouraged to see nursing homes as direct alternatives to long-stay hospitals, within the geriatric and mental health responsibilities. Much of the NHS accommodation was poorly sited, poorly appointed, difficult to staff adequately and received minimal input from specialist consultants (Benbow & Jolley, 1992; Benbow *et al*, 1994). The prospect of moving care from dormitories in distant mental hospitals to well-sited, well-furnished and well-staffed nursing homes, where they would be under the medical care of general practitioners, and be sponsored by the Department of Social Security (or their own capital and pension) was very attractive. Results of the residential boom are summarised in Box 15.1.

Box 15.1 Results of the residential boom

As the number of places in residential and nursing homes increased exponentially, the overall cost rose in a similar fashion, and far outweighed the apparent advantages to local authority and NHS budgets (Audit Commission, 1986; House of Commons Social Security Committee, 1991)

There was a 'perverse incentive' for older people to give up their independence and to go into care. This was counter to the philosophy of community care. Pressure came from family members keen to be assured of safety, and professionals keen to empty NHS beds as soon as possible so that they could be used for others in more urgent need of therapy

Older people with modest capital and pension resources found that their assets were taken from them to pay for care, which a few years previously would have been provided free by the NHS. Surviving spouses might be required to live in penury, and offspring find themselves denied an expected inheritance

As the cost of good quality care rose, the payment of benefits did not, putting pressure on families (where they existed) to find 'top-up' payments, or requiring older people to move to bottom-of-the-market homes

Continuity of medical care, particularly the contribution of geriatricians or psychogeriatricians to the multi-disciplinary team, was compromised

Training and the maintenance of skills of the medical, nursing and rehabilitative professions suffered

The optimal use of resources in the community such as care at home, day care, respite and long-term care, became impossible because of the fragmentation of responsibilities and competing roles of those involved in making clinical decisions

---

1990s

Local authorities

The National Health Service and Community Care Act (1994) addressed some of these issues. Following Sir Roy Griffiths' recommendations the open budget of the Department of Social Security was closed, ring-fenced and given over, with all responsibilities for purchasing care, to local authorities who had certain requirements (Box 15.2) (Griffiths, 1988; Department of Health, 1989).

This 'capped' expenditure terminated the exponential rise in cost to the public purse. It put services under pressure, but ensured that

---

Box 15.2 Local authority requirements

Identify people in need of care

Carry out appropriate assessments

Purchase care designed to meet their needs, taking into account the resources available

Review need, and how far current services were meeting that need, at regular intervals

Spend a fixed proportion of the budget on the independent sector

---

older people were properly assessed before major decisions were made about their care. The number of people going into care dropped and the number of viable residential and nursing homes reduced accordingly.

Health authorities

The responsibilities of health authorities in 'purchasing' long-stay care were re-examined, and it was confirmed that they have an absolute responsibility to ensure that patients, severely damaged by multiple, complex or unstable pathologies, are cared for within the NHS (Neill & Williams, 1992; Laing, 1993; Health Service Commission, 1994; Department of Health, 1995a, 1996; House of Commons Health Committee, 1995, 1996; Wistow, 1995; Joseph Rowntree Foundation, 1996). This means some health authorities have to reinvest in facilities. All authorities have been required to produce criteria for the use of their long-stay facilities (in liaison with social services departments) and put a procedure and appeal system in place.

The future

It is unlikely that the balance of beds will return to the pre-free market era of five continuing care beds per 1000 people aged over 65 in geriatric medicine, and two and a half beds per 1000 people aged over 65 in old age psychiatry.

The significance of NHS beds is wider than their capacity to care for individual patients. They emphasise the contribution of specialist health teams in offering advice, training and liaison to other caring teams; and facilitate the cohesive nursing of multi-disciplinary, multi-agency, multi-modal services for populations. Provision of a few beds may reduce the need for many people to enter long-term care in other ways.

Characteristics of residents

Age

The age profile of residents has shifted, almost exclusively, to the very old. Very few people now enter care in advance of the 80–85 year age band, and average ages continue to rise (Department of Health, 1994*b*, 1995) (Table 15.2). Younger residents are more likely to be suffering from severe disability arising from medical, or more often, mental illness.

Gender

In residential care women outnumber men in a ratio of roughly three to one. This reflects the phenomenon of women surviving beyond their husbands.

Marital state

Remaining married is a strong protector against entry to residential care. Only in long-stay hospital or, to a lesser extent nursing homes, are married people seen in any numbers, and then only among the more severely disabled. Married couples are traditionally determined to see each other through 'till death us do part', and they still do, though this phenomenon was threatened by the excess access to care available between 1985 and 1993.

Behavioural characteristics

Many residents are frail and unable to care for themselves. Townsend not only noted this but described a simple rating scale to quantify and compare the abilities of individuals and home populations (Townsend, 1962). Other scales have been developed and acquired popularity in general usage. The Crichton Royal Behavioural Rating Scale was constructed by Sam Robinson during his work with elderly mentally ill patients (Box 15.3). Wilkin added memory and bathing to reflect the most pertinent characteristics of people in care (Wilkin & Thompson, 1989).

Table 15.2 Age distribution in residential care homes for the elderly (%)

	1989	1995
<65	2	2
65–74	10	9
75–84	40	35
85+	47	55

Box 15.3 Important characteristics of people in care

Memory
Bathing
Mobility
Orientation
Communication
Cooperation
Restlessness
Dressing
Feeding
Continence

The use of such measures confirms that while residential care populations are, on average, more behaviourally dependent than older people living in private households, many very disabled or disordered older people still live in their own homes or with their families. The role of hospitals in caring for the very disabled has always been numerically small. The spectrum of disability and disorder is more severe in nursing homes than in residential homes. Long-stay hospital patients are even more damaged. There is a strongly held belief that the level of disability among residents has been increasing, progressively. However, follow-up studies using comparable scales, and a review of Townsend's findings, suggest that the changes over the past 40 years have not been that substantial (Wilkin *et al*, 1978; Davies & Knapp, 1981; Capewell *et al*, 1986; Hodkinson *et al*, 1988).

Physical health

More than half of admissions to residential and nursing homes occur after a period of care in hospital. The degenerative disorders (strokes, ischaemic heart disease, Parkinson's disease and arthritis) are common and often present in combination. Impairment of hearing and vision compound communication difficulties. The 'geriatric giants' of immobility, falls and incontinence, are often evident and respond to positive approaches. Decubitus ulcers are common and demand watchfulness and preventative work. Diabetes and other endocrine disorders often require daily supplements (Brocklehurst *et al*, 1978; Challis & Bartlett, 1987; Gosney *et al*, 1990; Peet *et al*, 1994). Residents maintain health but the incidence of intercurrent illness and decompensation of previously quiescent pathologies is higher among people of equivalent age at home (Nolan & O'Malley, 1989; Central Health Monitoring Unit, 1992; McGrath & Jackson, 1996).

Mental health

Dementia

The strongest determinant of need for residential care is dementia. The Newcastle community follow-up studies of the 1960s demonstrated that few people survived alone with dementia for more than a few months, and most moved into residential care (Kay *et al*, 1970). Mental hospital provision, although important for the few who were disturbed, was numerically dwarfed. This remains the case. At least half of people in care are suffering from dementia (Kay *et al*, 1962; Jolley, 1981; Harrison *et al*, 1990).

Depression

Depression is more common among residents than the general population, although the aetiology, characteristics and need for treatment require careful consideration (Mann *et al*, 1984; Ames, 1990; Stout *et al*, 1993). Some depressed residents have personality factors related to the difficulties encountered in late life, others have the features of 'biological' depression and benefit from antidepressants. It is important to avoid permanent placement in residential care when an individual might be better served by treatment of their depression and support in their own home. Similarly, caution is required in making the best provision for dysphoric individuals, who may find life within a home even less to their liking.

Long-standing mental illness

People with long histories of mental illness or those with learning disabilities are commonly placed in care with older people. Many towns found it possible to relocate the 'less damaged chronic psychotics' from the back wards of the local mental hospital into more-or-less specialised homes during the golden era of the 1960s and 1970s. Subsequent placements of similar people may continue this pattern of specialist homes, or take advantage of vacancies in any home willing and able to accept them. In similar fashion, individuals with lifelong learning disability may

---

Box 15.4 Characteristics of residents

Age: old and getting older
Gender: female, three to one
Marital status: usually widowed or single
Poor physical health
Disabled
Mental illness: over half have dementia

be placed in homes when their support system (often aged parents or older siblings) begins to falter. A feature of the chronic mentally disabled is their relative youth (60–70 years on admission) within a pool of much older people. This occurs because hostels for the younger mentally ill frequently require residents to move on when they reach retirement age, and they may be loathe to accept new admissions of older clients even when they are in their 50s (Jones, 1985; Jolley & Jolley, 1991*a,b*; Jolley & Lennon, 1991; Faulkner *et al*, 1992; Davidge *et al*, 1994).

Characteristics of homes

Ownership

Most residential homes (59%) are within the private sector and may be run as a family business or, more often, belong to a chain of homes under the umbrella of a large organisation (Faulkner *et al,* 1992; Department of Health, 1994, 1995; Joseph Rowntree Foundation, 1996). Charities have maintained a small contribution to the range (16%), often taking the lead in innovations of style and quality. Local authority stock has dwindled, sometimes by making over properties to local charitable trusts or by selling to the private sector. Nursing homes are very largely a private sector venture, many being run by one of a number of large national and international companies.

Distribution

Coastal resorts and other retirement areas have traditionally offered more homes than working towns and this pattern continues (Warnes, 1982; Davies & Challis, 1986; Larder *et al*, 1986; Fennell *et al*, 1988). In addition, homes cluster where there are suitable properties for conversion or cheap land available for new buildings. This means that the stock of homes, nationally and locally, does not relate to the need for such accommodation. People may be reluctant to move across town for their care. If they do, they may feel out of place as accents and topics of conversation are unfamiliar. These considerations are even more pertinent when moving to a new town to be near a relative or to take advantage of an available place in a favourite holiday resort.

Size

Although homes are regarded as 'homely' compared to the institutional alternatives, there is a wide range of size, from three beds to more than 100. The economics of a small home leave little room for profit, and only dedicated family businesses can operate in this way. Even then, most require 20 or more beds to be viable within the funding allowed to residents sponsored by the local authority (Jolley, 1992, 1994, *a,b,c*). Larger organisations may favour a complex of wings, with 20 to 24 beds in clusters of five or six, on one site (a total of around 140 beds). This allows for economies of scale in central facilities such as catering and laundry, flexibility in staffing, and for developing special environments within wings. This may include a special unit for the more behaviourally disturbed.

Specialised environments

The stratification of provision into residential homes, nursing homes and community hospitals is established. Within this framework, registration for work with the elderly, the mentally ill or the elderly mentally ill has been discussed earlier. There is a healthy move toward dual accreditation, allowing for a range of care within one home. This may be achieved by designated special wings or annexes, or on a named resident basis, allowing for a mixed environment. This reduces pressures for people to move on when their condition changes, and facilitates life together for husband and wife, who are differentially disabled. There is a modest market for homes dedicated to the care of people with requirements associated with background rather than current morbidity. Catholics, Methodists, Muslims, Jews, Asians, Afro-Caribbeans, ex-Service men and women, and even the medical profession may choose to travel, to pass time in the company of kindred spirits.

Staffing

Staffing levels are determined by registering authorities who also specify and inspect the availability of qualified nursing staff. Most hands-on care comes from unqualified carer staff, who are responsible to managers or qualified nurses. Even the qualified staff may have spent their training days in acute wards, or operating theatres, which hardly give them experience appropriate to their chosen careers.

Good nursing homes may include occupational therapy and physiotherapy skills within their staff, but few have speech therapy, psychology, dietetics or other remedial therapies. The characteristics of care staff differ between homes, and reflect the local economy as well as the aspirations, reputation and personal style of the home manager. Many staff have no formal educational, let alone health care or social care qualifications. In the best environments carers are drawn from local, mature women, who take up the work when their children become more independent. They enjoy the friendships and personal rewards of the work and gel into a stable team (Avebury, 1984; Phillips, 1988; Wagner, 1988; Chapman *et al*, 1994; Murphy *et al*, 1994; Relatives Association, 1994).

Less healthy scenarios (reported in the USA and London) see hard-pressed poor women striving to make ends meet by holding down more than one job at a time in an attempt to support themselves and their children. Their tolerance and devotion at work is limited, and they may drift from place to place, providing a pair of hands but never developing personal pride in the tasks, nor the shared confidence of team working to a common purpose. The need for generous and sensitive attention to the training and support of staff cannot be overestimated.

Other roles

Although the main role of a home is likely to be the safe keeping of people approaching their last months of life, other activities should be undertaken.

Assessment

Admission often occurs after a period of illness so that each new resident requires careful assessment and help in the tasks of regaining stability, confidence and skills. After a period of care, convalescence and rehabilitation they may become able to return home or move to a less supportive environment.

Respite

People who are vulnerable at home and only coping because of sustained care from others, may benefit from day care or periods of respite admission. Some homes offer both these options, others limit themselves to planned respite admissions.

Outreach

A number of agencies are now able to offer a full range of support, including outreach, to clients at home. This facilitates flexible arrangements, making optimal use of strengths, and covering for weaknesses when they threaten to show through. In other situations these differing aspects of care require coordination across a number of agencies.

Life within homes

The quality and style of life available to residents are also functions of a number of other elements (Social Services Inspectorate, 1990, 1993; Research Unit of the Royal College of Physicians, 1992; Royal College of Physicians and British Geriatric Society, 1992):

   (a) Design is important, in the personal space available to individuals, most of whom will prefer single rooms, and in shared or public rooms and facilities, such as bathrooms and toilets. Furnishings, wall coverings, floor surfaces, lighting as well as storage and personal possessions are all potent determinants of comfort, confidence and interest (Harding & Jolley, 1994).

(b) The programme of events gives shape, purpose and meaning to each day. These derive, in large part, from the personalities and behavioural abilities of the residents, both individually and in sum. For most, hours are spent in company with other residents. Staff interventions may be few, though they dictate the pace and structure of each day and may helpfully orchestrate the contributions of others.

(c) Frequent contact with children, friends and other relatives confirm for the individual that they are still part of that world which was theirs for so many years. They also serve to inform others in this inner world of styles and expectations, linked to a long-crafted reputation. Regular visits from other agencies including churches, schools, educational teams and volunteer visitors all add something to the fabric and richness of life, and are invaluable.

Physical health care (Box 15.6)

The cocoon of care in homes can distance them from medical, nursing and other therapeutic professionals, who should be involved in checking the progress of chronic illnesses, treating relapses and maintaining residents in the best possible health. Perversely, the danger may be greater in nursing homes because they are looked on as providing comprehensive care for health needs, as well as a safe roof and hotel accommodation. Residents may become invisible, and health care professionals convinced that they have no more to offer (Health Advisory Service, 1993).

General practitioners

Residents are under the care of a GP, who may or may not know them. Many homes rely on a nearby practice to accept new residents onto their

---

Box 15.5 Characteristics of homes

Ownership: now largely private
Distribution: coastal, or where large cheap buildings are found
Size: often large, over 100 beds
Staffing: mostly unqualified
Design: important for individual rooms, and shared areas
Events and activities: dictate the pace of life
Contacts with outside agencies: add to the fabric of life

list. The practice may be paid an honorarium to provide additional services, such as advice or training to staff, but it is not allowable within NHS contracting to employ them on a sessional basis to provide clinical sessions within the home. That means that many older people with multiple disabilities and pathologies are not reviewed regularly. Homes that encourage residents to be registered with one practice, risk the probability that their new doctors will not know them, may not receive good information about them, and may never establish a warm relationship. Homes that encourage retention of long-established GPs run the dangers of multiple medical input to one establishment, and delay or reluctance in visiting.

Specialists

Contact with physicians or surgeons may be made, or maintained, through out-patient appointments or domiciliary visits, although follow-up by routine visits to the home by geriatricians or their equivalent is rare, as is the use of day hospital. When patients are very ill, they may be admitted to hospital. There is a suspicion that admission is sometimes less readily offered to residents of homes than to people living independently and suffering from similar pathology.

Prescribing

One of the deficiencies of medical and nursing supervision which has attracted concern is the prescribing, delivery and monitoring of medication (Nolan & O'Malley, 1989; McGrath & Jackson, 1996). The modal intake of medicines per resident, in one study of homes, was five different compounds daily. Some residents were receiving up to 14 different medicines. Some medications have persisted from previous regimes and never been reviewed. Potential adverse effects by interaction abound.

Other services

District nursing responsibilities spread to residential but not nursing homes, but in the competition for scarce resources, residents may lose out in the allocation of nursing time and the provision of facilities such as incontinence classes and other aids. Occupational therapy, physiotherapy and other remedial skills are often very limited. People who are housed safely, and in reasonable comfort, still require informed and sustained rehabilitative programmes.

Death and the management of dying are important features of home life and should be approached actively for the benefit of staff and relatives, as well as residents. These frail friendships are repeatedly broken by final partings, and it is important to be sure that everyone is confident and competent in managing this most significant of transitions (Bender *et al*, 1990; Black & Jolley, 1990, 1991).

Mental health care (Box 15.8)

The residential care population is a concentrate of mental morbidity, dementia, mood disorders, chronic psychosis and a fertile, stressful environment for the emergence of new difficulties of adjustment reactions. Nevertheless, it is common for the mental health of residents to receive little attention beyond that of an interested and informed home manager and the individual concerns of families (Royal College of Physicians & Royal College of Psychiatrists, 1989). It is terribly easy for morbidity to be hidden, or to be seen but not appreciated for what it is, with limitations being attributed to age, deterioration and the approach of an inevitable demise.

The scale of the challenge is daunting (1400 people in over 60 homes in a town, such as Wolverhampton, with an elderly population of 40 000) but there is no doubt that specialist psychiatric services for older people should address the situation actively. The potential for improving the quality of life for individuals and groups of older people is considerable, as is the prospect for increasing the job satisfaction of staff in the homes, and the potential for obtaining optimal use of services of all kinds.

With appropriate staffing and a determined strategy it is possible to forge effective links with all the significant homes in a locality. In the pattern which concentrated 'elderly mentally ill' patients in particular homes, this was facilitated, at least for the residents of those homes. There was, however, always the risk that only the most troublesome were recognised by such arrangements, and the mild mannered, depressed or muddled majority who might benefit from attention never receive it. It may be feasible to include routine visits to homes in the work specification of community psychiatric nurses.

Box 15.6 Physical health care

Homes may easily become cocooned from health services
Residents tend not to be reviewed regularly by their GP
'New' GPs may have little information and poor rapport with
    residents
Maintaining 'old' GPs leads to multiple medical input
Polypharmacy is the rule, and five medications is most common
Hospital specialists rarely follow-up and may be reluctant to
    admit residents to hospital
There is often limited input from occupational therapists or
    physiotherapists

Another approach, which has advantages, is to add this responsibility to qualified staff based in long-stay or continuing care community hospitals which are an intrinsic part of NHS provision (Wilkin *et al*, 1982; Jolley, 1994*a*). This emphasises the role of such units as part of a spectrum of care, which can help other agencies involved in similar work, by offering expertise through liaison, training and exchange of good practices, rather than simply taking away the most difficult minority. It is important, however, to develop the expectation that the help available to the care homes will come from a full range of skilled professions (including consultant psychiatrists, clinical psychologists, psychiatric nurses, occupational therapists and others), and not just from one over-stretched community psychiatric nurse. With this multi-disciplinary approach, residents will have the benefit of a full competent assessment (Box 15.7)

Although homes are sometimes seen as 'the last refuge', they have tremendous therapeutic potential and, used properly, can achieve this very well for people vulnerable to mental disorders. People who have begun to fret and become frail because of progressive dementia can find reassurance and companionship, eat more, put on weight and contribute with encouragement to a communal life. Individuals who are prone to relapsing depression, despite strong support and the best of physical and psychological therapies, may find their present strengths become sufficient when the worries of organising every day food, warmth and structure are taken on by a home.

People with schizophrenia or paraphrenia can find a niche within the tolerant, confident, supported life of a home which sees itself as part of a wider spectrum of 'psychogeriatric' care. This means that florid symptomatology and the behavioural disorders that go with it can be

---

Box 15.7 Mental health assessments in residential or nursing homes

Full referral including background information
Gather further information from notes, staff and GP
Take a full history, mental state and physical examination
Speak to a relative or friend of the patient
Admission to day hospital or in-patient care may be necessary for further investigations
Management of troublesome behaviours are outlined in Chapter 6
Behavioural programmes can be effective
Other professionals may become involved, such as community psychiatric nurses, psychologists or social workers
Inform staff fully of assessment and interventions
Follow-up

Box 15.8 Mental health care

Mental health problems are often not detected
Psychiatric services have a key role to play
Effective links should be forged, e.g. regular community
    psychiatric nurse visits
Psychotropics may be poorly or overprescribed
Antidepressants may be underprescribed

---

minimised, reducing in turn the stresses and demands on the system of care (Jolley, 1994*b*).

There is particular interest in the use of psychotropic medicines. These may be poorly prescribed and under reviewed. Neuroleptics are sometimes prescribed with the intention of sedating patients. Their anticholinergic side-effects may worsen Alzheimer's disease. Antidepressants are often under prescribed. Residents may not be assessed because staff or doctors consider their depression to be understandable. Alternatively, residents may be overlooked as they cause no immediate concern.

Conclusion

Residential and nursing homes have an important role to play in the care and support of the most needy sections of society, including the old and the mentally ill. Recent history has shown that changes in Government policy can have a profound effect on these institutions. Resources should be focused on improving the health and quality of life of residents. This may allow residential and nursing homes to finally emerge from the shadow of the workhouse.

References

Age Concern (1991) *Under Sentence: Continuing Care Units for Older People Within the National Health Service*. London: Age Concern.

Ames, D. (1990) Depression among elderly residents of local authority residential homes: its nature and the efficacy of interventions. *British Journal of Psychiatry*, 156, 667–675.

Association of Directors of Social Services (1994) *Continuing Care: Continuing Concern*. Northallerton: ADSS.

Audit Commission (1986) *Making a Reality of Community Care*. London: HMSO.

Avebury, K. (1984) *Home Life*. London: Centre for Policy on Ageing.

Benbow, S. M. & Jolley, D. (1992) A cause for concern: changing the fabric of psychogeriatric care. *Psychiatric Bulletin*, 16, 533–535.

——, —— & Tomenson, B. (1994) Provision of residential care for vulnerable old people. *Journal of Mental Health*, 3, 235–240.

Bender, M., Lloyd, C. & Cooper, A. (1990) *The Quality of Dying*. Bicester: Winslow.

Black, D. & Jolley, D. (1990) Slow euthanasia? The deaths of psychogeriatric patients. *British Medical Journal*, 300, 1321–1323.

—— & —— (1991) Deaths in psychiatric care. *International Journal of Geriatric Psychiatry*, 6, 489–495.

Bond, J., Bond, S., Donaldson, C., *et al* (1989) *Evaluation of Continuing Care Accommodation for Elderly People*, Volumes 1–7, Health Care Research Unit Report No. 38. Newcastle upon Tyne: University of Newcastle upon Tyne.

Brocklehurst, J. C., Carty, M. H., Leeming, J. T., *et al* (1978) Medical screening of older people accepted for residential care. *Lancet*, 2, 141–143.

Capewell, A. E., Primrose, W. R. & MacIntyre, C. (1986) Nursing dependency in registered nursing homes and long-term care geriatric wards in Edinburgh. *British Medical Journal*, 292, 1719–1721.

Central Health Monitoring Unit (1992) *The Health of Elderly People. An Epidemiological Overview*. London: HMSO.

Challis, L. & Bartlett, H. (1987) *Old and Ill. Private Nursing Homes for Older People*. London: Age Concern.

Chapman, A., Jacques, A. & Marshall, M. (1994) *Dementia Care. A Handbook for Residential and Day Care*. London: Age Concern.

Copeland, J. R. M., Crosby, C., Sixsmith, A. J., *et al* (1990) *Three Experimental Homes for the Elderly Mentally Ill*. Liverpool: Institute of Human Ageing.

Davidge, M., Elias, S., Jayes, B., *et al* (1994) *Survey of Mental Illness Hospitals Monitoring the Closure of the Water Towers*. Birmingham: Inter-Authority Comparisons and Consultancy Health Services Management Centre, University of Birmingham.

Davies, B. & Knapp, M. (1981) *Old People's Homes and the Production of Welfare*. London: Routledge and Kegan Paul.

—— & Challis D. (1986) Matching Resources to Needs in Community Care. Aldershot: Personal Social Services Research Unit.

Department of Health (1989) *Caring for People: Community Care in the Next Decade and Beyond*. London: HMSO.

—— (1994) *Statistical Bulletin: Residential Accommodation Statistics 1994*. London: HMSO.

—— (1995a) *NHS Responsibilities for Meeting Continuing Health Care Needs*, SE(95)8/LAC(95)5. London: HMSO

—— (1995b) *Statistical Bulletin: Residential Accommodation Statistics 1995*. London: HMSO.

—— (1996) *Moving into a Care Home: Things you Need to Know*. Wetherby: Department of Health.

Faulkner, A., Field, V. & Lindesay, J. (1992) *Who is Providing What? Information about UK Residential Care Provision for People with Mental Health Problems*. London: Research and Development for Psychiatry.

Fennell, G., Phillipson, C. & Evers, H. (1988) *The Sociology of Old Age*. Milton Keynes: Open University Press.

Gosney, M., Tallis, R. & Edmond, E. (1990) The burden of chronic illness in local authority residential homes for the elderly. *Health Trends*, 22, 153–157.

Griffiths, R. (1988) *Community Care: Agenda for Action*. London: HMSO.

Harding, J. & Jolley, D. (1994) Design for Dementia. *Hospital Design,* November, 23–24.

Harrison, R., Savla, N. & Kafetz, K. (1990) Dementia, depression and physical disability in a London borough: a survey of elderly people in and out of residential care. *Age and Ageing,* 19, 97–103.

Health Advisory Service (1993) *Comprehensive Health Services for Elderly People.* London: HAS.

Health Service Commission (1994) *Failure to Provide Long-Term NHS Care for a Brain-Damaged Patient.* Second Report for Session 1993–1994, HC197. London: HMSO.

Hodkinson, E., McGafferty, F. G., Scott, J. N., *et al* (1988) Disability and dependency in elderly people in residential and hospital care. *Age and Ageing,* 17, 147–154.

House of Commons Health Committee (1995) *Long-term Care: NHS Responsibilities for Meeting Continuing Health Care Needs.* London: HMSO.

—— (1996) *Long-Term Care. Third Report: Future Provision and Funding.* London: HMSO.

House of Commons Social Security Committee (1991) *The Financing of Private Residential and Nursing Home Fees.* Fourth Report for Session 1990–1991, HC 421-1. London: HMSO.

Jolley, D. (1981) Dementia: misfits in need of care. In *Health Care of the Elderly* (ed. T. Arie), pp. 71–88. London: Croom Helm.

—— (1992) Nursing homes: the end of a great British tradition? *International Journal of Geriatric Psychiatry,* 7, 71–73.

—— (1994a) Independent means. *Care of the Elderly,* October, 373–376

—— (1994b) Realising a vision. *Care of the Elderly,* August, 306–307.

—— (1994c) The future of long-term care as a public health provision. *Reviews in Clinical Gerontology,* 4, 1–4.

—— & —— (1992) Developments in psychogeriatric services. In *Recent Advances in Psychogeriatrics II* (ed. T. Arie), pp. 117–135. Edinburgh: Churchill Livingstone.

—— & Jolley, S. (1991a) Psychiatry of the elderly. In *Principles and Practice of Geriatric Medicine* (2nd edn) (ed. J. Pathy), pp. 895–932. Chichester: John Wiley and Sons.

—— & Lennon, S. (1991) Urban psychogeriatric service. In *Psychiatry of the Elderly* (eds R. Jacoby & C. Oppenheimer), pp. 322–338. Oxford: Oxford Medical Publications.

Jolley, S. & Jolley, D. (1991b) Psychiatric disorders in old age. In *Community Psychiatry* (eds H. Freeman & D. Bennett), pp. 268–296. Edinburgh: Churchill Livingstone.

Jones, K. (1985) *After Hospital: A Study of Long-Term Psychiatric Patients in York.* York: Department of Social Policy and Social Work, University of York.

Joseph Rowntree Foundation (1996) *Meeting the Costs of Continuing Care.* York: Joseph Rowntree Foundation.

Kay, D. W. K., Beamish, P. & Roth, M. (1962) *Some Medical and Social Characteristics of Elderly People under State Care: Comparison of Geriatric Wards, Mental Hospitals and Welfare Homes,* Social Research Monograph 5. Keele: Keele University.

——, Bergmann, K., Foster, E. M., *et al* (1970) Mental illness and hospital usage in the elderly. *Comprehensive Psychiatry,* 1, 26–35.

Laing, W. (1993) *Financing Long-Term Care: The Crucial Debate*. London: Age Concern.

Larder, D. Day, P. & Klein R. (1986) *Institutional Care for the Elderly. The Geographical Distribution of the Public/Private Mix*. Bath: Centre for the Analysis of Social Policy, University of Bath.

Laslett, P. (1977) *Family life and Illicit Love in Earlier Generations*. Cambridge: Cambridge University Press.

—— (1989) *A Fresh Map of Life*. London: Weidenfeld and Nicholson.

Mann, A., Graham, N. & Ashby, D. (1984) Psychiatric illness in residential homes for the elderly: a survey in one London borough. *Age and Ageing,* 13, 257–265.

McGrath, A. M. & Jackson, G. A. (1996) Survey of neuroleptic prescribing in residents of nursing homes in Glasgow. *British Medical Journal,* 312, 611–612.

McLauchlan, S. & Wilkin, D. (1982) Levels of provision and of dependency in residential homes for the elderly. *Health Trends,* 14, 63–64.

Meacher, M. (1972) *Taken for a Ride. Special Residential Homes for Confused Old People: A Study of Separatism in Social Policy*. London: Longman.

Murphy, E., Lindesay, J. & Dean, R. (1994) *The Domus Project*. London: Sainsbury Centre for Mental Health.

Neill, J. & Williams, J. (1992) *Leaving Hospital. Elderly People and their Discharge to Community Care*. London: HMSO.

Nolan, L. & O'Malley, K. (1989) The need for a more rational approach to drug prescribing for elderly people in nursing homes. *Age and Ageing,* 18, 52–56.

Oldman, C. (1990) *Moving in Old Age. New Directions in Housing Policies. Social Policy Research Unit*. London: HMSO.

Pattie, A. & Moxon, S. (1991) *Community Units for the Elderly in York Health District. Evaluation and Research Support Unit*. York: Clifton Hospital.

Peet, S. M. Castleden, M., Potter, J. F., *et al* (1994) The outcome of medical examination for older applicants to Leicester homes for older people. *Age and Ageing,* 23, 65–68.

Pelling, M. & Smith, R. M. (1991): *Life, Death and the Elderly: Historical Perspectives*. London: Routledge.

Phillips, D. R. (1988) *Home from Home? Private Residential Care for Elderly People*. Sheffield: University of Sheffield Joint Unit for Social Services Research.

Relatives Association (1994) On being the relative of someone in a home. *The Journal of Care and Practice,* 3 (2 May).

Research Unit of the Royal College of Physicians (1992) *The CARE Scheme. Continuous Assessment Review and Evaluation. Clinical Audit of Long-Term Care of Elderly People*. London: Royal College of Physicians.

Rosenmayr, L. & Kockeis, E. (1963) Propositions for a sociological theory of aging and the family. *International Science Journal,* 15, 410–426.

Royal College of Physicians & Royal College of Psychiatrists (1989) *Care of Elderly People with Mental Illness. Specialist Services and Medical Training*. London: Royal College of Physicians.

—— & British Geriatrics Society (1992) *High Quality Long-Term Care for Elderly People*. London: Royal College of Physicians.

Social Services Inspectorate (1990) *Caring for Quality. Guidance on Standards for Residential Homes for Elderly People*. London: HMSO.

—— (1993) *Standards for the Residential Care of Elderly People with Mental Disorders*. London: HMSO.

Stone, L. (1982) *The Family, Sex and Marriage in England 1500–1800.* Harmondsworth: Penguin.

Stout, I., Wilkin, D. & Jolley, D. (1993) Psychiatric morbidity amongst 'able' residents of Part III homes. *International Journal of Geriatric Psychiatry,* 8, 949–952.

Thomson, D. (1983) Workhouse to nursing home: residential care of elderly people in England since 1840. *Ageing and Society,* 3, 43–70.

Townsend, P. (1962) *The Last Refuge.* London: Routledge and Kegan Paul.

Victor, C. R. (1994) *Old Age in Modern Society* (2nd edn). London: Chapman and Hall.

Wagner, G. (1988) *A Positive Choice.* London: HMSO.

Warnes, A. (1982) *Geographical Perspectives on the Elderly.* Chichester: John Wiley and Sons.

Wilkin, D., Evans, G., Hughes, B., *et al* (1982) Better care for the elderly *Community Care,* May, 22–25.

——, ——, ——, *et al* (1983) The implications of managing confused and disabled people in non-specialist residential homes for the elderly. *Health Trends,* 14, 98–101.

——, Mashiah, T. & Jolley, D. (1978) Changes in the behavioural characteristics of elderly populations of local authority homes. *British Medical Journal,* 2, 1274–1276.

——, Hughes, B. & Jolley, D. (1985) Quality of care in institutions. In *Recent Advances in Psychogeriatrics* (ed. T. Arie), pp. 108–118. Edinburgh: Churchill Livingstone.

—— & Thompson, D. (1989) *User's Guide to Dependency Measures for Elderly People.* Sheffield: University of Sheffield Joint Unit for Social Services Research.

Wistow, G. (1995) Paying for long-term care: the shifting boundary between health and social services. *Community Care Management and Planning,* 3 (3 June).

Wright, K. G., Cairns, J. A. & Snell, M. C. (1981) *Costing Care. The Costs of Alternative Patterns of Care for the Elderly.* Sheffield: University of Sheffield Joint Unit for Social Services Research.

16 Pharmacological treatments

Robert Baldwin and Alistair Burns

Pharmacokinetics • Pharmacodynamics • Dementia • Delirium •
Depressive illness • Mania • Schizophrenia • Sleep disorders •
Rapid tranquillisation • Conclusion

Pharmacokinetics

The pharmacological treatment of the elderly differs from that of younger patients, mainly because of altered pharmacokinetics and the higher proportion of patients with organic disorders. Pharmacokinetics describes the way in which drugs reach their target tissues.

Absorption

Absorption is not grossly affected in the elderly although there are reductions in gastric pH, area of absorptive surface, mesenteric blood flow and transport enzymes (Lader, 1994).

Distribution

Changes in distribution in the elderly include: reduction in lean body mass and increase in body fat (fat acts as a reservoir for psychotropics, increasing their half-lives); reduction in body water (increased concentration of water soluble compounds, e.g. alcohol); reduction in plasma proteins such as albumin (increased levels of free drug); and reduction in cerebral blood flow.

Metabolism

This is reduced and is particularly important with polypharmacy. Liver blood flow decreases (by up to a third in over 65-year-olds (Bender, 1965)) and liver microsomes are less efficient (with some exceptions).

Excretion

Excretion is decreased. Glomerular filtration reduces by up to a half by the age of 70 (Papper, 1978). Plasma creatinine may be unreliable, so creatinine clearance is the preferred test of renal function.

Pharmacodynamics

Pharmacodynamics describes the effects of drugs on body tissues. It is more difficult to study and is less well understood than pharmacokinetics. However, knowledge is increasing with the use of new technology such as positron emission tomography (see Chapter 12). Results about receptor numbers and characteristics do not always explain what is seen clinically, and these discrepancies may result from more complex changes (e.g. post-synaptic changes or receptor–effector system coupling).

Narcotics and sedative hypnotics

Generally there is an increased sensitivity to sedatives in the elderly. Fewer available receptors may mean that the same drug concentration results in increased receptor occupancy (Lader, 1994). The elderly are less sensitive to some drugs (e.g. isoprenaline).

Dopaminergic system

There are less dopaminergic cells in the basal ganglia. This contributes to an increased sensitivity to the extrapyramidal side-effects (excluding dystonias) of neuroleptics.

Cholinergic system

There are less cholinergic receptors. A cholinergic deficit is well established in Alzheimer's disease, and a number of medications (donepezil, rivastigmine, metritonate) have been developed to increase the availability of acetylcholine.

Noradrenergic system

Noradrenaline levels decrease with age. This may make the elderly more vulnerable to affective disorders.

Practical implications of these changes

'Start low, go slow' – changes in pharmacokinetics and pharmacodynamics mean that the elderly are generally two to three times more sensitive to many medications, including psychotropic drugs. It is important to reduce the dose and frequency of medications because a longer half-life means that it takes longer to reach a steady state.

Dementia

Pharmacological therapy is aimed at two areas in dementia: cognitive deficits and non-cognitive features (psychiatric symptoms and behavioural disturbances).

Cognitive deficits

Alzheimer's disease

Donepezil and rivastigmine, acetylcholinesterase inhibitors, are the first drugs aimed at improving cognitive function to be licensed in the UK, and others are likely to follow. Most medications targeted at cognitive function are based on the cholinergic hypothesis, with the common goal of increasing available acetylcholine. Three approaches have been described as:

  (a) Loading with acetylcholine precursors.
  (b) Cholinesterase inhibitors (i.e. inhibiting the enzyme which degrades acetylcholine).
  (c) Direct stimulation of the receptors.

Studies with precursors such as lethicin were initially successful but inconsistent results and a lack of efficacy have followed.

Anticholinesterases have been the most studied group of drugs with the most promising results. Donepezil appears to be less hepatotoxic and better tolerated than its predecessor tetrahydroaminoacridine. Trials have shown the drug to lead to an approximate six months delay in the course of the dementia, more evidence is required (Kelly *et al*, 1997).

Co-dergocrine mesylate is regularly prescribed in continental Europe and has been shown, in double-blind trials, to be effective at reducing symptoms of anxiety, depression, 'confusion' and 'impaired social care' (effects which can be of practical benefit to patients and carers). There is little evidence that it improves cognitive function. Negative results have been found in trials with thiamine and piracetam. Improvements in cognition have been described with desferrioxamine, indomethacin and N-acetylcarnitine (Burns, 1992).

Vascular dementia

There is some evidence that treating risk factors for stroke improves cognitive impairment. Reducing systolic blood pressure to between 135 and 150 mmHg improved cognitive function, but further reduction led to a deterioration (Meyer *et al*, 1986). Stopping smoking in normotensive patients with multi-infarct dementia was also beneficial. Prescribing 325 mg of aspirin per day can produce an improvement in cognitive function and cerebral perfusion (Meyer *et al*, 1989). Low dose aspirin (75 mg per day) reduces the risk of stroke and death in patients with pre-existing vascular disease (SALT Collaborative Group, 1991).

Dementia with Lewy bodies

The clinical features of dementia with Lewy bodies include episodic confusion, hallucinations and cognitive deterioration. Patients with dementia with Lewy bodies may have profound cholinergic losses. McKeith *et al* (1992) reported high mortality when prescribed neuroleptics. Furthermore, patients with Alzheimer's disease who respond to tetrahydroaminoacridine have Lewy bodies at post-mortem (Levy, 1993). In view of the fluctuation in cognitive state there are difficulties in attributing improvement to specific medication. Behavioural disturbances can be controlled with chlormethiazole and benzodiazepines.

Non-cognitive features

This term is generally applied to psychiatric symptoms and behavioural disturbances (for a review see Burns, 1993) (see Chapter 6). It is important to define accurately what features are being targeted.

Neuroleptics

Neuroleptics are moderately effective at reducing agitation and aggression. Schneider *et al* (1992) in a meta-analysis, found that 18% of patients with dementia and agitation may benefit from neuroleptics. Individual studies showed no significant change, but together there was a small effect in favour of neuroleptics. Also behaviour deteriorated when neuroleptics were stopped. There is no established difference between thioridazine and haloperidol. Lower doses are required than for treating psychoses in younger patients. In fact very low doses, such as 5 mg of thioridazine, or 0.125 mg of haloperidol, may be effective. There is a concern that the anticholinergic effects of neuroleptics may contribute to cognitive decline in some patients with dementia.

Choice of neuroleptic

This depends upon individual preference and experience. Thioridazine is often prescribed but has marked anticholinergic effects. Haloperidol is another common choice but can cause extrapyramidal signs and symptoms. Sulpiride is useful when avoiding parkinsonian side-effects. Chlorpromazine is not recommended because of hypotension, and promazine may be too weak. Regarding the newer agents, there are good theoretical reasons why clozapine may benefit patients with dementia with Lewy bodies. Risperidone and olanzapine may also be useful because of their side-effect profiles. Both clozapine and risperidone have been shown to be reasonably well tolerated and efficacious in psychosis in the elderly, and in the psychosis of Parkinson's disease (Kumar, 1997). The newer neuroleptics tend to be more expensive. Depot neuroleptics have been tried with some success and have the obvious advantage of improved compliance.

Other medications

A number of other medications have been used to control behavioural symptoms in dementia (Schneider & Sobin, 1994) (Box 16.1).

Box 16.1 Medications (other than neuroleptics) used for behaviour symptoms in dementia

Antidepressants have consistently been shown to be effective in alleviating affective symptoms in dementia. Monoamine oxidase inhibitors (type A and type B) are successful in improving memory and concentration, possibly by alleviating depressive symptoms. Selective serotonin reuptake inhibitors reduce aggression and irritability. They may be particularly effective in vascular dementia

Lithium has been shown in a few reports to control agitation, often dramatically, but the side-effect profile of the drug and the proven benefit of other drugs make it unlikely to become an agent of choice

Beta-blockers have been used in younger patients to control aggression, usually after brain damage

Carbamazepine has been reported to control aggression, although there has been no placebo controlled study that has shown any benefit

Benzodiazepines have a significant propensity to cause confusional states in the elderly, so their use is limited. However, from three recent studies, two have shown benzodiazepines to be more efficacious than thioridazine or haloperidol

Psychostimulants such as methylphenidate have only been shown to benefit patients in open trials. It is likely with the invention of newer drugs that these older agents will no longer be used

Buspirone have been reported, in two out of three cases of dementia, to have shown an improvement

Trazodone has been highlighted by the attention given to the serotonergic deficit in Alzheimer's disease. It has been shown to help with aggression, not just in dementia

---

Delirium

Delirium is caused by physical disease, and treatment is aimed at the underlying condition such as a urinary tract infection (see Chapter 3). Appropriate nursing and medical care are important, and include reassurance, the presence of familiar people and a quiet, well lit environment. Prominent behavioural disturbance may be managed with psychotropic medication. Haloperidol and thioridazine remain the drugs of choice. Conditions such as delirium tremens require detoxification regimes along conventional lines, with a corresponding dose reduction of around a half. Rapid tranquillisation may be required for serious behavioural problems which put the patient or others at risk.

Depressive illness

Antidepressants

Antidepressants can be classified into:
(a) Tricyclics: subdivided into traditional agents (amitriptyline, imipramine, dothiepin, doxepin, clomipramine, nortriptyline) and newer agents (lofepramine).
(b) Atypical antidepressants (trazodone, mianserin).
(c) The selective serotonin reuptake inhibitors (SSRIs) (fluoxetine, fluvoxamine, paroxetine, sertraline).
(d) Monoamine oxidase inhibitors (MAOIs), subdivided into traditional agents (phenelzine, tranylcypromine) and the newer reversible inhibitors of monoamine oxidase A enzyme (RIMA agents) (moclobemide).

Choice of antidepressant

Efficacy

The recovery rate of adult patients with depressive illness treated with an antidepressant is similar at any age, around 60–70%. There is no evidence that any drug or class of drugs is superior in terms of response rate to another (Katona, 1993). Some concern has been expressed that SSRIs may be less effective in severe depression, but there is no evidence supporting this in older patients.

Safety

There is little doubt that the newer agents are safer than traditional tricyclics in over dosage. However, the use of the newer medications should not lead to a complacent approach to managing suicide risk, which is high in the elderly.

Contraindications

Contraindications for tricyclics include a history of acute (but not necessarily chronic) glaucoma; prostatism; a myocardial infarct within the preceding three months; a tachy- or brady-arrhythmia; poorly controlled (but not necessarily stable) heart failure; or a clinically relevant cardiac conduction disorder (for example bi- or tri-fascicular block). Severe renal or hepatic insufficiency are contraindications to using an SSRI.

Side-effects

There are important differences in side-effects (Table 16.1). For the traditional tricyclics, anticholinergic effects are prominent and frequently troublesome, but are less marked with lofepramine. Postural hypotension is arguably the most troublesome and dangerous side-effect of the tricyclics. They commonly cause sedation, as does trazodone. Tricyclics may provoke delirium, especially in the setting of acute physical illness or dementia; amitriptyline is the worst offender.

With relatively minor variations, all the SSRIs cause nausea (5–15%), diarrhoea (10%), insomnia (5–15%), agitation or anxiety (2–15%), headache and weight loss. Many of these are transient and early phenomena. Also, dosages of SSRIs were originally too high, possibly exaggerating this profile. However, studies in the elderly have not found a lower rate of side-effects in SSRIs than the older tricyclics, but a different pattern (Katona, 1993). Sedation is least likely with fluoxetine and more likely with paroxetine, while fluoxetine may lead to anxiety and agitation. Fluvoxamine causes nausea, but has a lower incidence of insomnia. Paroxetine has a specific indication for the treatment of anxiety in association with depression.

Table 16.1 Side-effects of antidepressants (numbered 0 to 5 by increasing intensity of effect)

	Anticholinergic effects	Orthostatic effects	Sedation
Amitriptyline	5	5	5
Imipramine	4	5	2
Dothiepin	4	3	3
Mianserin	0/1	0/1	4
Lofepramine	1/2	1	1
Trazodone	0	1	3
Fluvoxamine	0/1	0	0
Sertraline	0/1	0	0
Fluoxetine	0/1	0	0
Paroxetine	0/1	0	1/2
Moclobemide	1	1	1/2

Moclobemide appears to be of equal efficacy to tricyclics and SSRIs in late-life depression. It has a low risk of the 'cheese effect', a short duration of action and half-life and is safe and seems well tolerated. Adverse effects include agitation, anxiety and insomnia.

Interactions

All antidepressants may antagonise anticonvulsant medication. Concomitant antipsychotics lead to increased levels of tricyclic drugs, and the plasma concentration of haloperidol may be increased by fluoxetine. There is an increased risk of lithium central nervous system toxicity if combined with SSRIs. Two SSRIs, fluvoxamine and paroxetine, may enhance the effects of warfarin. Plasma concentrations of lipophilic beta-blockers may be increased by fluvoxamine. Imipramine and possibly other tricyclics may lead to increased levels of diltiazem and verapamil. Anxiolytics and hypnotics may enhance the sedative effects of tricyclics. Cimetidine may raise plasma levels of moclobemide and the tricyclics. Although the risk of a hypertensive crisis is low, drugs with sympathomimetic effect and opiate-based drugs should be avoided with moclobemide.

If changing to a MAOI from fluoxetine five weeks must elapse, two weeks for paroxetine and a week for sertraline. Mixing an SSRI with a MAOI may cause the serotonergic syndrome characterised by excitement, confusion, rigidity, tremor, hyperthermia, tachycardia, hypotension and convulsions. Lastly, although rare, there have been a number of reports of SSRIs leading to, or exacerbating, parkinsonism or akathisia.

Compliance

Lack of compliance correlates with the number of other drugs prescribed and polypharmacy is frequent among older depressed patients. Memory is less efficient in depression and may impair compliance. The once daily dosage regime of most of the SSRIs is an advantage over tricyclics.

Cost

Costs are generally much higher for the newer medications. While arguments have been put forward that cost-benefit analysis favours the newer agents because of increased compliance, there is no relevant data with older, depressed patients.

Comorbidity

Tricyclics are less well tolerated by elderly medically ill patients (Koenig *et al*, 1989) than SSRIs (Evans, 1993). There is little evidence about the best way of treating depression comorbid with dementia. In a double-blind placebo controlled trial, using imipramine, Reifler *et al* (1989) found a significant improvement in mood in an elderly group of patients with Alzheimer's disease and depression. The mean dose was 80 mg daily, but it was noted that cognitive function remained stable only within a fairly narrow dose range. Other agents have been inadequately assessed in dementia. In one small open study, patients reported improvement in depression comorbid with dementia using 150–225 mg of moclobemide (Postma & Vranesic, 1985).

Treatment-resistant depression

This is defined as failure to respond to eight weeks of an adequate single agent therapy. There has been considerable interest in augmentation regimes, but little data about older depressives. Finch & Katona (1989) reported improvement and good tolerance with lithium augmentation in two-thirds of a small sample of patients resistant to either first line treatment or electroconvulsive therapy. Van Marwijk *et al* (1990) reported a similar improvement rate in a larger series, but encountered more side-effects, especially of lithium toxicity. Seth *et al* (1992), in an open study of eight refractory, mainly elderly, cases, reported improvement in all when given nortriptyline plus an SSRI. However, this combination may cause toxic plasma levels of the tricyclic.

Continuation therapy

Response to treatment often occurs later than in younger patients (Flint, 1992; National Insistute of Health Consensus Development Panel on Depression in Late Life, 1992). A minimum trial is six weeks, although a significant minority of patients respond up to eight or nine weeks after starting therapy (NIH Consensus Development Panel on Depression in Late Life, 1992). The standard six months of continuation therapy after resolution of depressive symptoms is probably too short for elderly patients (Flint, 1992); a year is more realistic. The main risk period for recurrence and relapse is the first two years (Flint, 1992).

Prophylaxis

Some clinicians argue for the long-term treatment of all patients who have had a major depression in later life. Few elderly patients remain symptom free during extended periods of follow-up (Baldwin & Jolley, 1986) and even one further episode of depressive illness occurring to an older person is time lost from an already short life expectancy. However, this is controversial.

Clinicians are faced with the choice of either maintaining patients on antidepressants indefinitely, or attempting to wean them off after about a year. As a guide, those patients who do best are characterised by having good health and an uncomplicated recovery from depression (Baldwin & Jolley, 1986). Both lithium (Abou-Saleh & Coppen, 1983) and dothiepin (Old Age Depression Interest Group, 1993) are reported to significantly reduce relapse rates in the medium term. For antidepressants the prophylactic dose should be as close as possible to the therapeutic one (Reynolds *et al*, 1993). However, weight gain associated with long-term tricyclic usage may be problematic; more work is needed on the role of the newer agents in prophylaxis.

Which antidepressant?

A meta-analysis of the efficacy and acceptability of SSRIs (Song *et al*, 1993) concluded that their routine use as first line agents in depressive illness was unwarranted. Tricyclic antidepressants can be recommended as a well-tried, effective and cheap treatment for depression in old age, provided the patient has no contraindications and is tolerant of side-effects. In practice, the newer agents constitute an important advance in the treatment of those elderly patients, not inconsiderable in number, who do not fulfil these conditions, especially the physically frail.

Mania

Acute treatment

Neuroleptic drugs are the mainstay of treatment in the acute phase. Haloperidol, which has an extremely wide dose range, is popular. Drugs with lower potency such as thioridazine or promazine can be prescribed to reduce the risk of extrapyramidal side-effects. Practical problems include falls caused by a mixture of parkinsonism and sedation in an overactive patient and anticholinergic delirium caused by prescribing neuroleptics and anticholinergic agents (benzhexol, orphenadrine, benztropine). Mania may then be erroneously diagnosed.

Lithium is an option for the less disturbed patient but serum levels should be lower than for younger patients, on average 0.4–0.6 mmol/l (Shulman *et al*, 1992). There is a little evidence that valproate or carbamazepine may be effective, but much further work is required, including research to produce definitive guidelines for lithium treatment in older people (Shulman *et al*, 1992).

Prophylaxis

Lithium is also used for prophylaxis. As with acute treatment, dosages will generally be half that of younger adults. Lithium toxicity is a risk and is associated as much with poor monitoring as with the presence of organic

---

Box 16.2 Key learning points

Non-cognitive features in dementia are amenable to treatment
with neuroleptics and non-neuroleptic drugs

In vascular dementia, removing risk factors and aspirin improve
cognitive function

Patients with Lewy body dementia are particularly sensitive to
neuroleptics

Remember inter-individual variation in drugs metabolism is
much greater in elderly than younger patients

All antidepressant and antipsychotic agents are equally effective
so prescribing decisions are largely based on side-effect profiles

The principles of prescribing to older patients are not different
but are complicated by issues of comorbidity, poorer
compliance and higher risk of side-effects

Suicide risk is not dealt with simply by prescribing a 'safer' drug

---

(not infrequently cerebral) pathology. Regular checks of renal and thyroid function and concurrent medication, particularly the inadvertent prescription of a diuretic, are essential.

Schizophrenia

Acute treatment

The principles of treating schizophrenia are similar at any age. Ageing results in reduced levels of dopamine and tyrolase hydroxylase, as well as lower counts of dopamine-rich neurons in the midbrain (Morgan *et al*, 1987). This raises susceptibility to neuroleptic-induced extrapyramidal symptoms.

Antipsychotic drugs can be classified into:

(a) Phenothiazines, aminoalkyl compounds (chlorpromazine), piperazines (trifluoperazine) and piperidines (thioridazine).
(b) Thioxanthenes (flupenthixol).
(c) Butyrophenones (haloperidol and pimozide, a butyrophenone derivative).
(d) Dibenzapines (clozapine).
(e) Other newer agents: sulpiride (a substituted 0-anisomide), risperidone (a benzisoxazole), sertindole and olanzapine.

The first three groups have similar pharmacokinetics and are metabolised in the liver and excreted by the kidney. Their elimination half-lives are in the order of 10–30 hours, although pimozide is much longer and clozapine and sulpiride somewhat shorter (5–15 hours). Clinical experience with clozapine, risperidone and olanzapine in the elderly is limited. However, the fact that these newer compounds may cause less extrapyramidal symptoms or tardive dyskinesia is of great significance to older patients.

Choice of neuroleptic

Effectiveness

All current antipsychotics are effective in late-onset schizophrenia.

Contraindications

Caution is necessary in patients with a history of myocardial disease (in particular with pimozide), hepatic disorder, prostatism and Parkinson's disease, but apart from agranulocytosis most contraindications are relative.

Side-effects

Choosing a neuroleptic depends largely on the anticipated side-effects. These are best understood by reference to neurotransmitter systems (Table 16.2):

(a) Antidopaminergic effects cause parkinsonism and akathisia. The former is a particular hazard in elderly patients. Lowering the dose, if practicable, is the first move; otherwise changing to a lower potency neuroleptic may help. Routine prescribing of anti-cholinergic agents to suppress such symptoms is not recommended as it may increase the risk of tardive dyskinesia in older patients (World Health Organization, 1990). Age is a major risk factor for tardive dyskinesia so that drug treatment should be reviewed regularly. Drug holidays can make the problem worse. Treatment of tardive dyskinesia is difficult, but sulpiride benefits some patients (Schwartz *et al*, 1990).

(b) Anticholinergic effects cause similar problems to those of the tricyclic antidepressants.

(c) Antihistaminic effects may lead to oversedation, especially when combined with other centrally active drugs, including antidepressants and hypnotics. Weight gain may occur with long-term use.

(d) Antiadrenergic effects may cause dangerous postural hypotension. Chlorpromazine is the worst culprit, it is not a drug of first choice for the frail elderly.

In addition, there are a number of idiosyncratic reactions of which the most important are the neuroleptic malignant syndrome, adverse liver effects (which are not confined to chlorpromazine) and agranulocytosis.

Table 16.2 Side-effects of antipsychotic drugs (+++ marked, ++ moderate, + mild, + minimal, 0 none)

	Anti-dopaminergic	Anti-muscarinic	Anti-histaminic	Anti-alpha-adrenergic
Chlorpromazine	++	+	++	+++
Thioridazine	+	++	++	++
Perphenazine	++	+	++	+
Trifluoperazine	+++	+	+	+
Haloperidol	+++	+	+	+
Pimozide	++	+	+	+
Sulpiride	+	+	0	0
Clozapine	+	+++	++	+
Promazine	+	+	+++	+
Risperidone	+++	0	++	+
Olanzapine	++	+++	++	+

Long-term use is associated with corneal particulate material which could carelessly be attributed to cataract in the elderly.

Interactions

Interactions which alter plasma antipsychotic levels may occur with: lithium, phenobarbitol, carbamazepine, phenyldantoin, cimetidine, propranolol and antidepressant drugs. Cost is a major issue with the newer agents such as risperidone and clozapine. Many clinicians have locally produced protocols for their use.

Treatment-resistant schizophrenia

Clozapine is reserved for refractory schizophrenia and is not contraindicated in older patients, although dosages are typically half that of younger adults, and hypotension can be problematic. Surprisingly, age has not been identified as a risk factor for agranulocytosis (Ball, 1992).

Maintenance therapy

Post's seminal work (1966) suggested that only a third of patients with late paraphrenia, followed over 14 to 21 months, remained symptom free. Regrettably, the advent of the newer antipsychotics and specialised services have not convincingly altered this prognosis (Howard & Levy, 1992). They suggested that compliance, and therefore outcome, may be improved by the use of depot neuroleptics and the deployment of community psychiatric nurses. All the current depot neuroleptics have been used in

---

Box 16.3 Good practice points

'Start low, go slow' when prescribing to elderly patients – to start in very low doses, syrups are sometimes available

Exclude Lewy body dementia, as far as possible, before prescribing neuroleptics to a patient with dementia

Examine a patient with dementia to exclude vascular disease – treatment of risk factors and/or aspirin may help

Gain experience with prescribing at least one of the tricyclics and one of the newer agents; become familiar with their dose ranges and side-effect profiles

Take a good drug and alcohol history – polypharmacy accounts for much iatrogenic morbidity

A therapeutic antidepressant trial in older patients should last at least six to eight weeks

A reasonable period for continuation treatment is 12 months.

Lithium dose ranges are lower in the elderly, generally 0.4–0.6 mol/l

---

elderly patients and there is little to suggest that one is superior to another, or that any is less likely to precipitate parkinsonism. Dosages will generally be half that of younger adults. Parkinsonism may occur quite suddenly after weeks of treatment and may take months to wear off, or may expose latent Parkinson's disease. Many clinicians avoid the longer acting depot agents (haloperidol decanoate, pipothiazine palmitate) in elderly patients.

Sleep disorders

Disturbed sleep in the elderly is a common complaint and often results in a request for sedative medication. It is important to recognise that sleep disturbances are very often secondary to a physical disorder (obvious symptomatic culprits being pain, dysuria and nocturia) or a psychiatric disturbance (such as depression or delirium). Attention to the primary problem often leads to restoration of the normal sleep pattern. It is important to be aware of iatrogenic causes of sleep disturbance, notably steroids, theophyllines and psychoactive medication, as well as alcohol. Specific sleep disturbances of snoring, sleep apnoea and neuromuscular disorders such as akathisia may be responsible.

Specific agents to treat sleep disorders include chlormethiazole, which is effective and widely used; the only side-effect being nasal stuffiness. Benzodiazepines are still the most commonly used drugs for sleep disturbance and the shorter acting the drug the better, temazepam being the best. Chlordiazepoxide and diazepam are longer acting and newer

Table 16.3 Medications prescribed for sleep disorders

	Starting dose	Maximum dose	Side-effects
Chloral hydrate	1–2 tabs (as 414 mg per tablet) nocte	Up to 5	Gastric irritation
Triclofos sodium	1–2g nocte	Same	Fewer gastrointestinal effects
Chlormethiazole	1–2 caps nocte	Up to 3	Nasal congestion
Zopiclone	1/2 tab nocte	Up to 2 tabs	New drug, caution in elderly
Temazepam	5–15 mg nocte	Up to 30 mg	As with other benzodiazepines

agents such as zopiclone require more research. Medications are summarised in Table 16.3.

Rapid tranquillisation

The elderly, in common with their younger counterparts, can become aggressive and agitated requiring emergency sedation. One has to exercise more caution with sedation as coexisting physical illness may interact detrimentally with prescribed medication. For example, heavy sedation in a person with a confusional state secondary to cerebral hypoxia could be fatal. Bearing this in mind, the principles of rapid tranquillisation are the same as in younger patients, although doses need adjusting accordingly. Intravenous treatment is rarely required and intramuscular injections usually suffice. Prolonged and sustained aggression is not as often a management problem and hence long-term treatment is rarely necessary. Haloperidol is particularly effective at controlling aggression

---

Box 16.4 Controversial issues

Donepezil may be helpful in alleviating the cognitive deficit in Alzheimer's disease. A careful diagnostic assessment and follow-up is necessary

The newer antidepressants are regarded by some, but by no means all, old age psychiatrists as drugs of first choice when prescribing to elderly depressives

There is a trend to life-long maintenance therapy in major depression of later life, but not all agree with this

and a suggested regime for management is: (a) haloperidol 1 mg orally every hour (1–5 mg intramuscularly in an emergency); (b) continue with 0.5 to 2.0 mg, eight hourly; when settled for 48 hours, reduce dose by 25%, continue with this until signs of aggression 'break through'; (d) aim to discontinue drug after a maximum of four weeks.

Conclusion

Care must be exercised when prescribing for the elderly. Changes in pharmacokinetics and pharmacodynamics mean that doses often need to be reduced and side-effects are more common. Good prescribing behaviour is summed up by the adage 'start low, go slow'. However, consideration must be taken not to treat mental illnesses in the elderly inadequately. In recent years, new treatments have become available for dementia, depression and schizophrenia. More studies, in the elderly, will be necessary to gain the maximum benefits for patients.

References

Abou-Saleh, M. T. & Coppen, A. (1993) The prognosis of depression in old age: the case for lithium therapy. *British Journal of Psychiatry,* 143, 527–528.

Baldwin, R. C. & Jolley, D. J. (1986) The prognosis of depression in old age. *British Journal of Psychiatry,* 149, 574–583.

Ball, C. J. (1992) The use of clozapine in older people. *International Journal of Geriatric Psychiatry,* 7, 689–692.

Bender, A. D. (1965) The effect of increasing age on the distribution of peripheral blood flow in man. *Journal of the American Geriatrics Society,* 13, 192–198.

Burns, A. (1992) Treatment by physical methods: medication. *Current Opinion in Psychiatry,* 5, 567–570.

—— (1993) Treatment of non-cognitive features of dementia. In *Treatment and Care in Old Age Psychiatry* (eds R. Levy, R. Howard & A. Burns), pp. 37–48. Petersfield: Wrightson Biomedical Publishing.

Evans, M. E. (1993) Depression in elderly physically ill inpatients: a 12 month prospective study. *International Journal of Geriatric Psychiatry,* 8, 587–592.

Finch, E. J. L. & Katona, C. L. E. (1989) Lithium augmentation in the treatment of refractory depression in old age. *International Journal of Geriatric Psychiatry,* 4, 41–46.

Flint, A. J. (1992) The optimum duration of antidepressant treatment in the elderly. *International Journal of Geriatric Psychiatry,* 7, 617–619.

Howard, R. & Levy, R. (1992) Which factors affect treatment response in late paraphrenia. *International Journal of Geriatric Psychiatry,* 7, 667–672.

Katona, C. L. E. (1993) Optimising treatment for the elderly depressive: new anti-depressants in the elderly. *Journal of Psychopharmacology,* 7 (suppl. 1), 131–134.

Kelly, C., Harvey, R. & Cayton, H. (1997) Therapies for Alzheimer's disease. *British Medical Journal,* 314, 693–694.

Koenig, H. G., Goli, V., Shelp, F., *et al* (1989) Antidepressant use in elderly medical inpatients: lessons from an attempted clinical trial. *Journal of General Internal Medicine*, 4, 498–505.

Kumar, V. (1997) Use of atypical antipsychotic agents in geriatric patients: a review. *International Journal of Geriatric Psychopharmacology*, 1, 15–23.

Lader, M. (1994) Neuropharmacology and pharmacokinetics of psychotropic drugs in old age. In *Principles and Practice of Geriatric Psychiatry* (eds J. Copeland, M. Abou-Saleh & D. Blazer), pp. 79–82. Chichester: John Wiley.

Levy, R. (1993) Is there life in the neuro-transmitter approach to the treatment of Alzheimer's disease? In *Treatment and Care in Old Age Psychiatry* (eds R. Levy, R. Howard & A. Burns), pp. 39–46. Petersfield: Wrightson Biomedical Publishing.

McKeith, I., Fairburn, A., Perry, R., *et al* (1992) Neuroleptic sensitivity in patients with senile dementia of Lewy body type. *British Medical Journal*, 305, 673–678.

Meyer, J., Judd, B., Tawaklna, T., *et al* (1986) Improved cognition after control of risk factors for multi-infarct dementia. *Journal of the American Medical Association*, 256, 2203–2209.

Meyer, J. S., Rogers, R., McClintic, K., *et al* (1989). Randomised clinical trial of daily aspirin therapy and multi-infarct dementia. *Journal of the American Geriatrics Society*, 37, 549–555.

Morgan, D. G., May, P. C. & Fich, C. E. (1987) Dopamine and serotonin system in human and rodent brain: effects of age and neurodegenerative disease. *Journal of the American Geriatric Society*, 35, 334–345.

National Institute of Health Consensus Development Panel on Depression in Late Life (1992) Diagnosis and treatment of depression in late life. *Journal of the American Medical Association*, 268, 1018–1024.

Old Age Depression Interest Group (1993) How long should the elderly take antidepressants? A double-blind placebo-controlled study of continuation/prophylaxis therapy with dothiepin. *British Journal of Psychiatry*, 162, 175–182.

Papper, S. (1978) *Clinical Nephrology*. Boston, MA: Little Brown.

Post, F. (1966) *Persistent Persecutory States of the Elderly.* Oxford: Pergamon.

Postma, J. U. & Vranesic, D. (1985) Moclobemide in the treatment of depression in demented geriatric patients. *Acta Therapeutica*, 11, 1–4.

Reifler, B. V., Teri, L., Raskind, M., *et al* (1989) Double-blind trial of imipramine in Alzheimer's disease patients with and without depression. *American Journal of Psychiatry*, 146, 45–49.

Reynolds, C. F., Schneider, L. S., Lebowitz, B. D., *et al* (1993) Treatment of depression in the elderly: guidelines for primary care. In *Diagnosis and Treatment of Depression in the Elderly: Proceedings of the NIH Consensus Development Panel Conference* (eds L. S. Schneider, C. F. Reynolds, B. Lebowitz, *et al*). Washington, DC: American Psychiatric Press.

SALT Collaborative Group (1991) Swedish aspirin low dose trial of 75 mg aspirin as secondary prophylaxis after cerebrovascular ischaemic events. *Lancet*, 338, 1345–1349.

Schneider, L., Pollock, D. & Lyness, S. (1990) A meta-analysis of controlled trials of neuroleptic treatment in dementia. *Journal of the American Geriatrics Society*, 38, 553–563.

—— & Sobin, P. (1994) Treatment for psychiatric symptoms and behavioural disturbances. In *Dementia* (eds A. Burns & R. Levy), pp. 519–540. London: Chapman and Hall Medical.

Schwartz, M., Moquillansky, L., Lanyi, G., *et al* (1990) Sulpiride in tardive dyskinesia. *Journal of Neurology, Neurosurgery and Psychiatry,* 53, 800–802.

Seth, R., Jennings, A. L., Bindman, J., *et al* (1992) Combination treatment with noradrenaline and serotonin reuptake inhibitors in resistant depression. *British Journal of Psychiatry,* 161, 562–565.

Shulman, K., Tohen, M. & Satlin, A. (1992) The significance of mania in old age. *Reviews in Clinical Gerontology,* 2, 39–43.

Song, F., Freemantle, N., Sheldon, T. A., *et al* (1993) Selective serotonin reuptake inhibitors: a meta-analysis of efficacy and acceptability. *British Medical Journal,* 306, 683–687.

Van Marwijk, H. W. J., Beeker, F. M., Nolan, W. A., *et al* (1990) Lithium augmentation in geriatric depression. *Journal of Affective Disorders,* 20, 217–223.

World Health Organization (1990) Heads of centres collaborating in WHO co-ordinated studies in biological aspects of mental illness. Prophylactic use of anticholinergics in patients on long-term neuroleptic treatment: a consensus statement. *British Journal of Psychiatry,* 156, 412.

17 Psychological treatments

Charles Twining

Practical applications ● *Psychotherapy* ● *Group therapy* ● *Family therapy* ● *Marital therapy* ● *Cognitive and behavioural therapies* ● *Anxiety management* ● *Grief counselling* ● *Therapies for dementia* ● *Carers and stress* ● *Conclusion*

The emergence of psychiatry of old age as a speciality has been paralleled by a rapid growth in the application of psychological treatments for the elderly. This chapter offers guidance to adapting treatments to meet the particular needs of older people. While it is necessary to sound a note of caution in case the gains sought are too great, on the whole the problem is overcoming resistance, not least among older people themselves, to the idea that psychological treatments are relevant and effective.

Practical applications

In some cases a psychological treatment may be the treatment of choice and the only treatment required. More often older people, especially those with serious psychological disorders, have a number of current problems. Psychological treatment then involves working in an orchestrated way with several other professionals, whose skills are also required. This is not always quite as good for the therapist's kudos as playing the solo part, but is generally better at meeting the patient's needs.

Psychological treatments may require adaptations for older clients (Box 17.1). Most of these are self-explanatory and allow for the effects of normal ageing and physical change. It is worth emphasising the importance of experience. The patient usually has more than the therapist! Rather than

---

Box 17.1 Adaptations for older clients

Take the therapy to the patient
Keep the session length flexible
Ensure achievable goals
Keep groups small
Allow for sensory impairment
Incorporate individual experience

---

teaching granny (or grandad) to suck eggs, it may be possible to help them rediscover a skill, and learn something yourself in the process.

Psychotherapy

Psychotherapy for older people has thrived despite the now famous statement by Sigmund Freud that older people are not amenable to psychoanalysis. He considered anyone over the age of 50 years as lacking "the elasticity of the mental processes on which treatment depends... old people are not educatable" (Freud, 1905). Thankfully, such overt ageism has largely been overcome, and psychotherapy is offered to older people and their carers. Psychotherapy covers the whole range of psychiatric problems, from adjustment disorders to Alzheimer's disease (see Box 17.2).

Dynamics

Psychotherapy is largely based upon a dynamic view of psychiatric (and some physical) illnesses. Although the word dynamic suggests activity where psychiatric symptoms arise, conflict often leads to a stalemate. Such a conflict might be between the drive to assert oneself and to make no trouble. The object of psychotherapy is to resolve the conflict and, in doing so, relieve symptoms and help the person function more effectively. This is achieved through words exchanged between the patient and the therapist, and the relationship which forms between them. Dynamic factors are important in old age psychiatry. Pitt (1982) identified dynamic factors in three-quarters of consecutive referrals to an old age psychiatric service.

Transference

The dynamic view is that disturbed relationships, past and present, contribute to illness. Psychotherapy seeks to improve these relationships by counselling, support and the use of transference. Transference occurs when the patient reacts to the therapist as a key figure from their past, such as a parent, sibling, child or spouse. The therapist can use transference by helping the patient become aware of subconscious feelings to these important figures. Although the patients are usually older than their therapists, this does not prevent them from being regarded as parent figures, as well as child (or grandchild) figures.

Dependency

One dynamic factor which may occur more commonly in later life is dependency. This may occur, for example, in people emotionally deprived in early life, who coped well as adults but in older age fear being neglected and unloved as they see their useful role slipping away. Goldfarb (1965) described the frantic search for help from a strong parent figure, which is frustrated because the demands are too clamorous.

In a colluding partnership, usually husband and wife but sometimes child and parent, one is seen by the other as strong but each is, in fact, dependent on the other. The 'strong' partner preserves an illusion of mastery through the weaker's reliance on them. A husband who finds a *raison d'être* in retirement in caring for his sick wife, may be threatened when she requires help from doctors. He may have a vested interest in her invalidism.

In these cases the therapist tries to establish a supportive relationship to meet the dependency needs of the patient, without being taken over, or turning the patient into a child. For some very old patients, supportive therapy may mean an involvement for life.

Confrontation

There is a place for pleasant personal remarks, warmth and friendliness in the therapist's approach to older patients which would be less appropriate with younger patients. Nevertheless confrontation may play an important part in therapy. Negative reactions to the therapist such as plaintiveness; exaggeration of symptoms; seeking help elsewhere; or lateness for appointments, should be explored. Skilfully handled these confrontations allow the patient to acknowledge resentment and aggression, and find relief that therapy can continue.

Life review

When the recital of symptoms becomes tedious and repetitive, it can be useful to move away from the illness to a consideration of the patient as

---

Box 17.2 Psychotherapy in later life

Psychotherapy in older age
Dynamic factors are usually identifiable in referrals
Resolution of conflicts may resolve symptoms
Transference may be altered as therapists are usually younger
Dependency, loss of sexuality and fear of death are important factors
Lifelong defences may decompensate with changes such as retirement
Confrontation may be a useful part of therapy
A 'life review' can help older patients integrate their experiences

a person with an interesting life history. Memories of the war are often evocative and revealing. Butler (1968) advocated a 'life review' to help older patients function by gaining strength from memories of adaptation and survival. The last of Erikson's (1959) eight stages in life, is the identity crisis of old age. Integrity (the capacity to value one's life experiences and oneself) is an antidote to despair.

Group therapy

For some patients group support, often in the setting of a day hospital, is a good means of meeting and working through problems including dependency needs. It is often less intense than one to one therapy, and less likely to lead to regression. Groups can help some older people with social functioning, especially those who have been isolated. Some special difficulties with group therapy in the elderly include deafness and somnolence. Avoiding meeting after heavy meals; using comfortable but supportive chairs; a well ventilated room; and a minimum of extraneous noise, help to keep everyone awake and able to hear. Meetings should not run for longer than half an hour.

Dobson & Culhane (1991) describe a therapeutic group run for older women. They emphasise the importance of having a clear purpose for a group and considering selection criteria carefully. In the early stages, rules such as not talking while others do, and valuing others' contributions, helped to harness good intentions. Finances, losses and reminiscences were powerful themes. The group ended after plenty of notice had been given, and a photograph taken on the penultimate session. The leader's responsibilities are defined in Box 17.3.

Family therapy

Most informal carers are close family members, and the problems shown by an older family member may reflect family pathology. Family therapy remains primarily associated with helping children, but there are now a

---

Box 17.3 Running a group (adapted from Dobson & Culhane, 1991)

Practical organisation: recruitment, starting, ending
Listening and encouraging
Protection from scapegoating
Focusing on common themes
Involving all in the group

number of established examples of its application to older people (Brubaker, 1985). The adaptations required are relatively minor, although they include all the general rules for involving older people in psychological treatments (Box 17.1). There may be problems with communication, for example deafness or poor vision, which can compound the effects of ageing in reducing information processing capacity. The overall effect is to make demanding tasks such as therapy very difficult. Physical or mental illness can be used to scapegoat the older person. Conversely, symptoms of physical illness can be accentuated or become an important vehicle for the older person's status and power (West & Spinks, 1988) (Box 17.4).

Benbow & Marriott (1997) listed the following ideas as being useful in family therapy with older adults:

(a) The family life cycle – looking at how families evolve. Key issues in later family life include retirement and becoming a grandparent.
(b) Cross-generational interplay – life cycle changes in different generations may not 'fit'. One generation may be more family orientated (e.g. during childbirth) while others are more outward looking (e.g. early retirement). Expectations may vary across the generations.
(c) Genograms – drawing a family tree is a useful way of collecting, organising and considering family information.
(d) Circular questions – these are in terms of relationships. Examples include, "If your mother says this, what does your brother do?" or "who in the family would this affect?"
(e) Reflecting teams – members of the multi-disciplinary team talk about the family while they listen, offering different perspectives.

The systemic approach derived from family therapy can also be applied to the care of older people in institutions (Jeffrey, 1986). Sometimes the

---

Box 17.4 Family therapy

Family problems are common in the elderly
Serious illness and impending death have major effects on the
    family
Carer stress is very common
Responsibility for older members can cause guilt in those not
    caring
Family myths may need to be explored
Illness can be used to bond the family together
Low key family meetings can be very useful
High expressed emotion includes criticism and overinvolvement

problems attributed to one or more residents are better addressed by looking at the social network and relationships in the home as a whole. Such networks are just as important in the community, and this approach can benefit older people and their carers (Pottle, 1984). It is certainly always worth considering family systems when dealing with complex problems in the elderly.

Marital therapy

"We've been together for 40 years and it doesn't seem a day too long" is, alas, not always the case. Couples who have barely tolerated each other during working life may find each other's company very difficult after retirement. Illness in one partner may result in guilt in the other. Marital therapy should not ignore the continuing sexual needs of many old people.

Cognitive and behavioural therapies

These approaches have aroused considerable interest in recent years. The most frequently reported developments have been with younger people (Williams, 1984), but there have been examples of applications to older people. These have been well reviewed, at least in relation to depression, and there is evidence that these approaches are effective (Morris & Morris, 1991). However, outcome studies have not indicated which particular forms of cognitive or behavioural therapy are most effective. Moreover there remains a lack of studies comparing these therapies with drug treatments or with combinations of approaches.

There is also a problem with generalising results. It is unlikely that a sample of elderly people with a history of at least four years of depression (Steuer *et al*, 1984) is the same as one recruited by media announcements and followed-up over the telephone (Scogin *et al*, 1989), or a group of depressed nursing home residents (Hussain & Lawrence, 1981). These groups may only have their ages and depression scores in common.

There are three reasons why cognitive and behavioural therapies are particularly suited to the elderly:

(a) Depression in later life is prone to relapse and there is evidence that cognitive and behavioural approaches have longer-term benefits. Patients may develop preventative skills.

(b) Older people are more susceptible to adverse side-effects from drug therapy, especially those who are physically ill or taking medications for other illnesses.

(c) Spontaneous remission is less likely in older depressed people (Lambert, 1976; Thompson *et al*, 1987).

Evidence suggests that depression often goes unrecognised or untreated when it occurs with physical illness (Koenig *et al*, 1992). Only 10% of their sample of depressed older men in hospital received some form of psychological therapy, and 44% received no treatment at all. They suggest that behavioural and cognitive techniques are a viable therapeutic option for the 50% of patients or more who have medical contraindications to antidepressants.

Anxiety management

The prevalence of phobic disorders is higher than might be expected, with a one month prevalence of 10% (Lindesay, 1991). Disability from phobias can be significant but specific treatment is rare. The majority of these patients suffer from a late-onset agoraphobia following a traumatic experience, typically an episode of serious physical illness. They have a higher than average contact with primary care services but tend not to be referred for specialist treatment (see Chapter 9).

While it may be necessary to adapt anxiety management for older people, it is just as effective as in younger patients. Older people may benefit from anxiety techniques such as relaxation therapy with tapes. By using headphones it is possible to deliver soothing instructions loudly, so overcoming all but the most severe hearing loss (Box 17.5).

Grief counselling

Although bereavement is not exclusively a problem of later life it is more common, and can mean the loss of an intimate relationship which has lasted many years. One ageist stereotype is that older people are better

---

Box 17.5 Anxiety management

Full assessment
Treat depression, or underlying physical cause
Identify when symptoms occur, precipitants and consequences
Educate the patient about anxiety, the physical manifestations
   and the treatment
Take baseline measurements
Identify contributing cognitions and challenge them
Identify contributing behaviours such as avoidance and plan
   exposure
Breathing exercises
Relaxation therapy

Box 17.6 Bereavement reaction (adapted from Viederman, 1995)

Stunned phase: lasting a few hours to several weeks
Mourning phase: intense yearning and distress; futility; anorexia, restlessness, irritability; preoccupation with the deceased; transient hallucinations; guilt denial
Acceptance and readjustment phase: may take several weeks to a year or more

---

at handling loss because it is expected, or because they have had more practice. In fact older people are not only more likely to experience loss, but the effects are cumulative in terms of risk for depression (Murphy, 1986). Being recently widowed is a major risk factor for mortality (Rees & Lutkins, 1967). Box 17.6 lists the phases of an uncomplicated bereavement (Viederman, 1995).

Losses can also reduce social support, either because friends and family have died, or because physical illness enforces isolation. Appropriate interventions include bereavement therapy and practical help to improve social networks. Important steps are recognising that something is wrong and encouraging the older person to accept help. Some of the principles of grief counselling are listed in Box 17.7 for a fuller text see Worden (1991).

Therapies for dementia

Reality orientation

Reality orientation is perhaps the best known specific psychological treatment for older people (Holden & Woods, 1988). Reality orientation aims to help patients with dementia by directly focusing on some of the deficits of the disorder, including disorientation and impaired short-term memory. It also helps to preserve skills.

Box 17.7 Principles of grief counselling

Offering support
Giving time to grieve
Help to express feelings
Reassure that feelings are normal
Identify abnormal coping

The approach can be divided into brief sessions (classroom reality orientation) and a pervasive approach influencing staff–patient interactions throughout the day (24-hour reality orientation).

Underlying both of these types of approach is the principle that staff enhance orientation by using identifying names and other information. This is supported by cues such as the commonly used reality orientation board, showing the date, weather, etc. (providing it is kept up to date!) and cues to everyday behaviour such as making tea or visiting a pub. Activities within formal reality orientation sessions include prompting basic information such as the names of group members; looking at current events; and using tactile, olfactory and other stimuli to encourage active cognition.

The enthusiasm with which reality orientation has been embraced by staff has sometimes exceeded the evidence for its effectiveness (Powell-Procter & Miller, 1982). There is evidence that reality orientation is beneficial, but the benefits tend to be modest, and only sustained with continued effort. There is little evidence to suggest that generalisation occurs (i.e. encouraging orientation for time does not lead to gains in orientation for place). There are also doubts about the suitability of reality orientation for use by informal carers at home.

Perhaps the biggest impact of reality orientation has been on staff attitudes, where it has resulted in staff improving the environments in which they work. When you orientate someone to their environment you become more aware of it yourself. There is little point in orientating someone to the day if all days are the same.

Reminiscence

Thinking about the past is not exclusive to older people. Younger people reminisce, although their memories may not extend back so far. Similarly, older people are not always reminiscing. Some avoid doing so because it is painful, others because they prefer the present. Nevertheless for many older people looking back is an important part of making sense of themselves and their lives. It allows the kind of integration that Erikson (1959) suggests is important as a developmental task of later life.

The ability to reminisce is preserved in early dementia. People with dementia are better at remembering what happened many years ago than what happened this week or earlier this morning. The act of reminiscence therefore offers a good way of engaging people with mild to moderate cognitive impairment without reminding them of their cognitive shortcomings. It is quite possible to use reality orientation and reminiscence in combination. Starting with reality orientation before progressing to reminiscence appears to offer better results (Baines *et al*, 1987).

Whether the activity of reminiscence, per se, can be considered a 'therapy' is open to question. Certainly reminiscence can have powerful emotional consequences and may be used with specific therapeutic targets in mind. However, it is neither a panacea nor is it always appropriate for older people. The overlap between reminiscence and post-traumatic stress disorder, requires more careful study. Certainly there are older people whose problem is not how to remember but rather how to forget memories from wartime or other past trauma. The effects of reminiscence, like reality orientation, are dependent on the environment. There is a more obvious effect in a less interactive environment (Head *et al*, 1990).

Validation therapy

Concerns about the specific effects of reality orientation in confronting dementia sufferers with their failings have crystallised around the development of an alternative therapy which is directed at emotional needs. There can, not surprisingly, be problems in reorientating people when the reality is upsetting. A common example given is of a disoriented person who wants to go home to his or her spouse, not remembering that they have died. Is reorientation the best solution in this situation?

Validation therapy focuses on the phenomenology of dementia at an emotional, rather than a factual level. It views the disoriented person as struggling to cope with a complex and confusing world. It is hypothesised that the content of 'confused' talk reflects the emotional meaning of past events. For example, worrying about getting home in time to meet the children may reflect that parenting was a time of reward and security. The response to the disorientation is directed at exploring what things were like for that person, and how this relates to how they are feeling now. It is suggested that even the most confused behaviour has some meaning for that person.

Validation therapy has begun to be reported but more investigation is needed (Jones, 1997). It remains to be demonstrated how validation therapy and reality orientation differ. Of course bad reality orientation can certainly be frustrating and even unkind. However, closer scrutiny of the practice of experienced therapists suggests that they are sensitive to the emotional content of 'confusion', and avoid inappropriate confrontation. We need to find the best responses to people with dementia.

Memory therapy

The emergence of specific approaches aimed at helping those with memory problems would seem to be of particular interest to those treating the elderly. On the whole, however, the work has been directed at younger brain damaged patients. This is because the conditions for memory therapy are not met so well in dementia. In particular the use of mnemonics or memory aids require insight into memory loss, as well as preserved language and psychomotor skills.

Older people with mild memory problems can make use of simple aids such as lists, alarms and placing notices and instructions in key areas. A useful list of such aids is given by Burnside (1988). However, these are of major significance in only a few cases. These tend to involve people with mild or relatively static memory problems, such as following a stroke. For those with progressive dementia prompts supplement, rather than replace, the presence of an alert carer.

Resolution therapy

Resolution therapy has been introduced as a companion to reality orientation (Stokes & Goudie, 1990). It shares with validation therapy the assumption that there is meaning in the behaviour and confused talk of patients with dementia. But, unlike validation therapy, it looks for that meaning in the 'here and now'. In other words it sees such behaviour or speech, as an attempt to make sense of what is happening now, or to communicate a current need. In order to try and understand these hidden meanings, the therapist must use reflective listening, exploration, warmth and acceptance.

Carers and stress

The carers of those suffering from dementia are often put under considerable strain (see Chapter 18). A third of relatives caring for someone with dementia show significant distress (Levin *et al*, 1989), and even higher rates than this have been reported. Distress is also found in those caring for an elderly person with a physical illness such as a stroke.

There is plenty of scope for improving the psychological well-being of carers and a genuine opportunity for primary prevention (George & Gwyther, 1988). This includes local support groups, individual therapy, education, practical advice and stress management. The Alzheimer's Disease Society and other organisations (see Appendix for a list of useful addresses) are very active in this area. Specific problems include

---

Box 17.8 Psychological therapies used in dementia

Reorientation therapy
Reminiscence
Validation therapy
Memory therapy
Resolution therapy

---

anticipatory grief and living bereavement. Living bereavement attempts to describe the difficulty of caring for someone whose personality has largely been lost.

Conclusion

More studies are needed to establish which patients benefit most from psychological treatments. It is difficult to generalise from research with selected older subjects with psychological problems in the absence of physical illness or social need. Such studies need to be complemented by naturalistic trials evaluating multi-disciplinary treatment. New pharmacological treatments for older people have to be evaluated, however it is equally important to evaluate psychological approaches.

References

Baines, S., Saxby, P. & Ehlert, T. K. (1987) Reality orientation and reminiscence therapy: a controlled cross-over study of elderly confused people. *British Journal of Psychiatry*, 151, 222–231.

Benbow, S. M. & Marriott, A. (1997) Family therapy with elderly people. *Advances in Psychiatric Treatment*, 3, 138–145.

Brubaker, T. H. (1985) *Later Life Families*. Newbury Park, CA: Sage.

Burnside, I. (1988) Nursing care. In *Treatments for the Alzheimer Patient* (eds L. F. Jarvik & C. H. Winograd), pp. 39–58. New York: Springer Publishing Company.

Butler, R. N. (1968) Towards a psychiatry of the life cycle: implications of sociopsychological studies of the aging process for the psychotheraputic selection. In *Aging and Modern Society* (ed. A. Simon). Washington, DC: American Psychiatric Association.

Dobson, H. & Culhane, M. (1991) Group work: family therapy. In *Psychiatry in the Elderly* (eds R. Jacoby & C. Oppenheimer). Oxford: Oxford University Press.

Erikson, E. (1959) *Identity and the Life Cycle*. New York: Norton.

Freud, S. (1905) On Psychotherapy. Reprinted (1953–1974) in *The Standard Edition of the Complete Psychological Works of Sigmund Freud* (trans. and ed. J. Strachey), vol. 7. London: Hogarth.

Goldfarb, A. I. (1965) The recognition and therapeutic use of the patient's search for aid. In *Psychiatric Disorders in the Aged*. Manchester: WPA/Geidy (UK Ltd).

George, L. K. & Gwyther, L. P. (1988) Support groups for caregivers of memory-impaired elderly: easing caregiver burden. In *Families in Transition: Primary Prevention Programs that Work* (eds L. A. Bond & B. M. Wagner). Newbury Park, CA: Sage.

Head, D. M., Portnoy, S. & Woods, R. T. (1990) The impact of reminiscence groups in two different settings. *International Journal of Geriatric Psychiatry*, 5, 295–302.

Holden, U. P. & Woods, R. T. (1988) *Reality Orientation: Psychological Approaches to the Confused Elderly* (2nd edn). Edinburgh: Churchill Livingstone.

Hussain, R. A. & Lawrence, P. S. (1981) Social reinforcement of activity and problem–solving training in the treatment of depressed institutionalised elderly patients. *Cognitive Therapy Research*, 5, 57–69.

Jeffrey, D. P. (1986) The systems approach to changing practice in residential care. In *Psychological Therapies for the Elderly* (eds I. Hanley & M. Gilhooly), pp. 124–150. Beckenham: Croom Helm.

Jones, G. M. M. (1997) A review of Feil's validation method for communicating with and caring for dementia sufferers. *Current Opinion in Psychiatry*, 10, 326–332.

Koenig, H. G., Veerainder, G., Shelp, F., *et al* (1992) Major depression in hospitalized medically ill older men: documentation, management and outcome. *International Journal of Geriatric Psychiatry*, 7, 25–34.

Lambert, M. J. (1976) Spontaneous remission in adult neurotic disorders: a revision and summary. *Psychological Bulletin*, 83, 107–119.

Levin, E., Sinclair, I. & Gorbach, P. (1989) *Family, Services and Confusion in Old Age*. Aldershot: Avebury.

Lindesay, J. (1991) Phobic disorders in the elderly. *British Journal of Psychiatry*, 159, 531–541.

Morris, R. G. & Morris, L. W. (1991) Cognitive and behavioural approaches with the depressed elderly. *International Journal of Geriatric Psychiatry*, 6, 407–411.

Murphy, E. (1986) Social factors in late life depression. In *Affective Disorders in the Elderly* (ed. E. Murphy). Edinburgh: Churchill Livingstone.

Pitt, B. (1982) *Psychogeriatrics. An Introduction to the Psychiatry of Old Age*. Edinburgh: Churchill Livingstone.

Pottle, S. (1984) Developing a network oriented service for elderly people and their carers. In *Using Family Therapy* (eds A. Treacher & J. Carpenter). Oxford: Blackwell.

Powell-Proctor, L. & Miller, E. (1982) Reality orientation: a critical appraisal. *British Journal of Psychiatry*, 140, 457–463.

Rees, W. D. & Lutkins, S. G. (1967) Mortality of bereavement. *British Medical Journal*, iv, 13.

Scogin, F., Jamison, C. & Godneaur, K. (1989) Comparative efficacy of cognitive and behavioral bibliotherapy for mild and moderately depressed older adults. *Journal of Consulting and Clinical Psychology*, 57, 403–407.

Steur, J. L., Mintz, L., Hammen, C. L., *et al* (1984) Cognitive–behavioral and psychodynamic group psychotherapy in treatment of geriatric depression. *Journal of Consulting and Clinical Psychology*, 52, 180–189.

Stokes, G. & Goudie, F. (1990) Counselling confused elderly people. In *Working with Dementia* (eds G. Stokes & F. Goudie), pp. 181–190. Bicester: Winslow Press.

Thompson, L. W., Gallagher, D. & Breckenridge, J. S. (1987) Comparative effectiveness of psychotherapies for depressed elders. *Journal of Consulting and Clinical Psychology*, 53, 385–390.

Viederman, M. (1995) Grief: normal and pathological variants. *American Journal of Psychiatry*, 152, 1–4.

West, J. & Spinks, P. (eds) (1988) *Clinical Psychology in Action: A Collection of Case Studies*. London: Wright.

Williams, J. M. G. (1984) Cognitive–behavioural therapy for depression: problems and perspectives. *British Journal of Psychiatry*, 145, 254–262.

Worden, J. W. (1991) *Grief Counselling and Grief Therapy: A Handbook for the Mental Health Practitioner* (2nd edn). London: Routledge.

Additional reading

Coleman, P. G. (1986) *Ageing and Reminiscence Processes: Social and Clinical Implications*. Chichester: Wiley.

Hanley, I. & Gilhooly, M. (1986) *Psychological Therapies for the Elderly*. Beckenham: Croom Helm.

Hanley, I. & Hodge, J. (eds) (1984) *Psychological Approaches to the Care of the Elderly*. Beckenham: Croom Helm.

Twining, T. C. (1988) *Helping Older People: A Psychological Approach*. Chichester: Wiley.

Woods, R. T. (1996) *Handbook of the Clinical Psychology of Ageing*. Chichester: Wiley.

18 Carers

Chris Gilleard

While it is recognised that caring for mentally and physically ill people can cause considerable stress, the precise nature of that stress, its causes and consequences remain unclear, despite a growing body of research.

Extent of carer stress

Early studies

Early studies on caring rarely included a comparison group of non-carers (reviewed by Baumgarten, 1989; Schulz *et al*, 1990). Without a control group it is difficult to determine whether care-giving is detrimental to health and well-being. Most carers are older people (average age around 60), who may experience problems of social isolation, poor health and unsatisfactory accommodation. These factors may contribute to impaired well-being, depression and difficulties in coping, quite independently from care-giving responsibilities. It was also unclear if caring for an older mentally ill person is more detrimental to health than caring for a younger mentally ill person, or an older person with physical illness.

Controlled studies

Controlled studies demonstrate that caring is stressful, as indicated by a wide variety of measures (see Box 18.1). Pruchno & Potashnik (1989)

Box 18.1 Measures of carer stress

Symptoms of psychological distress
Depressive symptoms
Psychotropic use
Medical care
Self-reported health
Immunological status
Stress scales
General Health Questionnaire scores

---

found that spouses looking after people with dementia were less likely to report good health; had higher rates of symptoms of psychological distress; higher rates of depressive symptoms; and were more likely to be taking psychotropic drugs, than age matched controls. Haley *et al* (1987) found that care-givers reported more depression; received more medication and health care; and reported poorer physical health.

Kiecolt-Glaser *et al* (1987) examined the immunological status of carers of Alzheimer patients and age- and gender-matched controls. They found several depressed immunological indicators in the carers, suggesting that prolonged strain had impacted on their physical health.

Importance of mental illness

Eagles and his colleagues (1987) found that the care-givers of elderly people with dementia scored higher on a strain scale than carers of elderly people without dementia. They did not differ on a measure of 'psychiatric morbidity'. This study is important because it involved carers recruited from a community survey, rather than from contact with services. The Hughes Hall Project for Later Life (O'Connor *et al*, 1990) provides some of the strongest evidence on the effects of care-giving for people with dementia. From a study group of over 2000 people, aged over 75, two groups of carers were identified: those caring for people with dementia and those caring for people without dementia. A measure of carer strain, but not scores on the General Health Questionnaire (GHQ: Goldberg, 1972) showed increasing strain with the severity of dementia. Gilleard (1984) found an overlap in the distress of carers of patients attending geriatric and psychogeriatric day hospitals in Scotland. In the psychogeriatric day hospitals, 63% of patients had dementia and 65% of carers scored 'psychiatric distress' on the GHQ. In the geriatric day hospitals only 8% of the patients had dementia while 46% of the carers scored distress. Carers in the two settings complained of similar behavioural problems.

Whittick (1988) compared the GHQ scores of middle-aged women caring for either a learning-disabled child or a parent with dementia. She found that the care-giving daughters reported significantly more distress than the care-giving mothers. Birkel (1987) found evidence of greater distress in the carers of mentally ill elderly people compared with the carers of physically ill, but mentally well elderly people. On the other hand, Liptzin *et al* (1988) found no difference in the reported burden between carers of depressed elderly clinic patients and carers of elderly clinic patients with dementia.

Although not always consistent, the evidence suggests that looking after people with dementia is a particularly stressful activity, which can impair health (Schulz *et al*, 1995). Psychiatric morbidity, especially depression, is more likely to occur in carers. There is less consistent evidence that caring affects the physical health of carers.

Causes of carer stress

Behavioural problems

A number of reviews (Morris *et al*, 1988; Baumgarten, 1989; Dunbar, 1995; Schulz *et al*, 1995) have concluded that behavioural problems contribute consistently and significantly to the level of stress experienced by carers. Several studies have reported positive correlations between the severity and frequency of problems and carer strain (Gilleard, 1984; Eagles *et al*, 1987; O'Connor *et al*, 1990).

It is difficult to establish which problems are most stressful for carers, as this may vary with the stage of dementia of the patient and the life course of the carer. O'Connor *et al* (1990) and Gilleard (1984) found strain to be most strongly associated with disturbed behaviour. Argyle *et al* (1985) found that behavioural disturbances (abuse, aggression, smearing and inappropriate micturition) and night-time disturbance were reported as being particularly difficult to cope with (see Chapter 6).

Poor communication

The importance of problems with communication has been reported in a number of studies (Greene *et al*, 1982; Gilleard *et al*, 1984; Argyle *et al*, 1985; O'Connor *et al*, 1990). This may explain why carer abuse is more common in patients with stroke and communication disorders (Homer & Gilleard, 1990).

Formal relationship

The significance of the formal relationship between carer and dependant has been examined in several studies of carer stress. Some studies have found that adult sons and daughters report more stress than wives or husbands (Gilleard *et al*, 1984; O'Connor *et al*, 1990) while others have found higher distress among spouses (Brodaty & Hadzi-Pavlovic, 1990; Baumgarten *et al*, 1992; Graftstrom *et al*, 1992).

A consistent finding is that husbands who care for a partner with dementia report lower stress and higher morale than wives (Zarit *et al*, 1986; Pruchno & Potashnik, 1989; O'Connor *et al*, 1990; Baumgarten *et al*, 1992; Mittelman *et al*, 1995). This may be explained by the coping strategies men use, and the assistance they receive (Gilhooly, 1987). Gilhooly found that male carers:

(a) Adopted a more behavioural and practical approach to care-giving.
(b) Were more able to distance themselves from their care-giving duties.
(c) Found help with care-giving more socially acceptable.
(d) Found help more readily available.

In addition, disinhibition associated with dementia may be more threatening to women than men. Personal violence from a husband with dementia, or excessive or inappropriate sexual demands, may be particularly stressful for wives who look after their husbands. Such experiences are largely absent in husbands caring for wives (Wright, 1991).

Home environment

The home environment may be an important factor in carer stress, especially in inner cities, where some couples find themselves isolated in multi-storey flats. Problems include poor support, endemic violence and cramped living conditions. While many clinicians automatically consider the adequacy of the home when making a domiciliary visit, it is remarkable that the contribution of housing conditions to care-giving stress has not been researched.

Premorbid closeness

Ratings of the quality and closeness of the premorbid relationship are negatively associated with carer stress (Gilleard *et al*, 1984; Morris *et al*, 1988). This may reflect the long-term effects of a positive emotional investment, or a retrospective view biased by present difficulties. One study favouring the former interpretation, found that premorbid relationship ratings did not change when carer stress was reduced by day hospital attendance (Gilleard *et al*, 1984).

Links have been established between a poor premorbid relationship, high expressed emotion in carers (Gilhooly & Whittick, 1989) and carer neglect (Homer & Gilleard, 1990). Clinically, the psychopathology of caring can often be traced to long-standing relationship disturbances, whether marital or parent–child. This is an area where family therapists can play an important therapeutic role (Richardson *et al*, 1994). A continuing sense of closeness between carer and dependant may sustain a sense of well-being in carers (Motenko, 1989).

One intriguing set of interactions are those between problem behaviours, premorbid relationships and distressed carers. While behaviour disorders are not simply the result of inter-personal and intra-personal pathology, it can be difficult for carers to separate problems caused by the 'mindlessness' of cortical decay from the 'wilfulness' resulting from expressed and unexpressed hostility in the relationship. The attributions made by carers are affected by the past, which continues to influence the manner in which difficulties express themselves in the home.

A number of factors, including the uncertainty surrounding dementia; the meanings to be attributed; the responsibilities to be taken on; and the extent to which the identity of the carer is challenged by the progress of mental decay, contribute to the stress of caring for someone with dementia.

Box 18.2 Factors associated with carer stress

Behavioural problems
Poor communication
Formal relationship
Home environment
Premorbid closeness

While research provides broad brush indicators (see Box 18.2), only good clinical practice can flesh out the complexities of meanings and misunderstandings that contribute to individual stress in care-giving.

Effects of carer stress

There are many potential effects of carer stress (Box 18.3). Importantly, carer stress can lead to the loss of supporting relationships. This is costly for society, dependants and carers.

Ways of reducing carer stress

There are several interventions that have been employed to reduce carer stress (Box 18.4), although few have been subject to careful controlled evaluation.

Respite care

Respite for carers tends to be provided as respite admissions or respite day care. However, a number of voluntary agencies offer 'sitting services', where a volunteer will stay at home with the dementing person while their relative has a break.

Despite some worrying findings (Rai *et al*, 1986) there is little evidence that respite hospital admissions lead to a deterioration in the health of

---

Box 18.3 Effects of carer stress

Increased use of expensive resources
Elder abuse
Withdrawal of carers from productive employment
Poor relationships between carers and services
Unhappy carers
An uncaring society

```
┌─────────────────────────────────────────────────────────────┐
│             Box 18.4 Factors which may reduce carer stress     │
│                                                                │
│   Respite care                                                 │
│   Home care support                                            │
│   Carer groups                                                 │
│   Individual counselling                                       │
│   Family therapy                                               │
│   Institutionalisation                                         │
│                                                                │
└─────────────────────────────────────────────────────────────┘
```

dependants (Seltzer *et al*, 1988; Selley & Campbell, 1989). Carers report significant benefits for themselves, such as better sleep, more free time and more socialising. Interestingly, over half of carers reported feeling sad or lonely while their relative is in hospital (Pearson, 1988). Although respite care is popular, controlled studies have failed to demonstrate clear-cut benefits for carers (Burdz *et al*, 1988; Lawton *et al*, 1989). The latter study was a comprehensive evaluation of respite care. Lawton *et al* concluded that the recipients of respite care resoundingly endorsed it, but neither their care-giving attitudes nor their physical and mental health varied according to the amount of respite they received (Lawton *et al*, 1989).

Studies of psychogeriatric day care also report high levels of consumer satisfaction (Panella *et al*, 1984; Diesfeldt, 1992). While no studies involving controlled comparisons have been conducted, there is evidence that some patients continue to live in the community as a result of reduced carer stress (Gilleard, 1987). The impact of in-home respite care has been less well examined, although some 'sitting services' are reported to have a favourable impact (Cloke, 1988; Turvey & Toner, 1991).

It seems that while respite receives high marks in terms of customer satisfaction, there is no direct evidence for its beneficial effects on the health of carers or patients (Knight *et al*, 1993).

Home care support services

Studies on the impact of augmented home care and case management have reported improvements in the well-being of carers (Challis *et al*, 1990). The problems of caring for someone with dementia are difficult to resolve through an enhanced 'package of care' model because of the psychological significance of the disease. However, the Lewisham intensive case management scheme showed that gains can be made. Less intensive interventions have failed to demonstrate this (Challis *et al*, 1996).

Not all studies are positive. Askham & Thompson (1990) found no evidence that the Guy's Age Concern Home Support Project led to greater carer well-being than 'services as normal'. Similarly, O'Connor *et al* (1991) found that an early home intervention service had no measurable benefits beyond accelerating the process of institutionalisation of some elderly people with dementia living alone. Levin *et al* (1985) examined the effects of domiciliary services on carer stress and the rates of institutionalisation. They found that respite and home help services were associated with reduced carer stress. Other cross-sectional studies have not confirmed this finding (Gilhooly, 1987; Dunbar, 1995).

Carer groups

While home care support services offer input to patients and carers, carer support groups target the specific needs of carers. Groups have traditionally formed around statutory services such as day centres, day hospitals, nursing homes or hospital wards, and around voluntary organisations like the Alzheimer's Disease Society. A number of studies testify to the value of these groups, at least in the short term. These studies highlight the importance of: educational input (Chiverton & Caine, 1989); emotional support (Zarit & Zarit, 1982); and behavioural and problem-solving skills training (Gendron *et al*, 1986).

It has not been established which carers benefit most, and from what groups, but carers probably vote (if choices are available) with their feet. Carers whose relative is in some form of institutional care may obtain as much benefit as those involved in active caring. It is important not to overlook carers whose dependant has recently been admitted into 'care' (Rosenthal & Dawson, 1992).

There is evidence from Sydney that small carer groups which focus on enhancing coping skills lead to significant reductions in distress and institutionalisation (Brodaty & Gresham, 1989). One intriguing finding was that the 'waiting list' control group, who entered the programme six months after referral, failed to benefit psychologically. Brodaty & Gresham suggest that early interventions are effective in teaching preventative coping strategies. This is consistent with findings elsewhere (O'Connor *et al*, 1991).

Individual counselling

Individual counselling may achieve greater stress relief than group programmes (Collins, 1988; Knight *et al*, 1993). Family therapy has been reported as a useful intervention (Ratna & Davis, 1984; Benbow *et al*, 1990), although there are no systematic evaluations to date (Richardson *et al*, 1994). The results of one of the few randomised controlled trials of individual and family counselling did demonstrate a significant impact on reducing levels of spouse-care depression (Mittleman, 1995). Selecting carers for individual counselling remains a clinical and resource decision.

Elder abuse

The ill treatment of older people is not new, but was not reported until 1975. Alex Barker, a psychiatrist and the first director of the Hospital Advisory Service, reported "granny battering". Elder abuse is now defined as "a repeated act against, or failure to act for, an elderly person, which causes distress or damage, and so prevents the living of a full life"(Fisk, 1997). Abuse takes many forms (Benbow & Haddam, 1993) (Box 18.5), and occurs in domestic and institutional settings.

In one study of older people admitted to respite care, 45% of carers admitted to carrying out some form of abuse. Important factors included alcohol, a poor previous relationship and reciprocal abuse (Homer & Gilleard, 1990). In the USA, Godkin *et al* (1989) found that 41% of abusing carers had mental health problems compared to 5% of non-abusers.

The USA has been quicker to recognise and act against elder abuse, and reporting elder abuse is mandatory in 80% of the USA. In the UK, reporting is not mandatory and social services have given it a lower priority than child abuse. However, most social services have guidelines, as have some NHS trusts. Age Concern and the British Geriatrics Society have fostered education, and there is an Elder Abuse Response helpline (0800 731 4141).

Fisk (1997) writes:

> "Abuse appears in many forms and for many reasons. Close relatives, professional carers and society at large make victims of the elderly by reason of greed, revenge, desperation or ignorance. We urgently need better methods of identifying those who have been abused; of counselling or removing abusers; and of preventing abuse."

Well-organised psychiatric services for old people should have high levels of suspicion and of compassion for abusive situations. Better services, which take full account of the strain on carers, may reduce abuse.

Conclusion

Caring for elderly mentally unwell people at home is difficult and often distressing. The distress is more commonly seen in carers who are already

---

Box 18.5 Forms of elder abuse

Physical violence
Verbal abuse
Neglect
Financial exploitation
Sexual abuse

in touch with services, which itself may be seen as a marker of potential breakdown of care. Children are at least as affected as partners, and daughters and wives more often than sons and husbands. Poor relationships usually get worse and the ill health of the carer or poor home conditions add to the difficulties. Behavioural (action oriented) coping strategies and reordering life's priorities (where possible) may improve the situation of carers. Practical assistance in the home via home helps improves carer well-being, although other domiciliary services have not been shown to have clear benefits. Similarly, respite care seems to help those who use it, although this is difficult to demonstrate in studies. Many carers of people with moderate or severe dementia only find relief when their relative goes into a home or hospital. Counselling may help carers who find this move a traumatic one. One must recognise that dementia remains for most carers a very personal tragedy.

References

Argyle, N., Jestice, S. & Brook, C. P. B. (1985) Psychogeriatric patients: their supporters' problems. *Age and Ageing*, 14, 355–360.

Askham, J. & Thompson, C. (1990) *Dementia and Home Care: A Research Report on a Home Support Scheme for Dementia Sufferers, Research paper no. 4*. London: Age Concern.

Baker, A. A. (1975) Granny battering. *Modern Geriatrics*, 5, 20–24.

Baumgarten, M. (1989) The health of persons giving care to the demented elderly. *Journal of Clinical Epidemiology*, 42,1137–1148.

——, Battista, R. N., Infante-Rivard, C., *et al* (1992) The psychological and physical health of family members caring for an elderly person with dementia. *Journal of Clinical Epidemiology*, 45, 61–70.

Benbow, S. M., Egan, D., Marriott, A., *et al* (1990) Using the family life cycle with later life families. *Journal of Family Therapy*, 12, 321–340.

—— & Haddad, P. M. (1993) Sexual abuse of the elderly mentally ill. *Postgraduate Medical Journal*, 69, 803–807.

Birkel, R. C. (1987) Toward a social ecology of the home-care household. *Psychology and Aging*, 2, 294–301.

Brodaty, H. & Gresham, M. (1989) Effect of a training programme to reduce stress in carers of patients with dementia. *British Medical Journal*, 299,1375–1379.

—— & Hadzi-Pavlovic, D. (1990) Psychosocial effects on carers of living with persons with dementia. *Australian and New Zealand Journal of Psychiatry*, 24, 351–361.

Burdz, M. P., Eaton, W. O. & Bond, Jr, J. B. (1988) Effects of respite care on dementia and non-dementia patients and their caregivers. *Psychology and Ageing*, 3, 38–42.

Challis, D., Chessum, R., Chesteran, J., *et al* (1990) *Case Management in Social and Health Care: The Gateshead Community Care Scheme*. Canterbury: Personal Social Services Research Unit, University of Kent.

——, von Abenbdorff, R., Brown, P., *et al* (1996) *Care Management and Dementia: An Evaluation of the Lewisham Intensive Case Management Scheme*, Discussion Paper 1242. Canterbury: Personal Social Services Research Unit, University of Kent.

Chiverton, P. & Caine, E. D. (1989) Education to assist spouses in coping with Alzheimer's disease: A controlled trial. *Journal of the American Geriatric Society*, 37, 593–598.

Cloke, C. (1988) New approaches in services for mentally ill older people. In *Mental Health Problems in Old Age* (eds B. Gearing, M. Johnson & T. Heller), pp. 45–53. London: Wiley.

Collins, P. (1988) *Caring for Confused Elderly People: Evaluation of an Experimental Carers Support Service*, PhD thesis, Department of Psychology, University of Birmingham.

Diesfeldt, H. (1992) Day care and dementia. In *Care Giving in Dementia: Research and Applications* (eds G. M. M. Jones & B. Mieson), pp. 314–323. London: Routledge.

Dunbar, M. (1995) *The Well-Being of Dementia Caregivers: A Series of Meta-Analyses with Empirical Confirmation*, PhD thesis, Department of Psychology, Open University.

Eagles, J. M., Craig, A., Rawlinson, F., *et al* (1987) The psychological wellbeing of supporters of the demented elderly. *British Journal of Psychiatry*, 150, 293–298.

Fisk, J. (1997) Abuse of the elderly. In *Psychiatry in the Elderly* (eds R. Jacoby & C. Oppenheimer) (2nd edn). Oxford: Oxford Medical Publications.

Gendron, C. E., Poitras, L. R., Engels, M. L., *et al* (1986) Skills training with supporters of the demented. *Journal of the American Geriatric Society*, 34, 875–880.

Gilhooly, M. L. M. (1987) Senile dementia and the family. In *Coping with Disorder in the Family* (ed. J. Orford), pp. 138–168. Beckenham: Croom Helm.

—— & Whittick, J. E. (1989) Expressed emotion in caregivers of the dementing elderly. *British Journal of Medical Psychology*, 62, 265–272.

Gilleard, C. J. (1984) Problems posed for supporting relatives of geriatric and psychogeriatric day patients. *Acta Psychiatrica Scandinavica*, 70, 198–208.

—— (1987) Influence of emotional distress among supporters on the outcome of psychogeriatric day care. *British Journal of Psychiatry*, 150, 219–223.

——, Belford, H., Gilleard, E., *et al* (1984) Emotional distress among the supporters of the elderly mentally infirm. *British Journal of Psychiatry*, 145, 172–177.

Godkin, M. A., Wolff, R. J. & Pillemer, K. A. (1989) A case comparison analysis of elder abuse and neglect. *International Journal of Aging and Human Development*, 28, 207–225.

Goldberg, D. P. (1972) *The Detection of Psychiatric Illness by Questionnaire (GHQ)*. Maudsley Monograph 21. London: Oxford University Press.

Grafstrom, M., Fratiglioni, L., Sandman, P. O., *et al* (1992) Health and social consequences for relatives of demented and non-demented elderly: a population based study. *Journal of Clinical Epidemiology*, 45, 861–870.

Greene, J. G., Smith, R., Gardiner, M., *et al* (1982) Measuring behavioural disturbance of elderly demented patients in the community and its effects on relatives: a factor analytic study. *Age and Ageing*, 11, 121–126.

Haley, W. E., Levine, E. G., Brown, S. L., *et al* (1987) The psychological, social and health consequences of caring for a relative with senile dementia. *Journal of the American Geriatrics Society*, 35, 405–411.

Homer, A. C. & Gilleard, C. (1990) Abuse of elderly people by their carers. *British Medical Journal*, 301, 1359–1362.

Kiecolt-Glaser, J. K., Glaser, R. & Shuttleworth, E. C. (1987) Chronic stress and immunity in family caregivers of Alzheimer's disease victims. *Psychosomatic Medicine*, 49, 523–535.

Knight, B. G., Lutzky, S. M. & Macofsky-Urban, F. (1993) A meta-analytic review of interventions for caregiver distress: Recommendations for future research. *Gerontologist*, 33, 240–248.

Lawton, M. P., Brody, E. M. & Saperstein, A. R. (1989) A controlled study of respite service for caregivers of Alzheimer's patients. *Gerontologist*, 29, 8–16.

Levin, E., Sinclair, I. & Gorbach, P. (1985) The effectiveness of the home help services with confused old people and their families. *Research, Policy and Planning*, 3, 1–7.

Liptzin, B., Grob, M. C. & Eisen, S. V. (1988) Family burden of demented and depressed elderly psychiatric patients. *Gerontologist*, 28, 397–401.

Mittelman, M. S., Ferris, S., Shulman, E., *et al* (1995) A comprehensive support program: Effect on depression in spouse-caregivers. *Gerontologist*, 35, 792–802.

Morris, L. W., Morris, R. G. & Britton, P. G. (1988) The relationship between marital intimacy, perceived strain and depression in spouse caregivers of dementia sufferers. *British Journal of Medical Psychology*, 62, 173–179.

Motenko, A. K. (1989) The frustrations, gratifications and well-being of dementia caregivers. *Gerontologist*, 29, 166–172.

O'Connor, D. W., Pollitt, P. A., Roth, M., *et al* (1990) Problems reported by relatives in a community study of dementia. *British Journal of Psychiatry*, 156, 835–841.

——, ——, Brook, C. P. B., *et al* (1991) Does early intervention reduce the number of elderly people with dementia admitted to institutions for long term care? *British Medical Journal*, 302, 871–875.

Panella, Jr, J. J., Lilliston, B. A., Brush, D., *et al* (1984) Day care for dementia patients: An analysis of a four year program. *Journal of the American Geriatrics Society*, 32, 883–886.

Pearson, N. D. (1988) An assessment of relief hospital admissions for elderly patients with dementia. *Health Trends*, 20, 120–121.

Pruchno, R. A. & Potashnik, S. L. (1989) Caregiving spouses: Physical and mental health in perspective. *Journal of the American Geriatrics Society*, 37, 697–705.

Rai, G. S., Bielawska, C., Murphy, P. J., *et al* (1986) Hazards for elderly people admitted for respite "holiday admissions" and social care "social admissions". *British Medical Journal*, 292, 240.

Ratna, L. & Davis, J. (1984) Family therapy with the elderly mentally ill: some strategies and techniques. *British Journal of Psychiatry*, 145, 311–315.

Richardson, C. A., Gilleard, C. J., Lieberman, S., *et al* (1994) Working with older adults and their families – a review. *Journal of Family Therapy*, 16, 225–240.

Rosenthal, C. & Dawson, P. (1992) Families and the institutionalised elderly. In *Care-Giving in Dementia: Research and Applications* (eds G. M. M. Jones & B. Mieson), pp. 398–418. London: Routledge.

Selley, C. & Campbell, M. (1989) Relief care and risk of death in psychogeriatric patients. *British Medical Journal*, 298, 1223.

Seltzer, B., Rheaume, Y., Volicer, L., *et al* (1988) The effects of in-patient respite care on patients and their families. *Gerontologist*, 28, 121–124.

Schulz, R., Visintainer, P. & Williamson, G. M. (1990) Psychiatric and physical morbidity effects of caregiving. *Journal of Gerontology*, 45, 181–191.

——, O'Brien, A. T., Bookwala, J., *et al* (1995) Psychiatric and physical morbidity effects of caregiving: Prevalence, correlates and causes. *Gerontologist*, 35, 771–791.

Turvey, T. & Toner, H. (1991) The evaluation of a home based respite service for dementia sufferers and their carers. *Generations*, 16, 14–17.

Whittick, J. E. (1988) Dementia and mental handicap: emotional distress in carers. *British Journal of Clinical Psychology*, 27, 167–172.

Wright, L. K. (1991) The impact of Alzheimer's disease on the marital relationship. *Gerontologist*, 31, 224–237.

Zarit, S. H. & Zarit, J. M. (1982) Families under stress: interventions for caregivers of senile dementia patients. *Psychotherapy: Theory, Research and Practice*, 19, 461–471.

——, Todd, P. A. & Zarit, J. M. (1986) Subjective burden of husbands and wives as caregivers: A longitudinal study. *Gerontologist*, 26, 260–266.

19 Law

Peter Jefferys

General principles ● *Legal rights of the mentally ill* ● *Financial affairs*
● *Compulsory admission* ● *Consent to medical treatment*

With one or two exceptions, law in the UK does not distinguish older people with mental disorder from younger people. However, the features of mental disorders in old age, particularly dementia, mean that some legal issues arise more often.

General principles

Individual circumstances

It is a fundamental feature of the law in the UK that it is the unique circumstances of the individual, at a particular point in time, that determines the relevance, or applicability, of specific legal action. For example, an individual may only be admitted to hospital on a compulsory basis under Section 2 of the Mental Health Act (1983) if three professionals attest to the unique circumstances. Similarly, an assessment of testamentary capacity (under common law) is specific to an individual at a particular point of time.

Psychiatric assessment

The reliability of a medical opinion about the mental capacity of an individual is largely determined by the quality of the psychiatric assessment. It should include information from others about an individual's history, behaviour and functioning, to complement the mental state examination. Psychiatric diagnosis is important because of its major contribution to predicting the natural history, and possible clinical, social and legal outcomes for individuals. For example, the risks of self-neglect or financial incompetence are considerably higher in dementia sufferers than in elderly people with anxiety neuroses. But diagnosis alone does not determine risk or legal competence. The risk of financial disaster will vary between sufferers from dementia, and be related to other variables such as social circumstances and personality. Similarly, one psychotically depressed elderly individual may be capable of consenting to medical treatment with electroconvulsive therapy and another not.

Civil rights

There are powerful ageist beliefs in our society about the incompetence of older people. These beliefs are sometimes associated with moves to protect an elderly individual from risk. There can be collusion between family or carers and health or social care professionals, in which the individual is not validly consulted. Decisions which are central to an individual's welfare and personal liberty, such as where they live, how their money is spent, what clothes they wear and in whose company they spend their time, may be made by others. The fundamental human right to be consulted may be overlooked.

In addition, decisions may deprive an individual of freedoms, and in misjudged cases amount to over-protection. Most older people, whether mentally disordered or not, prefer to choose whether to accept a degree of risk or lose some freedoms. It may be the responsibility of the psychiatrist to support the individual's right to make this choice.

Confidentiality

Doctors have a duty to preserve medical confidentiality, and this applies equally to older patients. Doctors must be able to justify, if necessary to the General Medical Council, any breach of this general rule. The doctor must be able to say why disclosure was in the 'best interests' of the patient. It may be necessary to specify the significant risk to the patient, or to others, that has persuaded them to break medical confidence. The practitioner is likely to be asked what efforts were made to gain consent from the patient or to justify the reasons for not seeking consent.

Capacity

The general test of capacity is an individual's capacity to perform the function in question. It usually depends on whether the individual can understand, in broad terms, what he is doing and the effects of doing it, rather that his capacity to perform the task well or easily. There are two general legal presumptions governing capacity: (a) the person is mentally competent unless proven otherwise; (b) competence (or incompetence) continues unless there is definite proof to the contrary (continuance).

The level of proof for capacity is 'on the balance of probabilities' rather than 'beyond reasonable doubt'. In other words, the degree of certainty required is that of the civil law rather than the criminal law. Capacity is a legal, not medical decision. In disputed cases the medical opinions and evidence are decided by the courts. Although considerable weight is placed on medical evidence, there is a precedent (Birkin *v.* Wing, 1890) where a judge preferred the evidence of a solicitor!

Reform

The Law Commission for England and Wales completed a major review of the law in relation to mental incapacity in 1995 (Law Commission, 1995) and presented a draft bill to the Lord Chancellor. The main focus of the bill is decision-making on behalf of people who lack mental capacity to make decisions for themselves. If some of their proposals are adopted in legislation, much of the current law for incapable people will change. Decisions about a person's individual welfare and medical care will be authorised via a new statutory authority, which will consolidate and modify existing powers for managing property and financial affairs. There are additional proposals to give powers to local authorities to protect vulnerable adults from abuse and neglect.

Best interests

The notion of 'best interests' has been part of accepted clinical practice, endorsed in common law, for some time. This means that, where an individual lacks capacity to make a decision, any act (or omission) taken on their behalf must be in their best interests. The Law Commission has provided a helpful check-list to assist decision-making in these circumstances. Consideration should be given to the:

(a) past and present wishes of the individual;
(b) need to maximise the person's participation in the decision;
(c) views of others as to the person's wishes and feelings;
(d) need to adopt the course of action least restrictive of the individual's freedom.

Box 19.1 General principles

Individual circumstances: determine the applicability of law

Psychiatric assessments: collateral information, history, mental state and diagnosis

Civil rights: at risk of being ignored in older people

Confidentiality: a doctor's duty and required by the General Medical Council

Capacity: broadly, understanding what you are doing, and the effects of your actions

Reform: a draft bill on mental incapacity

Best interests: acting for an incapable person

Legal rights of the mentally ill

Voting

A person is entitled to vote if he is on the Register of Electors, unless he is compulsorily detained in hospital at the time of election. The officer presiding at the polling station can bar someone if it appears to the officer that the person is of 'unsound mind', without the capacity to understand, in broad terms, what he is doing and the effects of doing it. This power is very rarely exercised.

Short-stay hospital patients are likely to be registered at their home address. Long-stay patients may register using the hospital address, unless it is a mental illness hospital or registered mental nursing home. Special provision in the Representation of the People Act 1983 allows informal patients in mental illness and learning-disability hospitals to register in the electoral registration district of previous residence. They must make a declaration indicating their intention to vote, which is attested by a member of the hospital staff.

Jury service

Eligibility for jury service is determined by being on the electoral register, and being under the age of 70. In addition, people receiving in-patient care or treatment for mental disorder are excluded, as are individuals subject to guardianship or whose affairs are under the Court of Protection.

Driving

Individuals in the UK are obliged to apply to renew their driving licence on a regular basis after reaching the age of 70, and are meant to disclose any medical conditions that might affect their ability to drive. Individuals are legally obliged to inform the authorities at any time, of any disability likely to cause the driving of a vehicle to be a source of danger to the public. This may include a progressive illness such as a dementia, which could be notified as a 'prospective disability' because its progress may lead to danger in the future. The outcome, in an early case, might be to issue a licence on a yearly basis, with reassessment before renewal.

Some older patients with dementia or psychotic illness may be unwilling or unable to accept medical advice to stop driving and tell the authorities. Where this is the case, and the doctor believes there is a likelihood of serious danger to the patient or others, the doctor should consider, very seriously, whether to inform the Driver and Vehicle Licencing Agency medical advisor in confidence, recognising that in less serious circumstances this would represent a breach of medical confidentiality, unacceptable to the General Medical Council.

Motor insurers are obliged to notify the Secretary of State if they refuse insurance on health grounds, and some insurers ask for medical certificates before renewing insurance cover with older people. If a doctor issues a certificate of fitness to drive contrary to established clinical practice and guidelines, he could be liable for damages if his patient was responsible for a driving accident. In all cases, doctors should document their opinion and the specific advice given to a patient and their family.

Marriage

The degree of understanding required to enter into a marriage contract is a very simple one, which requires a broad understanding of 'the duties and responsibilities normally entailing to a marriage'. Most older people, even with dementia, are likely to meet this criterion. This test, coupled with the intestacy rules, which allow a new marriage partner to claim the estate (because marriage revokes all previous wills), provide a potential bonanza for the fortune hunter seeking financial benefit from marriage to a mentally incompetent older person.

To prevent a marriage, a rarely used mechanism known as a 'caveat', or objection to the marriage, can be entered with the superintendent registrar (Marriage Act 1949, Section 29). The person seeking to oppose the marriage carries the burden of proof of lack of capacity. Medical opinion that a marriage would not be suitable for an individual is unlikely to persuade the registrar to deny a certificate.

A marriage can be made void if it can be proven that the bride or groom could not understand (at the time of the ceremony) the nature of the·contract being entered, and appreciate its basic responsibilities. Alternatively, a marriage may be void if an individual was suffering from a mental disorder 'of such a kind or to such an extent, as to be unfitted for marriage'. Neither is easy to prove, and proceedings must be instituted within three years of the marriage. Even in these circumstances, a marriage is still valid unless one of the parties successfully petitions for nullity (Matrimonial Causes Act, 1973).

If the Court of Protection carries responsibility for the financial and other affairs of a wealthy mentally incompetent individual, it has the power to make a fresh will, or to petition for nullity on the patient's behalf. The new will might disinherit the fortune hunting spouse. Nullity would have the effect of removing the automatic right of the spouse to share in the estate.

Divorce

The sole ground for divorce, following the Matrimonial Causes Act 1973, is that the marriage has irretrievably broken down. Mental disorder may be a relevant factor in certain circumstances. The most obvious might be where a couple are living apart, because one is being treated or cared for in hospital for mental disorder, on a long-term basis. If the separation has been for a continuous period of five years or more, a divorce can be granted irrespective of the mental capacity, or consent of the parties. If the respondent is able to understand the effect and consequences of divorce, and consents to it, the separation need only last two years.

A distinct ground for divorce (without a waiting time) is if the respondent has behaved in such a way that the petitioner cannot reasonably be expected to live with them. The patient's conduct need not be blameworthy, but simply negative in character, as in Thurlow *v.* Thurlow (1976). In this case it was argued that the husband's health was adversely affected by the burden of caring for his wife's severe neurological disorder, associated with gradual mental and physical deterioration. The Court of Protection also has the power to issue a petition for divorce on behalf of a mentally disordered patient.

Making a will

Testamentary capacity is the degree of understanding, required in law, to make a valid will. It must apply at both stages in will making, namely the giving of instructions for the preparation of the will and the executing or signing the will. It depends on the extent of the individual's understanding of the particular transactions concerned. As a consequence, greater mental capacity is likely to be required to make a complex will, by a wealthy individual, than a simple will by someone of limited means. No distinction is made between detained and informal patients. The essential test for testamentary capacity is that the individual should have, in simple terms: an appreciation of the nature of the act and its effects; an understanding of the extent of the property he or she is disposing; be able to receive and evaluate information from others; be able to distinguish and compare potential beneficiaries; and be able to arrive at some sort of judgement.

An individual suffering from fluctuating or relapsing mental illness, may have the capacity to make a valid will in a brief 'lucid interval'. Someone with symptoms of memory impairment, as part of dementia, may be able to concentrate sufficiently to make a valid will on a 'good' day. Individuals may make eccentric, cruel, foolish or improvident dispositions without invalidating their wills. The presence of delusions does not automatically negate testamentary capacity, although specific delusions about a close relative who would be a natural beneficiary are likely to do so.

In complex cases, when a will is drawn up for a seriously ill older person, or for someone receiving in-patient psychiatric treatment, solicitors are likely to request a psychiatric opinion or medical witness. Doctors should take care in these circumstances, following a judgement in Kennard *v.* Adams (1975), where the judge assumed that the doctor would not only make a formal assessment of capacity but also record his or her examination and findings.

Since 1969, the Court of Protection has been able to make a statutory will, where the patient is incapable of making a valid will for himself. The court is obliged to make a will, consistent with the one the patient would have made for himself, within reason, and with competent legal advice. In some circumstance, the outcome, reflecting the patient's likely views when of sound mind, may be far from impartial. In such circumstances, as with an ordinary will, it is open to members of the patient's family, if they are disinherited, to apply under the Inheritance (Provision for Family and Dependants) Act 1975 after the death.

A will is automatically revoked on marriage, but in other circumstances the standard required to revoke a will is the same as to make a valid will in the first place. In Re Sabatini (1969) the act of tearing up a will was not accepted as revoking it, because medical evidence showed the presence of severe dementia at the time.

Gifts

A family dispute may be triggered when a confused elderly person makes a 'gift' of property, such as jewellery, to another family member or even to a stranger. The judgement in Re Beaney (Deceased) (1978) set out the criteria for the capacity to make a lifetime gift. In this case, a widow with severe dementia, when admitted to hospital, 'gave' her home to a daughter. It was ruled that the extent of understanding required is relative to the particular transaction. So if the value of a gift were trivial, a low degree of understanding would suffice. But if the effect were to dispose of their only asset of value, the degree of understanding required is as high as that necessary for a will. Gifts by people with advanced dementia to charities, or seasonable gifts to relatives can be made by the holder of an Enduring Power of Attorney. They may specifically apply for permission to make more substantial gifts to the Public Trust Office or Court of Protection.

Contracts

The capacity of an individual to make a contract, like making a will, is determined by whether he understood the nature of the contract at the time. It is important to protect those who cannot help themselves, but the law also protects the other party who may have had no reason to believe that an individual was mentally capable. The general rule is that a mentally incapable person is bound by a contract he has made, unless there is proof that the other person knew of the incapacity. Even in these circumstances, the mentally incapable person must pay a reasonable price for 'necessaries' such as essential food and drink, and services such as accommodation.

Once a patient is under the jurisdiction of the Court of Protection any contract he makes does not bind the patient or his estate. Regrettably there is no legislative equivalent to the Race Relations Act 1974, or the Sex Discrimination Act, protecting mentally disordered or elderly people from discrimination in relation to housing, accommodation or financial services.

Arrest

The Code of Practice relating to mentally ill and learning-disabled persons, under the Police and Criminal Evidence Act 1984, indicates the steps to be followed by the police who detain and wish to interview such a person. Essentially, the Code of Practice requires the police to ask an independent 'appropriate adult' (such as a relative, social worker or health professional) to attend the police station and join any interview between the police and the mentally disordered person. The purposes of this presence are to:

(a) advise the person being interviewed;
(b) observe whether or not the interview is being conducted properly and fairly; and
(c) facilitate communication with the person being interviewed.

The appropriate adult must be given an opportunity to make representations about the need for continuing detention, and hear any charge made. In all circumstances, where a person brought to a police station appears to be suffering from mental illness (other than drunkenness alone) the custody officer must immediately call the police surgeon or, in urgent cases, send the person to hospital.

Serving as a witness

Successful prosecution of individuals who may have abused mentally ill older people may be undermined because of the difficulty in providing reliable evidence in the witness box. Even if the potential witness satisfies the judge beyond reasonable doubt that he can take the oath, their reliability may be challenged because of the presence of a mental illness. Other strong, corroborative evidence is likely to be needed.

Litigation

There are special provisions concerning mentally disordered people in terms of their representation and ability to make claims in any high court or county court proceedings. Actions cannot be brought, or defended, in the courts unless the mentally incapable 'patient' is represented by a 'next friend' (if the patient is the plaintiff, petitioner or applicant) or a 'guardian ad litem' (if the patient is the defendant or respondent). The

---

Box 19.2 Legal rights of the mentally ill

Voting: able to vote unless compulsorily detained
Jury service: not if over 70, or receiving treatment for a mental
   illness
Driving: must renew licence at 70 years of age, and inform the
   Driver and Vehicle Licencing Agency of any illness
Marriage: need to understand duties and responsibilities
Divorce: if marriage has broken down, or unreasonable to live
   with partner
Will: need to appreciate the act, effects, your estate and
   potential beneficiaries
Gifts: depends upon value of gift
Contracts: understand the nature of the act
Arrest: 'appropriate adult' present or police surgeon
Witness: reliability may be questioned
Litigation: 'next friend' or guardian may represent you

---

court approves the appointment and the official solicitor often acts for these patients. The criteria for incapacity, which is decided by the court, is mental disorder resulting in an inability to manage property and affairs.

Financial affairs

Capable person

Bank or building society accounts

A competent individual can arrange for a third party mandate to be drawn up, authorising someone else to use a bank or building society account on their behalf. It can be cancelled by the person holding the account at any time. Having a joint account has the advantage that a trusted relative or friend can have easy access to the funds. But it can get difficult if account holders disagree. There is less financial independence for those involved, with the potential hazard that one person can be individually liable for debts arising from a joint account incurred by the other account holder.

Social security benefits

An individual can select another person, called the authorised agent, to collect their social security benefits or state retirement pension. The order slip in the benefit book has to be signed each time.

Ordinary power of attorney

An individual (the 'donor') can appoint someone else to act on their behalf (an 'attorney') in relation to their financial affairs, using a power of attorney. The donor may limit its extent, both in time and in the range of transactions for which the attorney is authorised to act. Close relatives or friends are generally chosen. Although the legal form completed by the donor is usually simple, it is generally advisable to seek legal advice. A medical opinion about competence is an additional safeguard for people receiving psychiatric care. An ordinary power of attorney can be cancelled, at any time, by the donor or by the attorney. The main drawback is that the power is automatically cancelled if the donor becomes mentally incapable, for example, if they develop a significant dementia.

Incapable person

The presence of a mental disorder such as dementia or manic–depressive illness may cause a significant reduction in an individual's understanding and judgement, to the extent that they are mentally incapable of managing their own finances. There is no legal link between the presence of any specific mental illness, or the fact of being compulsorily detained (Mental Health Act) and the legal capacity to manage one's affairs.

Social security benefits

The appointeeship system enables someone else to receive and administer social security benefits or pension on behalf of the mentally incapable person. The local Department of Social Security office is informed that the individual is no longer capable. A confirmatory letter from a doctor may be requested as evidence, or a home visit may be made by a social security officer. When satisfied, the Department of Social Security appoints a suitable person (a relative, friend or caring professional) to receive and manage the benefits. The appointeeship can be cancelled if there is evidence that the appointee is not acting in the best interests of the individual. It is sometimes possible to make a similar appointee arrangement to manage some public service or private pensions. The appointeeship arrangements are likely to be insufficient safeguard for the mentally incapable individual with significant income from other sources, or where there are property or investments which require active management.

Enduring Power of Attorney Act

The Enduring Power of Attorney Act 1985 provides a procedure where power of attorney can continue after someone becomes mentally incapable. The power granted can be general or more limited, and can range from selling shares or property to paying bills. The individual and the proposed attorney sign an enduring power of attorney form which must be independently witnessed. The power is then 'live' and can be used by the attorney concurrently with the donor.

At the stage when the individual becomes mentally incapable, the attorney applies to register the enduring power with the Court of Protection. The individual and close relatives (who have to be notified) have an opportunity to object to the power being registered. Once the enduring power has been registered it cannot be revoked or cancelled by the donor. The Court of Protection can remove an unsatisfactory attorney. It is possible for the power of attorney to be shared between more than one person.

There was uncertainty after the new legislation came into operation in 1986, about whether individuals already suffering from dementia had the legal authority to create an enduring power. The test cases Re K. and Re F. (1988) have established that a power can be created, provided the individual understands in broad terms the nature and effect of the document at the time he executed it. This applies even when the person is incapable, by reason of mental disorder, of managing his property and affairs, and personally unable to carry out the transactions the attorney might undertake on his behalf. For example, an individual suffering from dementia in a more focused moment may create a valid enduring power which could be registered very shortly afterwards with the Court of Protection. Solicitors are advised that when a donor is of borderline capacity the power is witnessed, or approved, by a doctor who should record their findings.

The Law Commission of England and Wales has proposed an extension of this power to decisions about personal welfare and medical treatment. This requires new legislation.

Court of Protection

Where someone becomes incapable, by reason of mental disorder, of managing and administering their property and affairs, and they require active management, and they have not made an enduring power of attorney, application to the Court of Protection may be required.

History   The power and duty of the Crown to look after the property of lunatics and idiots was recognised in English law before the reign of Edward II. The function was delegated by the King to the Lord Chancellor, and later to other judges. Its role was redefined by the Mental Health Act 1959, which established the Court of Protection on a fully statutory basis, dealing only with the 'property and affairs' of a patient. It is an office of the Supreme Court headed by a judge (the Master). The court's powers and procedures are governed by Part VII of the Mental Health Act 1983 and by the Court of Protection Rules 1984. Its administrative functions are now carried out by the Public Trust Office, which has a Protection Division which deals with external receivers, and a Management Division which acts as receiver when no one else can be found.

Procedure   An application is made to the court, usually by a close relative of the person concerned, or by another relative, friend, business adviser or officer of the local authority. It must be accompanied by details of the individual's family circumstances and financial affairs. In urgent cases the court can proceed without a written application. A single medical certificate on a prescribed form is also required affirming that the patient is incapable, by reason of mental disorder, of managing and administering his property and affairs. In response to criticism about the quality of some medical certificates the court now provides notes prepared by the British Medical Association (1995) and Royal College of Psychiatrists to assist the doctor. In most cases it is advisable that certification is completed by a specialist. Objections to the process can be raised by relatives, or the patient at a formal hearing, at which a receiver is usually appointed.

A short procedure order can be made which allows the court to direct one of its officers, or some other person, to take a specific action, and is used, for example, when the patient's property is worth no more than £5000 and the appointment of a receiver is unnecessary because there is no continuing need for the court to be involved. It can be quick and inexpensive.

Relatives are usually appointed as receivers, but in complex cases, or where there may be a conflict of interest, professional people may be more appropriate. The receiver is accountable to the court for any decisions that are taken and is expected to visit the patient, and be consulted about significant changes in their care. The court monitors the performance of receivers. However, the receiver has no power to consent to medical treatment on the patient's behalf, nor to dictate where the patient should live (in contrast to a guardian under the Mental Health Act 1983).

Box 19.3 Court of Protection procedure

An application is made to the court, usually by a close relative

It must be accompanied by details of family circumstances and financial affairs

A medical certificate is completed on a prescribed form, stating that the patient is incapable, by reason of mental disorder, of managing and administering his property and affairs

This is usually completed by a specialist

Objections to the process can be raised by relatives, or the patient at a formal hearing

---

Box 19.4 Financial affairs of an incapable person

Social security benefits: Department of Social Security may make
an appointee to collect and manage benefits
Enduring power of attorney: powers continue if the person
becomes incapable
Court of Protection: appoints a receiver on behalf of an
incapable person

The court charges an annual fee for individuals under receivership in
proportion to the value of the persons assets, in addition to a
commencement fee. There is power to displace an unsuitable receiver
and for the court to revoke the authority if convinced by medical evidence
that protection is no longer required and an individual has regained the
capacity to manage their own affairs. If the court wants a specialist opinion
about a person's mental capacity, one of the court's medical visitors may
be asked to give one.

Compulsory admission

National Assistance Act 1948

Section 47 of the National Assistance Act 1948 provides a power to remove
an elderly person from their home, without their consent, and place them
in institutional care. The origins of this provision are in the public health
slum clearance programme, which was central to the activity of most
urban local authorities, from the end of the 19th century until the middle
of this. It is rarely used today.

The person concerned must be suffering from grave chronic disease,
or be aged, infirm or physically incapacitated. They must be living in
insanitary conditions and be unable to devote to themselves, or receive
from other people, proper care and attention. The magistrates order will
direct that person's removal to a suitable hospital or other place (such
as a residential home) to 'secure the necessary care and attention'.

The original procedure required a certificate from the public health
physician to the district local authority, who in turn applied to the
magistrates court, giving seven days notice to the individual. Because
many people died at home during the period of notice, an emergency
procedure was introduced in the National Assistance (Amendment) Act
1951. If a public health physician and one other doctor certify that removal
without delay is necessary, the former may apply direct to a magistrate

for an order to remove. Its duration is three weeks, but can be renewed by the local authority.

Controversy has surrounded Section 47, and partly as a consequence, some public health physicians will not use it. There is the limited protection of the civil liberty of the individual. The individual is not represented before the magistrates when an order is made, and cannot apply for revocation of a Section 47 order during the first six weeks after admission. The doctors involved do not need to have any special experience or knowledge of the elderly, or those with mental disorder. The safeguards in the Mental Health Act 1983 for mentally disordered individuals are stronger. In addition, the decision is based primarily on the opinion of the professionals concerned. Terms such as 'insanitary conditions' and 'ill treatment or neglect' are difficult to define, and depend ultimately on a value judgement about the balance between the individual's right to live as he wishes, even if such wishes are delusionary or extremely eccentric, and the need for protection from unnecessary suffering or danger.

Mental Health Act 1983

Sections 135 and 136

These provisions can be applied in an emergency to remove an individual from their home (Section 135), or from a public place (Section 136), and to take them to a place of safety for assessment. Both make provision for a fuller assessment at the latter venue by a medical practitioner and approved social worker, with the possible outcome of a detention under Part II of the Mental Health Act. Detention at the place of safety cannot exceed 72 hours, and medical treatment cannot be imposed under Part IV of the Act.

An approved social worker may apply to a magistrate for a warrant to enter (if need be by force), search and remove to a place of safety any person believed to be suffering from mental disorder. There must be reasonable cause to suspect he has been ill treated, neglected or kept other than under proper control, or is unable to care for himself and is living alone. The police constable exercising the warrant must be accompanied by an approved social worker and medical practitioner, and the latter should be able to advise the policeman on whether the person should be removed to a place of safety. The legal definition is quite wide (Section 136, 6); and includes residential accommodation, a hospital, a police station or any suitable place (such as the home of a friend), where the occupier is willing to receive the patient.

The police have similar powers, not requiring a certificate from a magistrate. In Section 136, a police constable may remove to a place of safety, for up to 72 hours, any person found in a public place and appearing to be suffering from mental disorder, and to be in immediate need of care and control.

Section 115

This section provides approved social workers with a power to enter and inspect premises where a mentally disordered person is living, if there is reasonable cause to believe that the patient is not under proper care. But the social worker is not empowered to force entry. If access is gained, the subsequent removal of the patient to hospital without their consent, would then require completion of medical recommendations, and application under Part II of the Act.

Sections 2, 3, 4 and 5

The circumstances and requirements of Part II of the Act apply equally to patients of all ages, and the advice in the Department of Health's memorandum on the Mental Health Act, and the Secretary of State's Code of Practice, is of general relevance. It is not appropriate to summarise the provisions here, but some misunderstandings that have arisen with elderly people are discussed:

(a) It is sometimes held that because dementia is associated with ageing, it is not a mental disorder or mental illness as defined in Section 1(2) of the Act, and individuals cannot be detained. This belief is false, as is the view that a Treatment Order (Section 3) cannot be applied to a patient with dementia because there is no effective medical treatment for dementia. Medical treatment is defined far more widely in the Act.

(b) Detention under the Mental Health Act may not be applicable in some situations where an individual suffering from physical illness and mental disorder requires hospital admission for assessment or treatment of a physical illness. Detention can only be used when the primary objective of hospital admission is the assessment or treatment of the mental disorder. Therefore, a woman with a stable, chronic depressive illness requiring hospital treatment for a fractured femur could not be compulsorily admitted under the Act. By contrast, a man with an acute confusional state triggered by a chest infection might be detained, even though the main specific treatment for both the infection and the confusional state was antibiotics.

Guardianship

The Percy Commission, which preceded the Mental Health Act 1959, proposed a modern form of guardianship which would enable community care to be extended to all groups of mentally disordered people. After 1959, patients could be received into the guardianship of a local social services authority or a private individual. A guardian had the powers which would be exercisable by the father of a child under 14, which certainly included power to consent to medical treatment. The power was not widely used, and there was wide discussion about alternatives during the period leading to the 1983 Act. A new type of community care order proposed by the British Association of Social Workers was rejected, and a much reduced guardianship power was incorporated into the 1983 legislation.

Powers   The guardian has power only to require the patient to live at a specified place, to attend for medical treatment, occupation or training, and to require access to be given at any place where the patient is living to people such as doctors and social workers. The patient cannot be compelled to undergo medical treatment, which he can refuse.

Procedure   A guardianship application must be made to the local social services authority by an approved social worker (or nearest relative) and be supported by two doctors. Medical recommendations must indicate the category of mental disorder present, and the evidence for it, and affirm that guardianship is necessary for the patient's own welfare or for the protection of others. The guardian may be either the local authority, or a private individual, and the latter must be acceptable to the local authority. The order has effect when accepted by the local authority, and initially lasts six months, but it is renewable. Nearest relative consent is required, and people placed under guardianship have a right to apply to a mental health review tribunal. An alternative route for guardianship is via the courts (using Section 37), with power given to a magistrate or higher court to make a guardianship order, subject to acceptance by the local authority and the provision of two medical recommendation. A responsible medical officer (RMO) may also make a guardianship recommendation for a detained hospital patient (Section 3 or Section 37), provided the local authority accepts it.

Comment   The limited use made of guardianship since 1983 reflects, in part, the limited power of the guardian. Although the guardian can insist that a patient attend a clinic for treatment, there is no power to force it on him should he refuse. There is no power to force entry if the patient refuses access. The Code of Practice (para 13.9) advises that it should not be used solely in order to transfer an unwilling person to residential care. There was no specific power to transport people against their will to day centres or new accommodation.

It was argued that guardianship had no teeth and was unworkable with people who are unprepared to recognise the guardian's authority. Not everyone accepted this view and there are examples of its positive value for some dementia sufferers, where real consent to living in residential care is absent, and care staff are legally supported by the guardianship authority. In the discussions arising from the Beverley Lewis case, where a learning-disabled woman cared for by her mother with schizophrenia died of neglect, the additional point was made that nearest relative consent is required and guardianship is therefore likely to provide long-term protection against neglect or abuse in the patient's own home by close family members.

Finally, because guardianship is essentially a social services function, it is acknowledged by the Mental Health Act Commission that some departments are reluctant to use it because of demands made on residential facilities or staff time. Fear that a social services department might be pilloried in the event of a disastrous outcome with a guardianship client, has also contributed to its cautious use. It is largely for these reasons that recent legislative change has not extended guardianship powers, but provided for a supervised discharge order where lead responsibility is with the doctor.

After-care and supervision

The limitations of the Mental Health Act 1983, coupled with shortcomings in communication and clinical practice, in ensuring safe supervision of vulnerable mentally ill people, following hospital admission has led to administrative changes and to amendments in the law. Although much of the drive to change practice and amend the law has come from pressure groups concerned with younger patients, the changes are relevant for vulnerable older people.

Care Programme Approach (CPA)

All NHS mental health providers are now expected to have systems in place to ensure that all patients discharged from hospital leave only after the risks of discharge have been fully assessed. There must be a plan setting out the after-care that will be provided, and a keyworker appointed with specific

---

Box 19.5 Compulsory powers

National Assistance Act: to place an elderly person in institutional care (rarely used)
Sections 135/6: to remove someone from home/public place to a place of safety
Section 155: to enter and inspect premises
Sections 2/3/4/5: to admit or detain someone in hospital
Guardianship: to enforce abode, attendance for training and treatment, access to professionals

tasks. Systematic review of the after-care should be arranged. The CPA encapsulates what should be good practice in old age psychiatry services.

Supervision register

This system was introduced to improve communication about patients who may present a substantial risk of harm to themselves or others. It involves the patient's doctor putting them on the register. It is an administrative decision, and like the CPA is part of NHS departmental guidance rather than the law. It is unlikely to be used often in old age psychiatry.

Extension of leave of absence (Section 17)

It has always been possible for a detained patient to live outside a hospital while on leave under Section 17 of the Mental Health Act. This allows the doctor to set conditions such as compliance with medication, with recall to hospital as a sanction for non-compliance. The recent Mental Health (Patients in the Community) Act 1985 has extended the period allowable, from six months to the time the hospital detention is set to expire. It has relevance for a small number of more vulnerable patients, particularly with functional psychosis.

Supervised discharge order

This new provision in the Mental Health (Patients in the Community) Act 1995 arises because of concerns voiced by the public about community management and treatment of people with serious mental disorder. Mental health professionals acknowledged the limitations of guardianship, and were concerned about people who stopped treatment and lapsed from supervision following hospital care. Although the most common group of patients subject to the new order are likely to be younger psychotic patients who present substantial risk of serious harm to others, it is likely be useful for some older patients with dementia, or suffering from chronic or recurrent psychosis.

Conditions   The RMO applying for supervised discharge has to make application while the patient (under Section 3, 37, 47 or 48) is still detained. The patient must be suffering from mental illness, psychopathic disorder, mental impairment or severe mental impairment. The doctor must state that there is substantial risk of serious harm to:

(a) the health or safety of the patient, or
(b) the safety of others, or
(c) a risk that the patient will be seriously exploited if the after-care services provided under Section 117 were not received.

Powers   The RMO can specify specific requirements, which echo those of guardianship. These could be: to live in a specified place; to attend a particular place at set times for medical treatment, etc; or allow access to his or her residence to anyone authorised by the supervisor.

In contrast to guardianship, there is now a power to convey the person, although no power to force entry to their home or to compel medical treatment (such as medication) without the individual's consent.

Process   The process is complicated, with the RMO taking the lead, but involving consultation with relatives, other agencies and a second doctor, as well as an approved social worker, who have to certify support for the RMO's application. The proposed after-care plan must be specified, and agreement from the case supervisor (such as a community psychiatric nurse or social worker) confirmed. The initial duration of an order is six months, and there are rights of appeal to the mental health review tribunal.

It remains to be seen how useful this power will be in the community management of the fairly small number of older people for whom it could apply. It is unlikely to be used to a significant extent for people with dementia and self-neglect, who would be safer in staffed accommodation.

Consent to medical treatment

Capable patient

Most elderly people are capable of giving valid consent to common medical treatments. The presence of an early dementia, or a depressive illness, need not adversely change capacity. The provisions of Part IV of the Mental Health Act 1983 acknowledge that even a detained patient may be capable of consenting to treatment. In the latter circumstances, the RMO certifies the individual's consent after negotiating it with him.

Section 58

This applies to a detained patient who does not consent to medication after three months, or electroconvulsive therapy. The RMO must seek a second opinion from a doctor appointed by the Mental Health Act Commission. After examining the patient and consulting with others, the appointed doctor has the authority to issue a Certificate of Second Opinion, which allows the imposition of the specified treatment to the capable patient.

The provisions in the Act allowing the imposition of treatment only apply to specified treatments for mental disorder, and not to unrelated treatment such as surgery for a fracture. There is no explicit legal provision for imposing medical treatment (other than for mental disorder) on a capable patient. However, the courts have recently decided that a broad view could sometimes be taken, so that treatment for mental disorder includes treatment for its consequences. In the case of B. *v.* Croydon District Health Authority (1995) it was decided that a detained patient with the capacity to refuse feeding, could nevertheless be treated against their will for extreme weight loss, because the physical condition was a consequence of their mental disorder. This has potential application for psychotically depressed patients refusing to eat.

Incapable patient

Statute law is generally unhelpful about the wide range of circumstances in which an incapable elderly person may require medical treatment. The two exceptions are:

(a) Section 58 of the Mental Health Act 1983 which allows treatment for mental disorder to be given to an incapable patient, provided a Certificate of Second Opinion has been issued.
(b) Section 62 of the same Act, which allows urgent treatment in certain circumstances to be given to detained patients.

In practice, many people with dementia are admitted to hospital or residential care without real consent. They may receive medication to relieve mental distress, or treat physical disorders, without either real consent, or detention under the Mental Health Act. Technically the interventions amount to assault. There is continued debate about the absence of statutory protection for the patient and professional staff in these circumstances.

It is fairly common for incapable elderly people to need surgical investigation, or treatment because of their physical morbidity. A common example is hip surgery for a person with dementia sustaining a fracture after a fall. No-one can give valid legal consent for the procedure. Consultation with relatives and others is good practice, but the legal defence of the operating surgeon against a claim of assault is the more nebulous 'duty of care'.

Much of the debate about medical treatment in mentally incapable people in recent years has been triggered by some cases concerning abortion, or sterilisation in learning-disabled people. Some of the legal points have relevance for old age psychiatry, although the medical treatments are different. The leading case is Re F. (Mental Patient: Sterilisation) (1990). This concerned the question of what treatment could (and should) be given in the absence of valid consent. The House of Lords held that there was no procedure for giving someone else the right to decide on behalf of a mentally incapacitated person, and that the court had no jurisdiction to approve or disapprove the giving of treatment. It was held that the court could grant a declaration that it would be lawful to proceed in the absence of consent, if the treatment was justified on the principle of necessity. This principle was further held to mean that

---

Box 19.6 Consent to medical treatment

Consent is required for medical treatment.
This applies to compulsorily detained mentally ill patients.
Incapable people are generally not covered by law.
Clinicians may act in the patient's 'best interests'.
Consent by relatives is 'good practice' only.
Complex situations may need to be decided in the courts.

---

the lawfulness of operating upon or otherwise treating a mentally incapacitated person depended upon whether such treatment was in a patient's best interest.

In practice, applying this judgement to treating the elderly mentally incapable patient, the doctrine of necessity means that the doctor is justified in providing treatment of a routine nature as well as more urgent treatment, provided it will ensure improvement of or prevent deterioration in health. If the patient is known to have objections to some specific treatment (before they became incapable) doctors may not be justified in proceeding.

In addition, it is expected that the doctor should act in accordance with a practice accepted as proper by a responsible and competent body of relevant professional opinion. In complex cases, independent confirmation and support of the medical treatment plan by other medical colleagues is likely to be a safeguard, by confirming lack of consent, and that the treatment is in the patient's best interests.

Most treatment decisions can be taken by the clinician, the patient and people providing care, but some decisions are so serious that the courts want each case brought before them, such as the withdrawal of hydration in the Bland persistent vegetative state case (1993). There will be other procedures where the courts may wish to become involved. Hospitals will need to take legal advice in cases of doubt.

References

British Medical Association (1995) *Assessment of Mental Capacity Guidance for Doctors and Lawyers*. London: BMA.
Law Commission (1995) *Mental Incapacity* (Law Commission Report no. 231). London: HMSO.

Airedale NHS Trust v. Bland (1993) AC 789.
B. v. Croydon District Health Authority (1995) ALL ER 683.
Kennard v. Adams C.L.Y. (1975) 3591.

Re Beaney (1978) 2 ALL ER 595.
Re F. (mental patient sterilisation) (1990) 2 A C 1.
Re K. and Re F. Law Reports, Chancery Division (1988) 310–16.
Re Sabatini (1969) 114 S.J.35.
Thurlow v. Thurlow (1976) Fam 32.

Additional reading

Age Concern (1986) *The Law and Vulnerable Elderly People.* London: Age Concern.

20 Research

Dee Jones

Basic principles ● *Types of study* ● *Ethical principles* ● *Stages in a research project* ● *Specific problems and challenges* ● *Future areas for research* ● *Conclusion*

Medical diseases and psychiatric disorders come together more frequently in older people. These conditions interact with each other, and with environmental and psychological variables to produce characteristic problems for management and treatment. This poses particular challenges for research. Old age psychiatrists need to test their assumptions about diagnoses, treatment and management, use the best research methods available and make their findings accessible.

Basic principles

Design

Every possible attempt should be made to reduce conscious and unconscious bias.

Sample size

Sample sizes should be calculated before research is initiated, as inappropriately small studies may lead to falsely negative findings.

Duration of study

The appropriate length of the study and time at which outcomes are measured, should be considered carefully as they can change over time. There may be a time-lag between treatment initiation and expected benefits (e.g. several weeks with antidepressants).

Timing of evaluations

Timing can cause methodological and ethical dilemmas. On the one hand it is desirable that all new treatments are initiated as soon as they are developed. On the other hand, some services do not work optimally at first and improve with practice (e.g. cardiac surgery). Early evaluation may give misleadingly negative results, preventing the use of beneficial treatments.

Outcome measures

These need to be valid, reliable and meaningful. Many evaluations can give falsely negative results because of insensitive outcome measures. A great deal of work remains to be done to improve outcome measures.

Types of study

Descriptive

Descriptive studies are undertaken to determine the frequency of a disease, the characteristics of people suffering from it, and where and when it occurs. Descriptive studies can either be cross-sectional (i.e. conducted at one point in time) or longitudinal (i. e. where observations are repeated at least once over a time period).

Analytic

Analytic studies investigate the determinants or factors associated with a disease. There are two types of analytic study: case-control studies and cohort studies; the former are retrospective and the latter prospective. A case-control study starts at the point of identifying a group of people with the disease and compares them with a control group. A cohort study compares a group of people exposed to the suspected determinant/factor with a group not exposed (Barker & Hall, 1991).

Experimental

Experimental studies are based on the classic scientific approach of formulating a hypothesis and conducting a controlled experiment to test it. This approach is considerably more difficult to adopt with humans than with animals or chemicals. Trials can be used to test hypotheses that have been generated from observational data, to quantify the effectiveness of certain treatments or to evaluate service provision. The randomised controlled trial, by using a study group and a control group which are identical in all respects apart from the factor or intervention in question, reduces the effect of confounding variables and clarifies whether or not associations are causal. Randomised controlled trials are often considered the gold standard of evaluative research.

Ethical principles

Truth-telling

It must be an overriding principle that patients are told the truth as often as possible. The use of placebos obviously pose many ethical questions. However, the importance of the placebo effect cannot be underestimated, particularly when alternative treatments are unavailable. There is evidence that informing people that they are on a placebo changes the outcomes (Hawthorne effect).

Informed consent

The aims of informed consent are two-fold: to guard the individuality and autonomy of patients within the health care system and to protect their rights of privacy and the right to be left alone. Informed consent requires full description of the proposed research project, and its intentions. However, on some occasions detailed description of the hypothesis may influence the research findings. It is generally agreed that patients should be fully informed of possible risks (minimal and maximal) and benefits. This information is often not available.

Confidentiality and privacy

Risks should be reduced as far as possible. All attempts should be made to maximise the personal privacy of all data collection records; names and addresses should be used as little as possible and certainly should not be stored on computers, alternative identifiers should be used. Many of these ethical aspects are particularly difficult in old age psychiatry and need careful consideration.

Right to refuse

Patients have an unquestionable right to refuse to participate in research as well as treatment. No professional has the right to breach the autonomy of an individual. Participants also have the right to withdraw from studies at any time, not only at their commencement. This obviously conflicts with the interests of researchers, who for good quality research require high response rates and low drop-out rates. These can usually be achieved with good communication.

The individual versus society

It is the role of clinicians and health care professionals to respond to the needs of individual patients, and their best interests must be paramount. On the other hand, epidemiological research is focused on communities, or groups of people, in order to maximise the benefit to society at large. At times these interests conflict.

Health care policy

The trial of a new drug is more likely to be regarded as research than is the initiation of a change in care policy, for example, the closing of mental hospitals. However, changes in health or social care delivery systems should warrant the same rigorous evaluation and monitoring as would a new drug. Scant attention has been paid to the ethics of experimentation in health and social care systems. It is still not required that new health care systems, changes to these systems or even reductions in services, be monitored or evaluated.

Stages in a research project

Definition of hypotheses and objectives

Before starting a research project it is crucial to develop a clear hypothesis and to formulate the research questions to be addressed. It is necessary to develop these before considering the design of a study, as they will dictate the aims and objectives of the project. Clear definitions are required for the disease and the interventions to be investigated. A thorough search of the literature will indicate the originality and value of the proposed project.

Seeking advice

Time invested in discussions with 'experts' from different professions (depending on the nature of the project) will pay handsome dividends. Seek advice at the outset. Poorly designed studies are no quicker to execute, analyse, interpret or write up, but are unlikely to find welcoming editors. Experts are often unwilling to assist in the analysis or interpretation of a poorly designed project.

Selection of a sample

Populations are usually large numbers of people in a defined context. These can be either unselected or groups selected because of: admission to hospital, attendance at out-patients or primary care, by socio-demographic or medical characteristics. A sample is a subset of a population in question, hence the use of a random sample. It is crucial that the sample is representative of the population, which is why random samples are often used. The findings of an appropriate sample should be generalisable to the population in question. The results of drug trials undertaken on young healthy medical students are unlikely to be applicable to an older population.

The size of the sample is also very important, particularly in experimental studies or if comparisons of subgroups are to be made. The appropriate sample size should be calculated early in the study design, with the advice of a statistician or epidemiologist. To maintain the representative nature of the initial sample, high response rates are essential at each stage. Losses through attrition (e.g. failure to trace, loss of notes, lack of contact, refusal to participate and loss to follow-up) will jeopardise the representativeness and consequently generalisability of the findings as non-responders are likely to have different characteristics from responders. Ideally non-response and loss to follow-up should not exceed 10%.

When a control group is required careful thought is essential; if the controls are inappropriate the results of an investigation are of minimal value. In analytic studies, to avoid confounding bias, the control group must resemble the study group in certain specified characteristics. Observations or measurements made on the control group must be directly comparable to those made on the study group. In randomised controlled trials the control and study group should be identical in all respects apart from the intervention.

Choice of instruments

Before commencing any research project it is necessary to decide what observations are to be made and which instruments are to be used; above all, wherever possible, those that are standardised (valid and reliable). To be valid an instrument must measure what it is intended to measure with high sensitivity and specificity. Accurate measurements are repeatable (i.e. remain the same when elicited more than once). There are two forms of observer bias/error to avoid or minimise: between-observer variation and within-observer variation. These can arise in laboratory tests, mechanical measures or questionnaires.

It is unwise to design original questionnaires but preferable to benefit from the mistakes and expertise of others. Wherever possible, aspiring researchers should employ previously used and validated questionnaires; this will, as well as saving a great deal of time and possible error, enable the results to be compared with those of others. There is an increasing number of such questionnaires and interview schedules available; social scientists, clinicians and epidemiologists working in the area in question can provide useful advice and guidance on the selection from the available menu. If standard questionnaires are not available again advice should be sought from experienced researchers. There is no virtue, only frustration, in repeating the mistakes others have made. Advice and guidance on the design of data collection sheets (for recording clinical data from notes etc.) will pay dividends. Particular care is required when designing and selecting questionnaires or interview schedules for older people.

Ethical approval

In the past most research was undertaken without formal ethical approval. This is no longer the case. All research projects need to be submitted to an appropriate ethical committee, even before applying for funding. Studies involving hospital and community may need to receive ethical approval from both committees. Generally, ethical approval is needed from each district in which a study is to be conducted. Hence a multi-centre study will require ethical approval from several districts.

Funding

The least complicated strategy is to conduct research that requires no extra funding but can be executed, with appropriate cooperation, within the available resources. The application for research funds will, even if successful, delay a project by at least six months. There are many different sources of funding: research councils, district health authorities, offices of research and development, research foundations, drug companies and charitable trusts and foundations. Information concerning each is usually available in medical libraries.

Execution

Collaborating colleagues, staff and study population need to be appropriately informed of the nature and purpose of the study. Colleagues and staff will need thorough initial and ongoing training to maintain standardisation. We all need to bear in mind that patients/members of the general population are under no obligation to participate in research activities; they do so only by grace and favour!

Analyses and interpretation

Advice on analyses at an early stage is essential, this can be gleaned from departments of (medical) statistics or epidemiology (public health). The presentation and discussion of findings with colleagues and other interested professionals is invaluable; they may be able to offer completely different perspectives on the findings and interpretations. A manuscript benefits enormously by being read and criticised by several people prior to submission to a journal.

Box 20.1 Stages of a research project

Definition of hypotheses and objectives
Seeking advice
Selecting of a sample
Choice of instruments
Ethical approval
Funding
Execution
Analyses and interpretation

Specific problems and challenges

Diagnostic criteria

Since Kay's seminal work (Kay *et al*, 1964) there have been at least 25 population surveys of depression in older people, most of which have been undertaken in the UK or USA. The results have differed enormously, reflecting the variation in criteria, instruments and populations selected. Standardised criteria in the form of ICD–10 (World Health Organization, 1992) and DSM–IV (American Psychiatric Association, 1994) are helpful, although neither has sections specifically for older people and problems have arisen with late-onset schizophrenia (see Chapter 10).

Diagnostic instruments

Many of the instruments which have been used are more suitable for hospitalised patients of younger age groups than community-based older populations. Many schedules were derived from the symptomatology of younger adults and hence many of the questions involve possible physical symptoms. Schedules such as the Geriatric Depression Scale have been developed to avoid these items where possible (Yesavage *et al*, 1983) (see Chapter 1).

Populations

Ideally, study populations should include people who are in residential care, as they tend to have a higher prevalence of mental illness. Inclusion or otherwise of residential or hospital patients can have a large effect on epidemiological studies. Similarly treatment outcomes may vary between these populations.

Association

People who are in residential care tend to have a higher prevalence of mental illness. The nature and direction of this association requires further investigation: are people selected for residential care because they are depressed or have dementia, or because they become so after admission? In the community, older people do not have an excess of depressive disorder (see Chapter 7).

Identifying patients

Many depressed older people are not identified in the community and very often no action is taken when it is identified to investigate or treat their mental illness (Gruer, 1975; Macdonald, 1986; Vetter *et al*, 1986). One way of improving the detection and treatment may be through using screening instruments and protocols. There is room for further work to develop the use of assessment instruments which can be used easily and reliably in the community by health visitors, practice nurses and other professionals, particularly in the light of the requirement upon general practitioners to assess those aged 75 years and over. Strategies for the multi-phasic assessment of older people in the community could enable earlier diagnosis and facilitate optimal management.

Physical illness

Many studies have shown associations between depression and physical illness (Vetter *et al*, 1986). For example, a high proportion of stroke sufferers develop depression (Robinson *et al*, 1984; Ebrahim *et al*, 1987). Depression is also more common among people with Parkinson's disease and Huntington's disease. Associations with many types of malignancies have been suggested and need further exploration. Raised rates of depression among patients after myocardial infarction have been well-documented, but reliable predictors have yet to be identified. Increased physical disability, dependency on others and reduction in active social life may also be important. Medications can also be responsible for the onset of depression (Ouslander, 1982).

Opinion varies as to whether depression can produce physical illness. Some research gives weight to the view that there is a raised mortality from cardiovascular disease in men within the first six months of their being widowed (Parkes *et al*, 1969). The lay view would certainly support this hypothesis. Anxiety, depression and insomnia have all been implicated in subsequent myocardial infarction in small studies (Kuller, 1978). Prospective studies with larger study populations may illuminate the relationship between physical and mental health.

Box 20.2 Possible reasons for the association between depression and physical illness (adapted from Murphy, 1992)

Depression may be a direct consequence of the cerebral organic effects of certain specified physical disorders.

Depression could be a consequence of treatments for physical illness.

Depression may result from a psychological reaction to physical illness and process of adaptation to future disability.

Depression may predispose to the onset of physical disease.

The behavioural consequences of depression may cause physical illness (e.g. self-neglect).

Social factors

The exploration of the involvement of social factors resulting in mental disorder in old age is of great importance because of the implications for prevention. Again, the lay public do not doubt these associations but more empirical evidence is needed concerning: poverty, social class, education, loneliness, social isolation, support networks, retirement, sensory impairment and life events. Significant associations have been demonstrated with some of these factors but a longitudinal approach is required to investigate causality.

Brown & Harris (1978) and Murphy (1982) identified the role in depression of life events such as bereavement, serious physical illness, financial loss and enforced relocation. However, not everyone experiencing these life events develops depression. Research is needed into the factors that protect some people from depression after life events. Murphy (1982) and others have indicated the ameliorating effects of social networks and close confidants.

Environmental interventions are important in dementia (see Chapter 6). The benefits of these types of strategies need to be carefully evaluated, particularly in residential settings where little work has been undertaken. New institutions provide opportunities for the evaluation of different types of architecture and design.

Drug studies

Medications have developed enormously in the past 10 years, with new antidepressants being introduced virtually every year. Reviews do not consistently favour one drug more than another (Veitch, 1982; Busse & Simpson, 1983). Selection is largely based upon cost, side-effects, compliance, toxicity in overdose and the individual experience of clinicians. Most drug trials in the past have been undertaken with younger adults; the results of which cannot be assumed to be valid for older populations. Optimum therapeutic levels are likely to be different in older people; some studies have indicated the benefits of lower doses in the elderly, while others argue that low doses may be less efficacious. General practitioners are increasingly prescribing the standard, once a day, doses of selective serotonin reuptake inhibitors. Antidepressants may cause dizziness and falls (Campbell *et al*, 1989); these and other adverse effects need to be investigated.

Studies to evaluate drug treatments are fraught with difficulties; patients need to be followed-up for a reasonable time, high compliance rates are difficult to achieve and many patients, because of a poor response or side-effects, require a change in medication. These factors necessitate large sample sizes. Most studies are too short in duration to investigate remission rates. Studies become even more complicated if combined treatments are evaluated (as they should be). To date, most evaluations of treatment have been undertaken in hospitals. More work is necessary in primary care where most older people with depression are seen.

Currently, the most hopeful drug therapies for mild to moderate Alzheimer's disease are the acetylcholinesterase inhibitors. Donepezil is the first one to gain a licence in the UK (Kelly *et al*, 1997), although tacrine was launched in the United States in 1993. These medications appear to delay deterioration in cognitive function and may delay nursing home admission (Knopman *et al*, 1996). Tacrine offers some potential benefit to about a third to a half of patients but a significant minority (a third) suffer side-effects and half of these cease the therapy (Knapp *et al*, 1994). Donepezil appears to have fewer side-effects. It is possible that the introduction of these medications, or newer ones to follow, may alter the management of Alzheimer's disease, with a new emphasis on early diagnosis.

Many drugs, including neuroleptics, have been used for the treatment of symptoms in dementia and there is a wealth of research potential in this area. Tricyclic antidepressants have been used with benefit in some patients with dementia and depression, but there is the possibility of increased cognitive impairment; other antidepressants need to be evaluated. Similarly, the anticholinergic component of many neuroleptics, prescribed for behavioural problems, may exacerbate Alzheimer's disease. Further work is needed to identify those patients who will benefit from which symptom-reducing medications.

Psychotherapy

Psychotherapy in conjunction with other treatments may benefit people living in the community or residential homes, or as hospital in-patients. However, there is a paucity of work evaluating such interventions. Clinical psychologists are increasingly working in the primary care sector; their effectiveness with patients who have mild or fluctuating depression, or who have been recently bereaved has yet to be established. Similarly, the role of cognitive therapy and self-help approaches needs evaluating in residential and primary care settings. These therapies are unlikely to gain wide use until they have been evaluated rigorously and shown to be effective.

Long-term outcome

Appropriate measures of long-term outcome for depressed older people and their carers need to be developed. Chronic disability and relapse are common (Post, 1972; Murphy, 1982); the identification of predictors for these conditions may allow the development of prevention packages, such as prophylactic management strategies for patients and their carers. Since social factors together with the severity and nature of the illness influence long-term outcome (Post, 1972), social interventions may be beneficial.

Measurement of outcome in dementia should be broad in nature, including not only memory, thinking and behaviour but also disability and quality of life, as assessed by patients and their carers. Effectiveness should be assessed long-term as well as in the short term.

Services

There has been little evaluation of after-care and service provision for people recovering from a depressive episode, or those with chronic depression. Some people only need support in the immediate post-discharge period, while others may require long-term help. Services are, to an extent, available for carers; this may be in the form of advice, day care or respite care. There is evidence that carers of depressed elderly people are often suffering from depression themselves (Jones & Peters, 1992) (see Chapter 18). The causality and direction of this association needs further investigation and preventive strategies need to be developed and evaluated.

A large proportion of people with Alzheimer's disease live in residential care, nursing homes or long-stay hospitals. Inadequate work has been undertaken to assess the quality of care in these institutions, and baseline standards have yet to be established. The design, organisation and running of homes have tangible consequences for the quality of life of people with dementia. Many residents, for example, are taking inappropriate medication or too many medications (Gosney *et al*, 1989). Institutions are ideal locations for introducing and evaluating new strategies for the management of people with dementia.

Services try to enable people to live in the community as long as possible and reduce the burden of care on carers (Department of Health, 1989). Studies have examined the effects of this policy upon carers and their quality of life (Levin, 1983; Gilhooly, 1984; Jones & Peters, 1992) (see Chapter 18). Any evaluation of management should include assessment of both patient's and carer's own quality of life (Howard & Rockwood, 1995) and use of community and institutional services. There is a lack of flexible, planned respite care. It is important to develop innovative forms of respite which are consumer-needs led; voluntary organisations have begun to address these needs. While there has been some evaluation of respite care there is more to do, on larger samples with controlled populations. Different models of supporting carers – as individuals, or in groups – need to be developed and evaluated. Such evaluations are best undertaken by multi-disciplinary groups, where the clinical perspective is crucial.

Memory clinics

In recent years, memory clinics have been developed in the USA and UK to assess and manage people with memory disorders. Since memory clinics

---

Box 20.3 Specific problems and challenges in old age psychiatry research

Treatment involves several types of intervention, often in combination

Treatment is commonly long-term and relapses occur

There are many interacting variables to take into account

Treatment involves all aspects of life including social, spiritual, functional and quality of life

Management and care involves other agencies and informal carers

Cultural contexts need to be taken into account

Treatments are often in combinations and therefore need to be evaluated in combinations as well as independently

---

involve several different disciplines, they provide particularly valuable environments to undertake research into diagnosis, treatment and management (Bayer *et al*, 1990). Some areas of the UK have invested in community memory teams to counter the perceived neglect of health and social services in this area. Rigorous evaluations will be required to compare the effectiveness of a specialised team with standard health and social services provision.

Future areas for research

There are many areas which offer the potential for new research, some of which are listed in Box 20.4. As society changes and new diagnoses and managements arise, so new areas of research will emerge. Competition for research grants is often intense but many organisations are realising that older people and their mental health have been relatively neglected.

Box 20.4 Future areas for research (SUCCESS)

Suicide: more common in older people but under researched

Users' opinions: encouraged by NHS reforms

Carers: belatedly recognised to be important

Crime abuse: the effects of abuse and the fear of crime on older people

Ethnicity: as ethnic minority groups in the UK age

Strategies: to prevent violence against or abuse of older people

Stabilising: Alzheimer's disease with medications

Conclusion

The multi-dimensional nature of old age psychiatry research requires collaboration with primary health care services, social service departments, community health and other hospital specialities (Jolley & Arie, 1978; Jolley & Jolley, 1991). Research expertise will increasingly need to be multi-disciplinary and include biological, epidemiological and social perspectives.

References

American Psychiatric Association (1994) *Diagnostic and Statistical Manual of Mental Disorders* (4th edn) (DSM–IV). Washington, DC: APA.

Barker, D. N. P. & Hall, A. J. (1991) *Practical Epidemiology*. London: Churchill Livingstone.

Bayer, A. J., Richards, V. & Philip, S. G. (1990) The Community Memory Project – a multi-disciplinary approach to patients with forgetfulness and early dementia. *Care of the Elderly*, 2, 236–238.

Brown, G. W. & Harris, T. O. (1978) *Social Origins of Depression*. London: Tavistock.

Busse, E. & Simpson, D. (1983). Depression and antidepressants and the elderly. *Journal of Clinical Psychiatry*, 44, 35–39.

Campbell, A. J., Borrie, M. J. & Spears, G. F. (1989) Risk factors for falls in a community-based prospective study of people 70 years and older. *Journal of Gerontology*, 44, 112–117.

Department of Health (1989) *Caring for People: Community Care in the Next Decade and Beyond*, Cmnd 849. London: HMSO.

Ebrahim, S., Barer, D. & Nouri, F. (1987) Affective illness after stroke. *British Journal of Psychiatry*, 15, 52–56.

Gilhooly, L. M. (1984) The impact of care-giving on care-givers: factors associated with the psychological well-being of people supporting a dementing relative in the community. *British Journal of Medical Psychology*, 157, 35–44.

Gosney, M., Vellodi, C., Tallis, R. C., *et al* (1989) Inappropriate prescribing in part III residential homes. *Health Trends*, 21, 129–131.

Gruer, R. (1975) *Needs of the Elderly in the Scottish Borders*. Edinburgh: Scottish Home and Health Department.

Howard, K. & Rockwood, K. (1995) Quality of life in Alzheimer's disease. *Dementia*, 6, 113–116.

Jolley, D. J. & Arie, T. (1978). Organisation of psychogeriatric services. *British Journal of Psychiatry*, 132, 1–11.

—— & Jolley, S. P. (1991). Psychiatry of the elderly. In *Principles and Practice of Geriatric Medicine* (2nd edn) (ed. M. S. J. Pathy). London: Wiley.

Jones, D. & Peters, T. (1992) Caring for elderly dependants: effect on the carer's quality of life. *Age and Ageing*, 21, 421–428.

Kay, D. W. K., Beamish, P. & Roth, M. (1964) Old age mental disorders in Newcastle upon Tyne. Part 1: a study of prevalence. *British Journal of Psychiatry*, 110, 146–158.

Kelly, C. A., Harvey, R. J. & Cayton, H. (1997) Drug treatments for Alzheimer's disease. *British Medical Journal*, 314, 693–694.

Knapp, M. J., Knopman, D. S., Soloman, P. R., *et al* (1994) A 30-week randomised controlled trial of high dose tacrine in patients with Alzheimer's disease. *Journal of the American Medical Association*, 271, 985–991.

Knopman, D. S., Scheider, L., Davis, K., *et al* (1996) Long term tacrine treatment: effects on nursing home placement and mortality. *Neurology*, 271, 985–991.

Kuller, L. (1978) Prodromata of sudden death and myocardial infarction. *Advanced Cardiology*, 25, 61–72.

Levin, E., Sinclair, I. & Gorbach, P. (1983) *The Supporters of Confused Elderly Persons at Home*, Report to the DHSS. London: National Institute for Social Work Research Unit .

Macdonald, A. J. D. (1986) Do general practitioners 'miss' depression in elderly patients. *British Medical Journal*, 292, 1365–1367.

Murphy, E. (1982) Social origins of depression in old age. *British Journal of Psychiatry*, 141, 135–142.

— (1992) Concepts of depression in old age. In *Oxford Textbook of Geriatric Medicine* (ed. J. Grimley Evans). Oxford: Oxford University Press.

Ouslander, J. G. (1982) Physical illness and depression in the elderly. *Journal of the American Geriatrics Society*, 30, 593–599.

Parkes, C. M., Benjamin, B. & Fitzgerald, R. G. (1969) Broken heart: a statistical study of increased mortality among widowers. *British Medical Journal*, i, 740–743.

Post, F. (1972) The management and nature of depressive illness in late life: a follow through study. *British Journal of Psychiatry*, 121, 395–404.

Robinson, R. G., Book-Starr, L. & Price, T. R. (1984) A two year longitudinal study of mood disorders following stroke: a six month follow-up. *British Journal of Psychiatry*, 144, 256–262.

Vetter, N. J. V., Jones, D. A. & Victor, C. R. (1986) A health visitor affects the problems others do not reach. *Lancet*, 32, 30–32.

Veitch, R. C. (1982). Depression in the elderly: pharmacological considerations in treatment. *Journal of the American Geriatrics Society*, 30, 581–586.

World Health Organization (1992) *The Tenth Revision of the International Classification of Diseases and Related Health Problems* (ICD–10). Geneva: WHO.

Yesavage, J., Brink, T., Rose, T., *et al* (1983) Development and evaluation of a geriatric depression screening scale: a preliminary report. *Journal of Psychiatric Research*, 17, 37–49.

21 Patient management problems

Rob Butler & Brice Pitt

---

*Assessment • Epidemiology • Delirium • Alzheimer's disease •
Vascular dementia • Management of dementia • Depression
• Mania • Anxiety disorder • Late paraphrenia • Alcohol dependence •
Personality disorder • Imaging • Services • Liaison • Residential
and nursing homes • Pharmacological treatments • Psychological
treatments • Carers • Law • Research*

Patient management problems are short descriptions of clinical situations, followed by a series of questions. They form part of the assessment for the MRCPsych Part 2 examination. In this chapter we have included a patient management problem for each chapter in the book. Fortunately, one of us has come across quite a few clinical situations over a long career in old age psychiatry. The answers are not intended to cover everything (the chapters are!) but are offered as a guide. Good answers tend to be systematic ones, which follow the time honoured order of gathering information; taking a history and mental state examination; performing a physical examination and investigations; involving the patient, relatives and carers (where possible and bearing in mind confidentiality); and offering social, psychological and biological interventions. We suggest that you attempt each problem after reading the relevant chapter.

Assessment

An elderly gentleman found wandering on the motorway last night, was brought to an accident and emergency department. The casualty officer says that he appears to be confused.

Q. What are the possible diagnoses?

A. Dementia, delirium, mania, depression, psychosis.

Q. How would you assess him?

A. This will involve a history, mental state and physical examination. Gain as detailed a history as possible. Speak to informants, such as the person who brought him in, the casualty officer and the nurses in casualty. Talk to the patient and see if he is carrying any information. Examine his appearance for signs of long-term dirtiness. Undertake a mental state examination, including a detailed cognitive examination and a Mini-Mental State Examination (MMSE; Folstein *et al*, 1975). On physical examination record his temperature, pulse and respiration rate, and examine his level of consciousness, respiratory, cardiovascular and neurological systems, including signs of injury or intoxication. Investigations include routine blood tests, mid-stream urine chest X-ray and CT scan, if there is any evidence of a neurological lesion.

Q. *You find that the patient is unable to give a coherent history and has a MMSE of 13/30. There is no collateral history, no obvious physical signs and routine tests are negative. How would you manage him?*

A. Try to find out more information. Ring the police and social services to see if they have a missing person matching his description. Consider acute admission to hospital, or emergency admission to respite care if the patient agrees. Also, an overnight ward may be suitable.

Q. *The patient is unwilling to be admitted. What are the possible management situations?*

A. Letting a confused man leave the department would put him at risk and would not be advised. He may be reassured and gently persuaded to come into hospital by repeated calm explanations of the situation from a sympathetic member of staff. Otherwise he may need compulsory admission under the Mental Health Act 1983.

Epidemiology

Q. *Using the same, standard epidemiological techniques, researchers found a prevalence of dementia in the elderly of 4.2% in New York and 2.8% in London (Gurland et al, 1983). What factors could account for the difference?*

A. 1. Interview or sampling biases such as different social class, age structures or proportion living in residential accommodation.
    2. The screening instrument favouring educational or cultural sub-groups.
    3. A true difference – attributable to possible risk factors such as exposure to 'bath tub gin' drink during prohibition in New York.

On closer inspection of the data, it becomes apparent that the difference extends over the whole range of cognitive scores, and not just to those below the cut-off score for dementia.

Q. *How does this affect the possible explanations?*

A. It could still be explained by the use of a screening instrument which favoured London educationally or culturally. Alternatively, a real difference may exist as the result of factors which generally lower cognition in New York.

Delirium

Mrs Fraser is a 75-year-old lady who fractured her neck of femur and had it pinned. She was grossly disturbed last night on the orthopaedic ward, keeping all the other patients awake. This morning she is shouting and refusing to take medication.

Q. What are the diagnostic possibilities?

A. Delirium, dementia, mania, schizophrenia.

Q. How would you establish the diagnosis of delirium?

A. From a full history (which includes information from the nursing staff), mental state and examination. You need to establish whether she was mentally well before the operation. She may have a fluctuating level of consciousness and cognitive impairment.

Q. What are the most likely causes of her delirium?

A. There may be an underlying cognitive impairment. Causes of delirium include anaesthesia, blood loss, pulmonary embolus, wound infection, chest infection, urinary tract infection, electrolyte disturbance, medication side-effects, post-operative analgesia, alcohol withdrawal, stroke, cardiac event and fat embolus.

Q. What are the most important principles of management for a delirium?

A. 1. Treat the underlying cause or causes.
    2. Maintain adequate hydration and nutrition.
    3. Rest, reassurance and reorientation.
    4. Nurse in the same room, with the same staff (if possible), and have relatives or friends present.
    5. Neuroleptics such as haloperidol or thioridazine may be prescribed acutely, in small doses to reduce agitation. Alternatives include benzodiazepines and chlormethiazole.

Alzheimer's disease

A general practitioner (GP) rings you to say he has a deputation from a local housing estate complaining that Mrs Smith, 85, living alone, is in a state of serious neglect, and is causing considerable nuisance by wandering out at night, getting lost and banging on doors. The GP thinks she is suffering from dementia and would like her to be admitted to hospital urgently on a section.

Q. How would you manage the situation?

A. Gather information from her GP and other sources, including details of her past medical and psychiatric history. Speak to others involved in the situation including her relatives, friends, carers and the head of the deputation. Make a joint home visit with her GP, someone who knows her, or alone.

Q. How could you prepare yourself for a home visit if you felt she may be reluctant to see you?

A. Telephone her first, being as pleasant as possible and offering a time to suit her. Her next of kin, neighbour or social worker may be able to offer advice on the best approaches to visiting her, or agree to come with you.

She allows you in. There is a faint smell of urine. The dwelling is cluttered and there is clothing close to electric fires. The milk is off. She scores 21 out of 30 on the MMSE. Although she is polite, she says she does not want any interventions, such as meals on wheels or home help.

Q. What action would you take?

A. Her GP may want to investigate a possible urinary tract infection. Call a case conference, convened by a social worker, involving next of kin, other family members, neighbours, her GP and any other involved professionals. Discuss how to achieve a balance between her rights and the risks she faces. Consider using the Mental Health Act 1983, but only use it if alternatives fail, and she is considered a danger to herself. A community psychiatric nurse (CPN) or another person may develop a relationship with her and be able to encourage her to accept services. You will need to follow-up her situation and place her on a dementia register if there is one locally.

Vascular dementia

Mr Milford, a retired solicitor aged 82, is reported by his wife to have become cantankerous and confused over the last few months, especially at night. He was always been irritable but is now said to be abusive, raising his fists and swearing at the slightest prevarication.

Q. What diagnostic possibilities occur to you?

A. Dementia, alcohol misuse, marital tension, depression, delirium.

You are asked to see Mr Milford at his home after a bad night; his wife says she is at her wit's end and something must be done. You find him to be pleasant, courteous, smartly dressed, clean shaven and able to converse. He has no recollection of the alleged disturbance, but implies that his wife has become rather pernickety of late. His MMSE score is 24 out of 30.

Q. How would you seek to clarify the diagnosis?

A. From a history, mental state and physical examination. Interview Mr Milford and his wife, assessing their relationship and their mental states. Consider admitting Mr Milford to day hospital for a more thorough assessment and observation over a period of time. Look for risk factors for vascular dementia such as smoking, a family history of heart disease or a history of myocardial infarct, diabetes mellitus or transient ischaemic attacks. Repeat cognitive assessments at different times of day to pick-up 'sundowning'. Physically examine Mr Milford, looking for signs of cerebrovascular disease, such as hypertension and peripheral vascular disease. On neurological examination test for frontal lobe signs including the pouting and grasp reflexes. Arrange for investigations and a CT brain scan.

Q. The diagnosis is vascular dementia. What are the principles of management for these aggressive outbursts?

A. 1. Suggest he has activities during the day, such as attending a day centre. Ask occupational therapy for ideas to employ his residual cognition as fully as possible.
   2. Support and offer help and advice to his wife, including marital counselling if necessary.
   3. A neuroleptic such as haloperidol 0.5 mg once a day increased up to four times daily may reduce his level of agitation, but you must monitor for side-effects.

Management of dementia

Mr Green, 78, a widower, former grocer and councillor, lives alone. Children in the neighbourhood report that he has been exposing himself from his front room window. He strenuously denies this. Cognitive assessment shows no gross abnormality, but his flies are open and he tells rather inappropriate dirty jokes.

Q. What is the differential diagnosis?

A. Frontal lobe dementia, alcohol dependence, hypomania.

Q. What would be the management?

A. Take a full history, mental state and physical examination. The assessment would include gathering information from his GP, hospital notes and forensic history. A programme of assessment and supervision might include help with his dressing, such as an *aide-*

mémoire "have you done up your flies?". If he has difficulty in fastening buttons or pulling a zip, velcro might be used to fasten the flies. A fuller structured day might keep him occupied and relieve boredom. Attendance at a day centre or hospital, complemented by visits from community staff would help. If he is able to acknowledge a sexual drive behind his self-exposure, counselling, or in an extreme situation, anti-androgens or benperidol could be considered.

Depression

Mr Montgomery, 84, was admitted to a psychiatric ward from his sheltered flat because he cut his wrist with a safety razor blade. There was not much blood loss, but he had severed a tendon.

Q. *How would you assess his suicide risk?*

A. Take a full history and mental state examination. This would include collateral information from his warden and GP. Ask Mr Montgomery why he did it and whether anything had changed. Find out if he had left a note, how soon before it came to light and had he told anyone. Ask about a family history of psychiatric illness, or past psychiatric history including deliberate self-harm. Find out how he views his present life situation and what his intentions are for the future. Does he have a mental illness such as depression, alcohol dependence, schizophrenia or dementia?

Q. *You decide that this was a failed attempt at suicide in the presence of an agitated depression and he still wants to die. What management would you offer?*

A. You would want to keep him in hospital, even if this involved using the Mental Health Act 1983. On the ward he would initially have close observations. A full assessment would include finding what management has been successful in the past. On the ward, a more sedative antidepressant such as lofepramine would be prescribed, as well as a small dose of a neuroleptic such as thioridazine to reduce his agitation. Electroconvulsive therapy would be considered if his depression was psychotic, he remained a high suicidal risk or if he failed to eat or drink.

Mania

Mrs Luke, 71, is a new arrival at the Everest Old People's Home on a one-month trial. She has been placed there by the social services, as an emergency, because of confused behaviour and self-neglect. The manager complained that she is noisy, talks nineteen to the dozen, is rude, disinhibited, flirtatious, greedy, takes her nightie off in the living room and is up all night.

Q. *What is the differential diagnosis?*
A. Mania, delirium, dementia, drug misuse.

Q. *What features of the history are consistent with hypomania?*
A. Pressure of speech, disinhibition, poor sleep and over-activity.

Q. *The GP tells you she has a history of depressive illness. How would you manage her?*
A. Make a full assessment including history, mental state and physical examination. Admission to hospital will depend upon how well the home can manage her. Day hospital attendance is an alternative. If her diagnosis is mania, then consider prescribing a neuroleptic such as thioridazine. Lithium may be appropriate for prophylaxis, although it can also be prescribed for acute episodes. Explain to the staff the implications of Mrs Luke's diagnosis, emphasising that it is a treatable condition which explains her behaviour and that you will follow-up.

Anxiety disorder

Mr Evans, 69, never married, has not left his sheltered flat since he had a heart attack three years ago. His new GP does not want to continue prescribing the lorazepam 1 mg three times daily, which he has been taking for three years.

Q. *What is the differential diagnosis?*
A. Anxiety disorder, depressive illness, agoraphobia, anxious personality disorder, benzodiazepine dependence, physical illness such as angina.

Q. *You have reached the diagnosis of a late-onset agoraphobia. Are there any benefits to stopping the benzodiazepines?*
A. Apart from tolerance and dependence, benzodiazepines may have interactions and side-effects such as unsteadiness and falls, which may be more problematic in older age. Most older people can withdraw from benzodiazepines successfully.

Q. *He would like to stop taking the lorazepam, and you agree. How would you do this?*
A. Alter the lorazepam to an equivalent dose of a long-acting benzodiazepine, such as diazepam. Reduce the dose gradually over

several weeks, based upon regular reviews. Offer help for any underlying problems. Support includes day hospital admission, individual or group psychotherapy, relaxation therapy and monitoring by a CPN or psychologist.

Late paraphrenia

The housing welfare officer has been told by Miss Jones that she hears her neighbours talking to her through the radio and what they say distresses her.

Q. *What possible diagnosis occurs to you?*

A. Late paraphrenia, schizophrenia, depression, dementia, poor hearing, no mental illness – she is being persecuted by the person next door.

Q. *How would you assess her?*

A. With a history, mental state and physical examination. Speak to her housing officer, GP and other involved individuals to gain as full a history as possible. Visit her at home with her GP, someone who knows her or alone.

Q. *What special features might you notice in her flat?*

A. Lots of locks and precautions against voices such as loudspeakers. She may whisper and insist you only talk in another part of the flat.

Q. *You have made a diagnosis of late paraphrenia. How would you manage her?*

A. Following a full assessment you may consider doing little more than excluding treatable conditions, such as ear wax, and improving her social isolation as much possible. Sometimes a cure for paraphrenia can be worse than the condition in its milder forms. She should be offered medication but she may well refuse it. She may be more willing to take it if she develops a good relationship with her GP, yourself, a CPN or staff at the day hospital. Hospital admission should be considered, especially if she is neglecting herself, not eating adequately, threatening her neighbours, or putting herself at risk of eviction or criminal charges.

Alcohol dependence

Mr Evans, 72, unmarried, has lived in sheltered accommodation since a stroke six months after his retirement at 65. He is reported to be abusive, uncooperative, complaining all the time about his home help, bathing attendants, wardens and social worker. At a domiciliary visit he is smelling of alcohol. There are bottles of beer and whisky under his bed.

Q.   *What is the likeliest diagnosis and how would you manage the situation?*
A.   The likeliest diagnosis is alcohol dependence. The management would include finding out how much he is drinking, how he is supplied and the cost (if he is unable to leave his home alone, how does he obtain his alcohol?). He will need a full assessment, including physical examination and investigations looking for alcohol damage. If he acknowledges his problem with alcohol he may agree to a programme of detoxification, followed by support. Should he be admitted to a residential home he may have less access to alcohol.

Personality disorder

The housing authority has been approached by Miss Dawson's neighbours, because Miss Dawson, aged 68, causes a nuisance through her persistent feeding of pigeons. She was contacted by the housing authority and told that she would face eviction if this behaviour continues. One week later she is feeding the birds as before. The housing officer wants a psychiatric assessment, with a view to finding an alternative to eviction. Miss Dawson has agreed to see a psychiatrist at her home.

Q.   *What possible diagnosis do you entertain as you go to see her?*
A.   No mental illness (non-conformity or eccentricity), dementia, personality disorder.

Q.   *An assessment reveals no evidence of a mental illness. How would you manage her?*
A.   A realistic appraisal may conclude that what cannot be cured, must be endured. However, a further appeal should be made to her to avoid eviction. Inform the housing officer that you have found no evidence of mental disorder, and although she is unlikely to change her behaviour, an eviction order will simply move the problem to another area. A home help or other sympathetic worker may be able to develop a relationship with her and influence her behaviour that way. She may agree to attend a day centre.

Imaging

Mr Brotherton, 84, living in Torquay, has been in the habit of going for a swim with his widowed daughter every day. She reports that in the last three months he has been unsteady as he emerged from the water, and occasionally incontinent of urine during their car drive back to his home. He is also becoming mentally slow and forgetful.

Q. *What possible diagnoses do these symptoms suggest?*

A. Normal pressure hydrocephalous, vascular dementia, stroke, tumour.

Q. *How would you confirm the diagnosis? What treatments might be available?*

A. A full assessment including mental state, history and physical examination. The typical triad for normal pressure hydrocephalous is dementia, incontinence and ataxia. A CT scan will show enlarged ventricles in hydrocephalous or may reveal a tumour. Both conditions may be amenable to surgery. Hydrocephalous is treatable, with a shunt from the ventricle into the vena cava or the peritoneal cavity.

Services

Mr Jones, 86, suffering from moderate dementia, is looked after by his wife who needs to have a cataract operation. Two days before the operation, a caring geriatrician admits him to his ward as a social admission, but the next morning Mr Jones is extremely agitated, searching for his wife, and insisting they have not been separated in more than 50 years. He demands that he is allowed home.

Q. *You are asked to transfer him to a psychogeriatric ward for containment. What are your options?*

A. Assess him on the geriatric ward and try to persuade him to stay. Find out how long his wife will be in hospital, what support he needs at home and whether alternative arrangements can be made, such as staying with relatives. His wife's operation may need to be postponed. An assessment for Section 2 of the Mental Health Act 1983 and sedation should be avoided if possible.

You visit Mr George on the ward, and confirm he is confused, agitated and very keen to return to his wife. He scores 15 out of 30 on the MMSE. You are unable to persuade him to stay while his wife has the operation. You therefore arrange for him to return home to his wife, and the operation to be delayed. He rapidly settles, but she still needs the operation.

Q. *What better arrangements might be made?*

A. Day surgery may be possible, but the couple would need support. A full domiciliary assessment, including activities of daily living and social worker assessment, will establish what support is required at home. He may be gradually introduced to other sources of support such as home help, a day centre or a home carer. It may be necessary to provide full domiciliary care including a live-in carer during his wife's hospital admission.

Liaison

Mr George, 75, is unpopular on the geriatric ward where has been admitted for treatment for a chronic leg ulcer, diabetes and vascular disease. His wife says she cannot deal with him as he is demanding, intolerant of pain and stubborn about not using crutches. There is a strong feeling on the ward that he is attention-seeking. On questioning him, you find he was a pilot in the Second World War involved in the Dresden raid. Subsequently he was a teacher, until he retired 10 years ago. In 1965, he had an agitated depression and was suicidal. His depression responded well, on that occasion, to electroconvulsive therapy and amitriptyline.

Q. *What is the differential diagnosis?*
A. Agitated depression, anxiety disorder, dementia, cerebrovascular disease, frontal lobe personality change, post-traumatic stress disorder.

Q. *He has a depressive illness. What information and advice would you offer the ward to facilitate his management?*
A. Explain to the staff that he is depressed, and that his behaviour is not attention-seeking but is a part of a treatable illness. Explain that sympathetic listening and reassurance from the staff will play a vital part in his therapy. They should also monitor important indicators of the mental state including appetite, weight and sleep. Prescribe an antidepressant such as lofepramine and explain the effect this will have. Arrange for Mr George to be reviewed regularly by the old age psychiatric team, with a member of the nursing staff present, until he recovers.

Residential and nursing homes

Mr Simon, a widower of 86, has mild dementia and moved to sheltered housing because he wandered at night. After four months he still wanders and occasionally goes into the rooms of other residents, sometimes climbing into their beds. Their complaints have made the social worker suggest he moves to a residential home. His son, however, who visits at least once a week, feels that his father is happy there and has not had time to settle in.

Q.   *Give one advantage and one disadvantage of Mr Simon remaining where he is, for himself, his son, and his social worker.*

A.   Advantage for Mr Simon – he is spared another move. Disadvantage for Mr Simon – his wandering puts him at risk. Advantage for his son – he feels his father is happier living where he is. Disadvantage for his son – he will remain under pressure from other residents and their families. Advantage for his social worker – he does not have to seek more costly care. Disadvantage for his social worker – he remains under pressure from the sheltered accommodation staff.

Q.   *What measures would help him to remain in the sheltered flat?.*

A.   Treat any underlying medical or psychiatric problems. A CPN may be able to advise staff on how to avoid confrontation with Mr Simon, while accepting an element of risk for him. A programme of activities could be arranged within the housing development and at a day centre. A neuroleptic, such as thioridazine or haloperidol, may be helpful for agitation, but should not be used to damp down his overall activity.

Pharmacological treatments

Mrs Forsyth, aged 77, has a history of variable confusion for the past seven months. She also experiences visual hallucinations and intermittent clouding of consciousness.

Q.   *What is the differential diagnosis?*

A.   Lewy body dementia, subdural haematoma, alcohol misuse, brain tumour.

She has been visited by the GP who prescribed thioridazine 50 mg twice daily. She is now in a state of being barely able to walk because of extreme muscular stiffness and shaking. She can barely speak, and drools.

Q.   *Which of your diagnoses does this favour and what are the main features of this condition?*

A.   Lewy Body dementia. Visual hallucinations, dementia, clouding of consciousness, sensitivity to neuroleptics and Parkinsonian symptoms.

Psychological treatments

Mrs Jenkins has a history of bipolar affective illness. In recent years she has been almost constantly unhappy, dissatisfied, negative and self-critical.

Her physical health is good for her 82 years, but she complains of inertia and fatigue, and spends much of the day in bed. She is financially well off, has a pleasant home and a generally cheerful, long suffering husband. She has been treated with tricyclics and monoamine oxidase inhibitors, and is now taking paroxetine 40 mg daily and lithium carbonate with a serum level of 0.7 mmol/l.

Q. *Her GP refers her to the old age psychiatry department, with a view to her having psychotherapy for her refractory depression. What forms of psychological treatment might be available?*

A. Counselling and support, brief dynamic psychotherapy, marital therapy, cognitive–behavioural therapy or analytical psychotherapy.

Q. *You feel that counselling would be insufficient. You can identify no dynamic or marital stresses amenable to therapy, but you are struck by her persistent pessimism and self-criticism (although of less than delusional intensity). Along what lines would you offer cognitive–behavioural therapy?*

A. The therapist needs to be trained in cognitive–behavioural therapy and able to offer the time for treatment. It may be yourself or one of your colleagues, such as a psychologist or CPN. Mrs Jenkins should be willing to have the therapy. The therapy is explained to her and a series of appointments made. She will need to complete a diary, and her 'home work' will involve prioritising her negative thoughts, with examples from her daily thinking and behaviour, and exploring and challenging them with her therapist.

Carers

Mr Stevens, aged 78, a former bus driver, suffered a right hemiplegia 10 months ago. He is now ambulant but emotional, irritable, erratic and forgetful. His wife of 44 years is mentally alert, but stressed by his bad tempers, his wandering (he sometimes has to be brought back by the police) and his turning on the gas without igniting it. She says that she must have a break.

Q. *What help could you offer her?*

A. Counselling and support. Relative support group and information from the local Alzheimer's Disease Society. Respite care from a day carer, day centre, day hospital, residential home or hospital.

Q. *You decide that she needs respite, and social services find him a place in a nursing home for two weeks. Ten days after his admission you are asked to see her again because she is in a state of great distress.*

Her husband is with her, she removed him from the home after six days. Why might this be?

A. 1. Her husband missed her greatly, clamoured to come home and was eventually allowed to do so.
    2. She had not realised that she would have to make a financial contribution and felt she could not afford it.
    3. Mr Stevens settled into the home, but his wife was distressed by the inactivity of the residents, and the excessive prevalence of senility. She could not bear to leave her husband there.
    4. After two days, she found that she missed him dreadfully, felt very anxious alone, so bought him back for her own comfort.

Q. *You decide that support should be provided at home and that she needs expert counselling. What should the counsellor seek to address?*

A. The counsellor needs to be able to offer her the chance to express her feelings in a safe environment. Particular issues may include those of attachment, dependency, guilt and ambivalence. She may need to be guided through the loss of her husband as she knew him.

Law

Mrs Lockwood, aged 87, was admitted to the geriatric ward suffering from pneumonia and a heel ulcer. Her Mental Test Score (MTS; Hodkinson, 1972) on admission was four out of 10. You are told that she wants to alter her will in favour of her nephew, who visits frequently. The geriatricians are concerned and want your advice.

Q. *What would your assessment take into consideration?*

A. Her cognitive functioning may have improved as her pneumonia got better and needs to be reassessed. You need to establish her testamentary capacity (i.e. that she knows the extent of her estate and which people have reasonable expectations from her will). You should establish if her reasoning for changing her will is affected by mental illness or by pressure from her nephew. Undue influence may invalidate a will.

Q. *She tells you she has been looked after very nicely by the ward and she wants to leave £1000 for a new music centre. Does this change your position?*

A. No. Accepting a large donation to the ward would only be considered if she could afford it, and she was fully aware of the nature of the donation and the repercussions to her own finances. Mania needs to be excluded as a possible diagnosis.

Research

Mrs Granger, aged 67, complains of a failing memory. This is confirmed by her husband, who has made her an appointment at the memory clinic. You make a diagnosis of early Alzheimer's disease and inform her husband. He asks for this information to be withheld from his wife, but wants her to be considered for a drug trial of a new anti-dementia drug.

Q. *Should you tell her, and can she enter the drug trial?*

A. Yes and no. Mrs Granger has the right to know her diagnosis and cannot give informed consent to participate in a drug trial unless she is fully aware of her diagnosis, and its implications. When and how to tell someone their diagnosis is a sensitive issue and should take into account the cultural and family feelings.

Q. *How might you tell her diagnosis?*

A. Explain the situation to her husband and gain his support. Break the news to her in a sympathetic and unhurried manner, offering plenty of time for questions. Confirm to her that she has an impaired memory and this goes beyond what is normal for her age. Explain that the likeliest cause is Alzheimer's disease, although the diagnosis can only be confirmed with the passage of time. Say that with Alzheimer's disease, progress can be slow, with a plateau. Offer further counselling and support, including details of the Alzheimer's Disease Society. Inform her that there is medication that may delay the disorder and that research is likely to yield other medications. She will be able to plan her own future including establishing a power of attorney and making a will. If she drives she is obliged to inform the Driver and Vehicle Licencing Agency of her diagnosis.

References

Folstein, M., Folstein, S. & McHugh, P. (1975) Mini-Mental State. A practical method for grading the cognitive state of patients for the clinician. *Journal of Psychiatric Research*, 12, 189–198.

Gurland, B., Copeland, J., Kuriansky, J., *et al* (1983) *The Mind and Mood of Aging: Mental Health Problems in the Community Elderly in New York and London.* New York: Haworth Press.

Hodkinson, H. (1972) Evaluation of a mental test score for assessment of mental impairment in the elderly. *Age and Aging*, 1, 233–238.

Appendix

Useful addresses

Action on Elder Abuse, Astral House, 1268 London Road, London SW16 4ER. Tel: 0181 764 7648

Alzheimer's Disease Society, Gordon House, 10 Greencoat Place, London SW1P 1PH. Tel: 0171 306 0606

Age Concern, Astral House, 1268 London Road, London SW16 4ER. Tel: 0181 679 8000

Carers National Association, 20–25 Glasshouse Yard, London EC1A 4JT. Tel: 0171 490 8818

Christian Council on Ageing, Epworth House, Stuart Street, Derby DE1 2EQ. Tel: 01355 390484

Cruse Bereavement Care, Cruse House, 126 Sheen Road, Richmond, Surrey TW9 1UR. Tel: 0181 940 4818

Help the Aged, 16–18 St James's Walk, Clerkenwell, London EC1R OBE. Tel: 0171 253 0253

MIND, Granta House, 15–19 Broadway, Stratford, London E15 4BQ. Tel: 0181 519 2122

Index

Compiled by Caroline Sheard

Page numbers in italic refer to tables and/or text in boxes